INTERNATIONAL ENCYCLOPEDIA OF PHARMACOLOGY AND THERAPEUTICS

Sponsored by the International Union of Pharmacology (IUPHAR)

(Chairman: B. UVNÄS, Stockholm)

Executive Editor: C. RADOUCO-THOMAS

Section 14

NEUROMUSCULAR BLOCKING AND STIMULATING AGENTS

Section Editor

J. CHEYMOL

Paris

VOLUME I

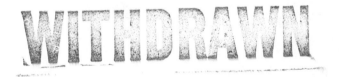

INTERNATIONAL ENCYCLOPEDIA OF
PHARMACOLOGY AND THERAPEUTICS

NEUROMUSCULAR BLOCKING
AND
STIMULATING AGENTS

VOLUME I

CONTRIBUTORS

F. BOURILLET	LISE ENGBAEK
D. BOVET	J. I. HUBBARD
W. C. BOWMAN	A. R. MCINTYRE
A. S. V. BURGEN	I. G. MARSHALL
C. CHAGAS	L. SOLLERO
J. CHEYMOL	G. SUAREZ-KURTZ
R. COUTEAUX	O. VITAL-BRAZIL
J. E. DESMEDT	P. G. WASER

PERGAMON PRESS
OXFORD · NEW YORK · TORONTO · SYDNEY
BRAUNSCHWEIG

Pergamon Press Ltd., Headington Hill Hall, Oxford

Pergamon Press Inc., Maxwell House, Fairview Park, Elmsford,
New York 10523

Pergamon of Canada Ltd., 207 Queen's Quay West, Toronto 1

Pergamon Press (Aust.) Pty. Ltd., 19a Boundary Street,
Rushcutters Bay, N.S.W. 2011, Australia

Vieweg & Sohn GmbH, Burgplatz 1, Braunschweig

First edition 1972

Library of Congress Catalog Card No. 70–189280

Printed in Great Britain by A. Wheaton & Co., Exeter

08 016277 0

CONTENTS

SUBSECTION I

THE NEUROMUSCULAR JUNCTION

SUBSECTION II

INHIBITORS OF THE NEUROMUSCULAR JUNCTION

A. NATURAL INHIBITORS

Contents

CONTENTS OF VOLUME II

LIST OF CONTRIBUTORS

BOURILLET, FRANÇOIS, Assistant à l'Institut de Pharmacologie, Faculté de Médecine, 21 rue de l'Ecole de Médecine, 75—Paris 6e, France. (Vol. I, Chaps. 5, 8, 12).

BOVET, DANIEL, Professor of Psychobiology, University of Rome, Italy. (Vol. I, Chap. 11).

BOWMAN, WILLIAM C., Professor of Pharmacology, University of Strathclyde, Royal College, George Street, Glasgow C.1, U.K. (Vol. I, Chap. 13; Vol. II, Chap. 16).

BURGEN, ARNOLD, Director, National Institute for Medical Research, London, NW.7. (Vol. I, Chap. 7).

CHAGAS, CARLOS, Professeur à l'Institut de Biophysique, Avenue Pasteur 458, Universidade Federal do Rio de Janeiro, Rio de Janeiro, Brasil. (Vol. I, Chap. 15).

CHEYMOL, JEAN, Professeur de Pharmacologie, Faculté de Médecine, 21 rue de l'Ecole de Médecine, 75—Paris 6e, France. (Vol. I, Chaps. 1, 5, 8, 12).

COUTEAUX, RENE, Professeur, Laboratoire de Cytologie, Faculté des Sciences, Quai Saint-Bernard, 75—Paris 5e, France. (Vol. I, Chap. 2).

DESMEDT, JEAN EDOUARD, Professeur au Laboratoire de Physiopathologie du Système nerveux et Unité de recherche sur le cerveau, Université libre de Bruxelles, 115 bd. de Waterloo, Bruxelles, Belgium. (Vol. I, Chap. 4).

ENGBAEK, LISE, Doceut, Institute of Neurophysiology, University of Copenhagen, Juliane Maries Vej 36, Denmark. (Vol. I, Chap. 14).

HUBBARD, JOHN I., Professor and Chairman, Department of Biological Sciences, North-western University, Evanston, Ill., U.S.A. (Vol. I, Chap. 3).

MARSHALL, IAN G., Lecturer, University of Strathclyde, Department of Pharmacology, Royal College, George Street, Glasgow C.1, U.K. (Vol. I, Chap. 13).

MCINTYRE, ARCHIBALD, R., Senior Consultant in Pharmacology and Toxicology, University of Nebraska, Medical College, Omaha, Nebraska 68105, U.S.A. (Vol. I, Chap. 9).

SOLLERO, LAURO, Professeur de Pharmacologie, Instituto de Ciencias Biomedicas, UFRJ, 458 Ave. Pasteur, Rio de Janeiro, Brasil. (Vol. I, Chap. 15).

SUAREZ-KURTZ, GUILHERME, Professeur de Pharmacologie, Instituto de Ciencias Biomédicas UFRJ, 458 Ave. Pasfeur, Rio de Janeiro, Brazil. (Vol. I, Chap. 15).

VITAL-BRAZIL, OSWALD, Professeur de Pharmacologie, Faculdade de Ciencias Medicas, Universidade Estadual de Campinas, Caixa Postal 1170, Etat de Sao Paulo, Brasil. (Vol. I, Chap. 6).

WASER, PETER G., Professeur Dr., Pharmakologisches Institut der Universität, Gloriastrasse 32, Zürich, Switzerland. (Vol. I, Chap. 10).

PREFACE

For the convenience of the reader, it has seemed appropriate to divide Section 14 into two volumes.

The first volume groups together the chapters relating to the study of the neuromuscular junction and its inhibitors, both natural and synthetic, with those dealing with their pharmacodynamics and their metabolism.

In the second, after a study of the peripheric stimulants, the chapters concerned with the clinical and therapeutic study of the modifiers of both the normal and pathological functioning of the neuromuscular synapse are grouped together.

Lastly, the final chapter enables all those who are interested in general biology to compare the myoneural junction of the vertebrates with that of the insects and the crustaceans.

J. Cheymol

CHAPTER 1

INTRODUCTION

J. Cheymol

Paris

WHY publish a book on the neuromuscular junction when in the same issue of *The International Encyclopedia of Pharmacology and Therapeutics* there is another volume covering in general terms "The physiology and pharmacology of synaptic transmission"?

There are several reasons for this, each of which is enumerated:

AT THE ANATOMICAL LEVEL

The motor end-plate is the simplest form of synapse, the most exposed, "the most vulnerable synapse known" (Estable, 1959),* and the most accessible to investigation. Both the nervous and the muscular tissues are in intimate contact at this point owing to the absence of a myelin sheath, the whole structure being covered by neurilemma only, like a lid.

AT THE PHYSIOLOGICAL LEVEL

Whereas many nervous synapses receive a number of both excitatory as well as inhibitory inputs and in consequence are very difficult to study, the motor end-plate—a simple relay between the directing nerve and the effector muscle—lends itself easily to observation and to experiment. Several eminent research workers have devoted themselves to the study of this particular synapse.

This relative simplicity has made possible investigation into the details of the physicochemical phenomenon of neuromuscular transmission, in which various enzymes, acetylcholine, Na^+, K^+, Ca^{++} and Mg^{++} ions, electrical currents and probably other factors as well are involved.

* Estable, A. (1959) Curare and Synapse, in D. Bovet, *Curare and Curare-like Agents,* Elsevier, Amsterdam, p. 357.

Four recent research techniques have enabled striking advances to be made in this field. Let us simply enumerate them:

the *electronmicroscope* has allowed examination to be carried to the ultrastructural level;

the *microelectrode* has made possible the intracellular recording of the most minute electrical phenomena;

iontophoresis enables the intracellular application of minute amounts of pharmacologically active substances, identical or antagonistic to the chemical mediators, at the physiological dose level;

radioactive isotopes allow the movements of ions, responsible for the membrane potentials, to be followed and the receptors to be localized.

AT THE PHARMACOLOGICAL LEVEL

Although nearly a century has elapsed since Claude Bernard's original work with curare on the neuromuscular junction, contemporary pharmacologists continue to explore this fruitful field of study in its many aspects:

the investigation into an understanding of the fundamental process of neuromuscular transmission—for example, the link between the action potential and the release of acetylcholine;

the preparation of naturally occurring substances of known composition, isolated from the *Chondrodendron* and *Strychnos* species;

an appreciation of the role of the quaternary ammonium group (the presence of one or more such groups in a molecule almost certainly determines whether it shows a curarizing action);

the development of sensitive and specific tests, qualitative as well as quantitative, by which this effect can be followed and understood;

the great interest in the historic, folkloric (strange Indian poisons) and practical aspects (in, for example, anesthesiology, etc.).

Thanks to "scalpels pharmacologiques", research is advancing on two fronts, namely:

(i)   An understanding of the structure of neuromuscular inhibitors which possess an optimum spacing between their quaternary ammonium groups (true gold number equals 14 or 20 Ångströms) has enabled a topographical model of specific receptors to be devised. Do the cholinesterases correspond to the cholinergic receptors? A vital question!

(ii) An understanding of the biochemistry of proteins, in which anionic and esterophilic sites are responsible for linkage with the transmitter, involves experiments in which the relatively unstable acetylcholine

2

is substituted at the giant motor end-plate of *Gymnotus*, by that of the more stable labeled curare-like substance.

AT THE PATHOLOGICAL LEVEL

The aetiology and hence the treatment of myopathies, in particular myasthenia, is still uncertain. This current state of affairs justifies the inclusion of separate chapters.

AT THE THERAPEUTIC LEVEL

Neuromuscular blocking agents have enabled operations previously lasting minutes to extend over hours, as well as inducing temporary relief by the abolition of contractures (tetanus, spastic states, etc.).

Finally, what relationships can be drawn between the anatomy and physiology of the neuromuscular junction of insects, crustacea and of higher animals? This study is far from being entirely academic. Has it been established that the lethal action of the powerful organophosphorous insecticides is by virtue of their anticholinesterase property, as established in higher animals? A better understanding of the basic mechanism would enable a more rational employment of these insecticides, so useful in the protection of man's food, and a move in the direction of less dangerous substances for the consumer.

All these facts and many others which are contained in this volume dictated the need for a separate article. The authors hope that basic scientists and clinicians will find the information they need in these two volumes (Vol. I, Chaps. 1–15; Vol. II, Chaps. 16–21).

Subsection I

THE NEUROMUSCULAR JUNCTION

CHAPTER 2

STRUCTURE AND CYTOCHEMICAL CHARACTERISTICS OF THE NEUROMUSCULAR JUNCTION

R. Couteaux

Paris

2.1. INTRODUCTION

The neuromuscular junctions where transmission of the impulse from a motor nerve to striated muscle takes place are characterized by a very short distance separating in these regions the plasma membrane of the motor axon from the plasma membrane of the muscle fiber, by the absence of other cytoplasms between these membranes, as well as by a certain number of structural and cytochemical peculiarities exhibited by the nerve fiber and the muscle fiber in the junctional region.

These are the only regions of the muscle where the interrelationship between the motor axons and the muscle fibers is so direct. Everywhere else the sheaths which surround the axons separate them from the muscle fibers.

The nerve fiber and the muscle fiber exercise an inductive influence one on the other in the region of their junction. During their development this leads to a sort of localized differentiation, which gives to the terminal portion of the nerve fiber and to the adjacent region of the muscle fiber their own morphological character.

The neuromuscular junction comprises both cytoplasms and nuclei belonging to cells of very different types: nerve cells, muscle cells, Schwann cells, and connective cells.

The special character of the nerve cells and the muscle fibers in the region of the junction adds further to the complexity of this ensemble composed of four tissues.

Although the nervous and muscular cytoplasms are intimately linked at the point of the junction, they constitute regions which are completely distinct one from the other both anatomically and physiologically, each being limited by a plasma membrane and an extracellular basal lamina. The juncture of the nerve fiber and of the muscle fiber takes place between the two basal laminae and leaves a distance of some hundred Ångströms between the two plasma membranes. These two regions correspond to the presynaptic and postsynaptic portions of the junction.

One of these portions, the presynaptic, trophically depends on the nerve cell, whilst the other, the postsynaptic, depends on the muscle fiber. However, as regards the maintenance of their particular character in the synaptic zone each also depends one on the other and the proof for this may readily be shown for the postsynaptic portion. After section of the motor nerve, the disappearance of the nerve terminal takes place approximately at the same time as that of the distal segment of the motor axon and leaves apparently intact the muscle fiber including the postsynaptic portion of the junction. However, this portion soon demonstrates morphological and histochemical changes which finally lead to the disappearance of the characteristics which makes it a differentiated zone of the muscle fiber.

Induced by the action of the motor nerve fiber during the development this differentiation thus still remains dependent, for its maintenance, on the influences exerted by the nerve fiber.

The intimate union of the two portions of the junction has naturally been the source of great technical difficulties in localizing the phenomena for which they are both, respectively, the site.

Similar difficulties have been counted in the localization of the chemical constituents, and particularly the enzymes, and these difficulties have not yet been entirely overcome. It is not always easy to technically achieve the required precision to distinguish two sites only separated by a few hundred Ångströms.

The trophic interdependence of the two portions, nervous and muscular, of the junction also greatly complicates the study of the pathogenesis in neuromuscular diseases, since a lesion which initially is confined to one of the two zones, presynaptic or postsynaptic, of the junction more or less rapidly leads to an alteration of the other portion.

Only a very general approach to the neuromuscular junction will be considered here. More detailed information can be found in recent reviews and papers dealing with the morphology and cytochemistry of the neuromuscular junction (Andersson-Cedergren, 1959; Coërs and Woolf, 1959; Lehrer and Ornstein, 1959; Robertson, 1960; Birks *et al.*, 1960; Couteaux, 1960; Zacks, 1964; Csillik, 1965; Coërs, 1967).

2.2. STRUCTURE OF THE NEUROMUSCULAR JUNCTION

2.2.1. GENERAL ASPECTS OF THE NEUROMUSCULAR JUNCTION

For this general description of the neuromuscular junction, we have chosen the motor end-plate of reptiles and mammals.

The motor axon, the terminal branches of which are embedded in the peripheral sarcoplasm of a muscle fiber, usually loses its myelin sheath just before the beginning of the first branches.

Beyond the final myelin segment, the Schwann cells are represented by cells which are intimately linked with branching processes and which form the teloglia.

The sheath of Henle, which extends the system of lamellar sheaths of the nerve up to the motor end-plate, is formed of flattened and uninucleated cells of an endothelium reinforced by collagen fibrils. In spreading out at its termination, this sheath resembles an overturned funnel covering the entire motor end-plate and whose ends are attached to the muscle fiber.

Appropriate staining methods reveal the existence within the terminal branches of small mitochondria localized primarily along the axis of the branches.

The methods of silver impregnation enable the demonstration that the neurofibrils of the myelinated portion of the motor axon continues within the interior of the nerve ending. The neurofibrils often terminate in a swelling in the form of an olive, a curle or a ring.

At the surface of the muscle fiber, the terminal branches of the nerve occupy cavities, the synaptic gutters. The depth, shape and size of these gutters are very variable from species to species; they are cut into the flattened heap of the sarcoplasm, containing an abundance of nuclei and mitochondria, which Kühne has termed the sole.

The nuclei observed at the motor end-plate belong to cells of very different character. Some, attached to the terminal branches of the nerve, are nuclei from teloglial cells. Others, which contain rather large nucleoli, belong to muscle fibers. In addition to these two groups of nuclei are nuclei of endothelial cells of blood capillaries (these are often closely linked to the motor end-plate) and the nuclei of the sheath of Henle.

With the aid of certain postvital stains and enzymatic histochemical techniques, it is possible to render visible to the light microscope the "interface" between the terminal axoplasm and the sarcoplasm. In a section cut across a motor end-plate, this interface appears as a thin line to which is attached, on the sarcoplasmic side, lamellae. These are extended in the form of ribbons which constitute the subneural apparatus. In a transverse section examined under the light microscope, these subneural lamellae appear as rodlets, about one micron in length, and which are always orientated perpendicular to the surface of apposition of the axoplasm and the sarcoplasm. The juxtaposition of these rodlets on the deep face of the terminal branches results in an aspect resembling a palisade at the frontier between the nerve ending and the muscle fiber (Fig. 1).

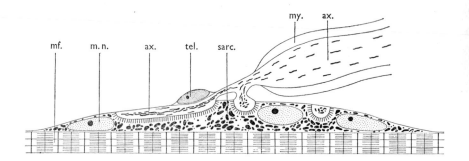

Fig. 1. Schematic drawing of a motor end-plate as seen through a light microscope (Couteaux, 1958). *ax.*, axoplasm with mitochondria; *my.*, myelin sheath; *tel.*, teloglia (terminal Schwann cells); *sarc.*, sarcoplasm with mitochondria; *m.n.*, muscle nuclei; *mf.*, myofibrils. The terminal nerve branches are lying in synaptic gutters. Immediately under the interface axoplasm–sarcoplasm, the ribbon-shaped subneural lamellae, transversely cut, may be seen as rodlets.

On the motor end-plate seen full-face, the lamellae of the subneural apparatus, which run under the terminal branching, give an overall appearance comparable to a finger print. From one point to another of the subneural apparatus, these lamellae have a very variable orientation and very unequal length.

2.2.2. FINE STRUCTURE OF THE NEUROMUSCULAR JUNCTION

Examination of the neuromuscular junction with the electron microscope has permitted the validation of a number of conclusions and interpretations which previously were based on studies with the light microscope and the use of stains more or less selective for certain organelles (nuclei, mitochondria, neurofibrils, and plasma membranes). On the other

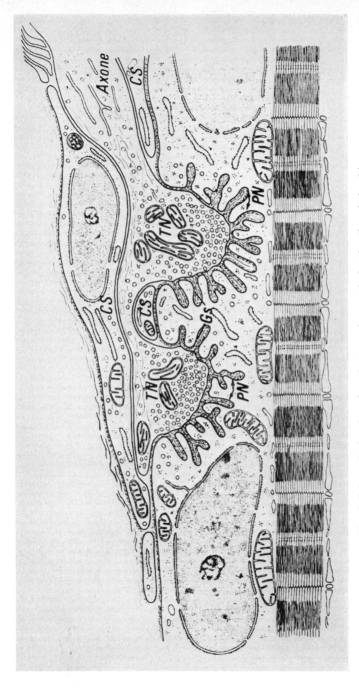

Fig. 2. Schematic drawing of an electron micrograph showing the relationship between the terminal nerve branches (T.N.), cut in cross-section at the motor end-plate, and the terminal Schwann cells (C.S.), the synaptic gutters (GS) and the subneural folds (PN) of the post-synaptic membrane. (After Porter and Bonneville, *Structure fine des cellules et des tissus*. Edit. Favard, Ediscience, Paris, 1969.)

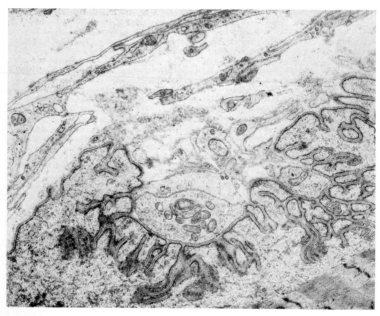

FIG. 3. Human motor end-plate (*M. peronoeus brevis*). A cross-section of synaptic gutters showing the terminal nerve branches, the teloglial caps (covering them), and the folds of the subneural apparatus. (Electron micrograph by M. Fardeau.)

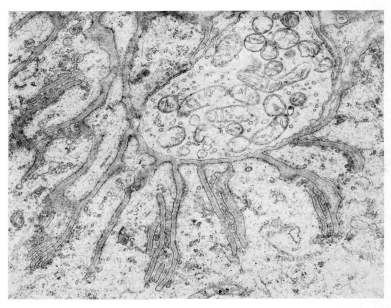

FIG. 4. Human motor end-plate (*M. peronoeus brevis*). Cross-section of a synaptic gutter. (Electron micrograph by M. Fardeau.)

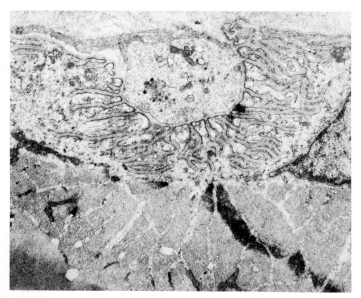

FIG. 5. Human motor end-plate (*M. peronoeus brevis*) showing in cross-section the particularly numerous subneural folds, radiating from a synaptic gutter. (Electron micrograph by M. Fardeau.)

hand, it has filled a number of important omissions and supplied some completely new facts (Figs. 2–5).

The electron microscope has shown that the terminal branches contain not only mitochondria and neurofilaments, approximately 10 nm in diameter, grouped in bundles which correspond to the neurofibrils of the light microscope, but also "synaptic vesicles". These are some 30 to 60 nm in diameter and generally grouped in the deeper region of the nerve terminal branches, near the boundary which separates them from the sarcoplasm. Often glycogen particles are intermixed with these vesicles. It is of note that the microtubules, about 25 nm in diameter, observed within the motor axon usually terminate just before the terminal branching.

In the synaptic gutter which it occupies, each branch is in contact by its deeper part with the muscle fiber and by its superficial part with a teloglial cell. This is a thin layer of cytoplasm which covers the nerve terminal branch along its entire length, but leaves it uncovered on the side of the synaptic gutter.

The plasma membrane or plasmalemma which limits the nerve terminal branch as well as the plasmalemma which limits the sarcoplasm are covered by a basal lamina both within the synaptic gutter and outside it. These basal laminae seem to be separated from the plasmalemmas by a layer some 10 to 20 nm in size and which is not opaque to electrons under the conditions of fixation and "staining" used in electron microscopy at the present time (fixation with OsO_4 or by an aldehyde, followed in the latter case by a postfixation by OsO_4; embedding in araldite or epon; staining with phosphotungstic acid or by uranyl acetate and lead citrate). The basal laminae, nervous and muscular, fuse intimately together at the bottom of the synaptic gutter. As a result of this configuration, the presynaptic and postsynaptic membranes remain separated by a basal lamina even in the region of the junction where they are the closest one to the other. The space, partly occupied by the basal lamina, between the presynaptic and postsynaptic membranes where these two are apposed one to the other corresponds to the synaptic cleft. This is 30 to 50 nm in size, and it is across this that the transmission of the excitation from the motor axon to the muscle fiber takes place. The portions of the plasma membranes, nervous and muscular, which are situated above and below this cleft play a particularly important role in synaptic transmission. This is both because of their position and also certainly because of their specialization. The synaptic vesicles are generally amassed against the "suprasynaptic" membrane of the axon plasmalemma. The specialization of the subneural or subsynaptic zone of the muscular plasmalemma is clearly demonstrated by its enzymatic activities. In a number of vertebrates, particularly in reptiles and mammals, it constitutes the lamellae of the subneural apparatus which has been described above in the general terms observable with the light microscope and the ultrastructure of which will be discussed below.

The subneural folds. The first observations of the neuromuscular junction carried out with the electron microscope (Palade and Palay, 1954; Reger, 1954, 1958; Robertson, 1954, 1956b) immediately made it possible to interpret with certainty the lamellae of the subneural apparatus as the folds of the membrane which limits the sarcoplasm at the junction.

The depth of these folds, when observed in transverse section, is usually slightly less than 1 mcm, but in man may sometimes reach larger values and even exceed 2.5 mcm (Harven and Coërs, 1959).

Each of the subneural folds (this term is preferable to "junctional folds" which could equally apply to the folds formed by the muscle plasmalemma at the site of the muscle–tendon junction) is formed not only by the muscle plasmalemma, but also by the basal lamina which accompanies the muscle plasmalemma in its invagination and carpets the concavity of the fold. At each fold, the space delineated by the plasmalemma opens into the synaptic cleft. For this reason the synaptic cleft is often separated into the primary synaptic cleft, the space between the nerve and muscle plasmalemmas, and the secondary synaptic clefts, the spaces delineated by the folds of the muscle plasmalemma.

Judged by its appearance after the currently used methods of fixation and staining, it would seem that the structure of the plasmalemma and that of the basal lamina is the same in the synaptic and non-synaptic parts of the muscle fiber. However, the criteria available to us at present are insufficiently sensitive for the comparison to be really conclusive. The only difference which is evident at present concerns the connections of the basal lamina with the fibrils of the adjacent connective tissue. Thus whilst the ordinary basal lamina of a muscle fiber is usually reinforced on the outside with fibrils of various size, all fibrils, even the thinnest, are completely excluded from the primary and secondary synaptic clefts.

Although it is not possible, at least with present-day electron micrographs, to detect a significant difference between the structure of the basal lamina which covers the muscle fiber at the subneural apparatus and that in the non-synaptic zones, this is not the case on the internal side where the plasmalemma appears doubled by an opaque stratum some hundreds of Ångströms in thickness.

After fixation with OsO_4 or by an aldehyde and secondarily by OsO_4, this layer seems to make union with the plasmalemma. However, after fixation with potassium permanganate, only the subneural plasmalemma seems to be stained and shows a thickness apparently equal to that of the ordinary plasmalemma, i.e. less than 10 nm. Thus in the subneural region of the muscle fiber there is no real thickening of the plasmalemma but rather a differentiation of the sarcoplasm immediately neighboring this membrane. This sublemmal stratum does not have a uniform electron opacity. In the external portion, it seems as opaque as the plasmalemma, but the opacity progressively diminishes from the exterior towards the interior and ends in merging with that of the ordinary sarcoplasm. Thus it is impossible to recognize by a difference of opacity the internal limit of the sublemmal stratum. In addition, on its inner side it often possesses a fringed appearance which renders its delineation even more difficult. On the human motor end-plate after fixation with OsO_4, a fine striation has been observed in the sublemmal stratum (Fardeau, personal communication). It is of note that micropinocytotic images, which are presented quite frequently by the ordinary plasmalemma of a muscle fiber, are not observed in the region of the plasmalemma lined with the sublemmal stratum.

This stratum is present at all regions of the muscle plasmalemma which borders the primary synaptic cleft, but it disappears in certain zones of the subneural folds, particularly in their deeper regions. In the regions of the folds where the sublemmal stratum is interrupted, numerous micropinocytosis vesicles and sections of tubules are found close to the plasmalemma. These tubules seem to belong to the sarcoplasmic reticulum.

Mention should equally be made of the presence, in the subneural region of the muscle fiber, of a layer of special sarcoplasm. This layer is divided into slices by the subneural fold and possesses structural particularities which have recently been studied in the frog (Couteaux and Pécot-Dechavassine, 1968). Between the subneural folds, which in the frog are aligned transversally in relation to the direction of the nerve branch, bundles of filaments may be observed which are also transversally orientated. These are particularly clearly seen after primary fixation with an aldehyde. These subneural filaments, some 5 nm in size, are particularly found in the central region of each sarcoplasmic "interfold".

As is the case with the sublemmal stratum, the existence of these filaments indicates the differentiation of the subneural sarcoplasm.

In concluding this brief description of the subneural apparatus, mention will be made of the selective staining of this apparatus obtained by Sávay and Csillik (1958), by treating the fresh muscle with a solution of lead nitrate and then with a solution of sodium sulfite. Csillik (1965) has shown that all the sarcoplasmic membrane has an affinity for lead. This applies equally to the non-synaptic region as the synaptic region. The marked reaction of the subneural apparatus results mainly from folding of the membrane at the apparatus. It would also appear that the reaction shows qualitative differences in the synaptic and non-synaptic regions. Nakamura *et al.* (1966) and Namba and Grob (1967) have obtained similar results not only with lead but also with other divalent metals (tin, cadmium, zinc and copper), either by immersing the fresh muscle in solutions of the metallic salts or by intramuscular injection of these solutions *in vivo*. It also seems from their experiments that the affinity of the subneural apparatus for these metallic ions is independent from the cholinesterase activity of the subneural apparatus.

The primary and secondary synaptic clefts. One of the most important problems raised by the study of the neuromuscular junction is that of the ultrastructure and the chemical constitution of the primary and secondary synaptic clefts between the nerve and muscle plasmalemmas.

It has previously been mentioned that the basal lamina observed at the surface of the plasmalemmas of the motor axon and of the muscle fiber also exists at the primary and secondary synaptic clefts, and that there is morphological continuity between the basal, synaptic and non-synaptic, laminae (Robertson, 1956b). There is also continuity between the non-opaque layers which separate the basal laminae of the plasmalemmas in the synaptic and non-synaptic regions.

All data concerning the basal lamina, even non-synaptic, of the muscle fiber in relation to the plasmalemma could be important in defining the nature of the synaptic cleft. At the present time, there is unfortunately only very imprecise data on the structure and constitution of these laminae. Situated above the plasmalemma of cells of various types, they have been given the much too general and certainly only provisional name of basal laminae.

Some authors have expressed the opinion that some of the electron opaque areas described from electron micrographs as basal laminae, situated above the plasmalemma of cells of various types, are, in reality, artefacts. In the particular case of the striated muscle fibers, there is no doubt of the existence of this lamina, as a structure pre-existing the fixation and staining. One of the main arguments that may be advanced in favor of this point of view is of an experimental nature. Birks *et al.* (1959) have shown that in the muscles of the frog where a high degree of atrophy followed denervation, the basal lamina was a stable structure. This showed a certain independence of the plasmalemma during the atrophy of

14

the muscle fiber. The lamina does not shrink as does the plasmalemma and thus becomes too large relative to the reduced volume of the fiber. In severely atrophied muscle, it forms a complicated system of longitudinal folds.

The basal lamina of the muscle fiber may thus be considered as a real structure; its nature is, however, still ill-defined. The same applies to the layer not opaque to electrons situated between the plasmalemma and the basal lamina.

The main data at present available on the chemical nature of the basal lamina and other extracellular layers found on the surface of the cells, and in particular on the surface of the plasmalemma of the striated muscle fiber, will be outlined below.

In a number of publications dating from 1946, McManus has shown that the basal laminae of a number of cells are stained by periodic acid—Schiff's reagent (PAS positive reaction). These results were rapidly confirmed by Lillie, Hotchkiss and subsequently by numerous authors.

Schiebler (1953), who studied cardiac muscle, found that the "sarcolemma" was always stained by PAS.

It seemed very likely that the staining of the basal lamina by PAS was due to the presence of a mucopolysaccharide linked to protein (Leblond *et al.*, 1957; Goldstein, 1959). The observations carried out on the motor end-plate (Noël, 1957; Zacks and Blumberg, 1961b) where the nerve cell, Schwann cells and muscle cell membranes were "PAS positive" material have enabled a similar conclusion to be drawn. In the studies just mentioned, which were carried out with the light microscope, the resolving power of the instrument did not make it possible to state with any certainty what proportion of the PAS positive staining was due to the various layers observable with the electron microscope, i.e. the basal lamina, the plasmalemma and the intermediate layer not opaque to electrons.

Two series of studies carried out with the electron microscope make it possible to suppose that the material stained by PAS on the cell surface is not exclusively situated in the basal lamina, but also in a layer closely linked to the plasmalemma. These studies are, first, those of Bennett (1963) leading to the still hypothetical notion that the plasmalemma of all animal cells is covered with a thin layer of amorphous material which is rich in carbohydrates, the "glycocalyx". Secondly, Gasic and Berwick (1963) have established that the cells of an ascites tumor are covered with a layer which is rich in carbohydrates and that sialic acid exists on the surface of these cells.

The histochemical studies of Rambourg *et al.* (1966), with the light microscope and those of Rambourg and Leblond (1967) with the electron microscope have shown that it is probably a general fact that a "cell coat" rich in carbohydrates exists on the surface of cells which are in close contact with the plasmalemma. This cell coat contains acidic groups which could be those of sialic acid.

Benedetti and Emmelot (1966, 1967) have shown, using preparations of isolated membranes of liver cells, that sialic acid is situated on the external surface of the plasmalemma, and was probably linked to the glycoproteins of the cell coat.

By combining the action of ruthenium red, the classical stain for pectine of plant tissues, with that of OsO_4, Luft (1966) rendered opaque to electrons a layer surrounding the striated muscle fibers. This layer was closely linked to the plasmalemma, as is the cell coat. It was, however, thicker than the latter and extended even beyond the basal lamina.

Finally, three groups of authors (Pease, 1966; Marinozzi, 1967; Rambourg, 1967) were able, by modifications in the techniques using phosphotungstic acid (PTA) to demonstrate on the surface of the plasmalemma, a thin layer which Rambourg considers as equivalent to the "cell coat" or "glycolemma". The richness of the latter in carbohydrates has been demonstrated by other methods (Rambourg and Leblond, 1967). It would seem that the hydroxyl groups of the polysaccharides and the glycoproteins are responsible for this reaction with PTA (Marinozzi, 1968; Rambourg, 1968).

Since the basal laminae described by Robertson on the surface of the muscle fiber (1956a) and at the neuromuscular junctions (1956b) owe their electron opacity to the "staining" by PTA, it may be surprising that the cell coat is not also rendered visible on the electron micrographs of this author. It should be realized that the conditions under which Robertson uses PTA are very different from those adopted by Pease, Marinozzi and Rambourg in their respective techniques. Among these important differences was that Robertson treated the tissue with PTA after fixation with OsO_4 and then embedded in n-butyl methacrylate. Marinozzi and Rambourg, on the other hand, treated the tissues with PTA after fixation with aldehydes and embedded in glycol methacrylate (GMA). Pease stained the sections on grids after embedding in hydroxypropylmethacrylate (HPMA) the tissues which were not fixed but the water of which had been removed by glycol (inert dehydration). It appears likely that the differences in opacity to electrons described by Robertson have a very different histochemical significance from the staining recently obtained with the same reagent but using very different conditions.

By using his method (PTA at pH 0.3) on the motor end-plates of the cat tongue Rambourg (personal communication) found that the primary and secondary synaptic clefts were completely stained by the PTA. It would thus appear that glycoproteins are distributed throughout the entire space delineated by the nerve and muscle plasmalemmas. These glycoproteins probably correspond both to the cell coat and to the basal lamina without it being possible to state precisely what proportion belongs to each of these layers.

At the primary synaptic cleft the nerve and muscle basal laminae are always joined one to the other without there being the slightest space between them. This is not the same, however, in the case of the secondary synaptic clefts where both sheets of the basal lamina which penetrate to the interior of each fold are not in general completely joined one to the other, but between them in certain regions of the fold a space remains. This space is much less opaque to electrons than the basal lamina and thus gives the impression of being a free space.

If one examines a transverse section of the subneural fold of a mammalian motor end-plate, particularly in man, two or three segments may be distinguished within the subneural fold. These follow one to the other from the surface to the depth of the fold and differ one from the other by a number of characteristics, in particular their thickness, the relationship between the two sheets of the basal lamina and the structure of the sarcoplasmic zone adjacent to the plasmalemma.

At the entrance to the fold the two sheets of the basal lamina are often joined together and become disconnected in the following segment which is slightly thicker than the initial one.

The space delineated by the sheets of the basal lamina in the second segment constitute a sort of flattened canaliculus which crosses the fold longitudinally and opens in the extracellular medium by slot-shaped orifices which are placed on either side of each nerve branch.

It is in this slightly dilated region of the folds where anastomoses are established between them in various types of neuromuscular junctions, notably in man. Due to these anastomoses the canaliculi form a sort of network below each nerve terminal branch.

If the space which it surrounds is filled by a fluid substance or is only more hydrated than the basal lamina such a system of canaliculi may naturally play an important role in the normal functioning of the neuromuscular junction since it places into direct communication the synaptic clefts with the extracellular medium. This also allows the more ready penetration of pharmacological agents into the synaptic clefts.

17

The fold is often terminated by a more narrow segment where the two sheets of the basal membrane are again joined. Along these terminal segments the sublemmal stratum does not generally exist, but the micropinocytosis vesicles are in contrast usually numerous on the deeper face of the plasmalemma.

When the subneural folds are particularly numerous and well developed, as is often the case with the human motor end-plate, each of these give rise, in the deeper regions of the subneural apparatus, to two or more secondary folds which are close together and which separate the micropinocytosis vesicles. Due to a number of experimental results it may be considered as established that the primary synaptic clefts, although they are occupied by the basal laminae and by the "cell coats", are highly permeable both to ions and molecules of very various kinds. These ions and molecules can enter into the primary synaptic cleft or emerge from it through the slot-shaped openings situated between the nerve branch and the muscle fiber along the edges of the synaptic gutter.

It may thus be supposed that independently from the possible resources of the canalicular system previously described the secondary synaptic clefts also possess a high degree of permeability since they possess a basal lamina and a "cell coat" which are similar both in their structure and in the abundance of glycoproteins to those present in the primary synaptic cleft.

2.3. CYTOCHEMICAL CHARACTERISTICS OF THE NEUROMUSCULAR JUNCTION

The particular morphological characteristics of the nerve ending and of the subneural apparatus which distinguish them both from the motor axon and from the normal sarcoplasm are associated with cytochemical peculiarities concerning the distribution of cholinesterases, of nonspecific esterases, of choline acetyltransferase and of acetylcholine. The distribution of carboxylic esterases will first be discussed.

2.3.1. DISTRIBUTION OF CHOLINESTERASES AND OTHER CARBOXYLIC ESTERASES

When assuming that in the transmission of a nerve impulse from a motor nerve to the striated muscle the depolarization of the sarcoplasmic membrane is determined by the local liberation of acetylcholine (Dale *et al.*, 1936; Brown *et al.*, 1936) one must postulate at the motor end-plate a mechanism for inactivating the acetylcholine liberated during the refractory period.

It is to search for this hypothetical mechanism, a condition necessary for attributing to acetylcholine a role as a mediator, which has led to the discovery of a high enzymatic concentration at the junction between a motor nerve and a striated muscle.

Amongst the various processes capable of causing rapid inactivation of acetylcholine it was natural to first envisage a hydrolysis by cholinesterase since it was known from the work of Plattner and Hinter (1930) that these enzymes were widely distributed in animal tissues.

The studies carried out in this direction with the aid of varied techniques, which will be reviewed later, have been remarkably fruitful. They have revealed in the region of the neuromuscular junction an accumulation of acetylcholinesterase (AChE-E.C. 3.1.1.7, acetylcholine acetylhydrolase). This would explain the hydrolysis, with the required rapidity, of the acetylcholine liberated during the synaptic transmission.

Other carboxylic esterases have also been detected in appreciable quantities in the region of the neuromuscular junction. These are nonspecific cholinesterases (CHE.ns-E.C. 3.1.1.8, acetylcholine acylhydrolase) and nonspecific esterases (E.ns).

2.3.1.1. *BIOCHEMICAL METHODS*

The first important biochemical studies on the distribution of cholinesterase activity in striated muscle were carried out using manometric techniques of Barcroft-Warburg on tissue homogenates. Marnay and Nachmansohn (1937) showed on the sartorius of the frog that there exists in the region of the motor innervation of this muscle an enzymatic concentration considerably more elevated than in the motor nerve or than in the aneural region of the muscle. They attributed this difference to the high concentration of the enzyme in the motor terminals of this muscle in the frog.

With this interpretation the enzymatic concentration in the region of the motor terminals appeared to be sufficient for the hydrolysis during the refractory period of the acetylcholine liberated during the nerve impulse transmission. These results have been confirmed by the findings of Feng and Ting (1938) on the muscles of the toad.

The first attempt to find on mammalian striated muscle the differences in the concentration of cholinesterase found on the sartorius of the frog was carried out on the internal and external gastrocnemii of the dog by Marnay, Nachmansohn and Couteaux (in: Marnay and Nachmansohn,

1938). In spite of the small number of results obtained the data were quite conclusive. However, the first really significant results, enabling the conclusions obtained on the end-bush of amphibia to be extended to the mammalian motor end-plate, were those obtained on the internal gastrocnemius of the guinea pig (Couteaux and Nachmansohn, 1939, 1940, 1942).

In these latter studies it was possible to determine the distribution of cholinesterases and to establish that there existed a relationship between this distribution and that of the motor end-plates. This was made possible by combining manometric determinations with histological studies. By measuring cholinesterase activity in a series of sections made with a freezing microtome with suitable orientation a curve may be drawn of the distribution of this activity in the muscle and to compare it with the curve of distribution of motor end-plates. The correlation between these two distributions may be accurately determined by alternating the biochemical determination of enzymatic activity with the staining of the nerve terminals by silver techniques in serial sections obtained from the same muscle.

Since the motor end-plate only represents a minute fraction of the total volume of muscle one could deduce from differences in the observed activity between regions of the muscle in which the motor end-plates were present and regions in which the motor end-plates were absent that the enzymatic concentration is probably extremely high at the motor end-plates themselves.

Knowing the number of motor end-plates in a muscle one could measure indirectly the enzymatic activity of a single motor end-plate. Marnay and Nachmansohn (1938) thus calculated on the sartorius of the frog that 1.6×10^9 molecules acetylcholine could be hydrolyzed by a single motor end-plate in 1 msec.

Studies subsequently carried out with micromanometric methods on segments of muscle fibers which had been isolated by means of micromanipulators so that each contained a single motor end-plate have enabled a much more direct measurement to be made of the enzymatic activity of a motor end-plate (Brzin and Zajicek, 1958; Giacobini and Holmstedt, 1960; Brzin and Majcen-Tkacen, 1963). The muscles used in these latter experiments were the diaphragm and the gastrocnemius of the mouse, the rat, or the rabbit. The figures obtained for the number of molecules hydrolyzed in one msec ranged according to the species and muscle between 2.9×10^7 and 3.7×10^8. Using microcolorimetric methods Buckley and Nowell (1966) obtained a similar figure (1.79×10^7) on the rat diaphragm. Finally, Namba and Grob (1968) have carried out studies on the anterior tibial muscle of the rat and have prepared muscle membrane fractions in which the motor end-plates were completely separated from the muscle fibers. The cholinesterase activity of these preparations was, per unit of nitrogen, 26.9 times higher than that of muscle homogenates and these authors found 2.69×10^8 molecules of acetylcholine hydrolyzed by the motor end-plate in 1 msec.

The high cholinesterase activity of the neuromuscular junction was first attributed to the nerve terminals themselves. Studies carried out on the variation in the cholinesterase activity of striated muscle after section of the motor nerve have led to a very different interpretation of the distribution of this activity. The degeneration of the nerve endings which follows section of the motor nerve did not lead to a disappearance of the large difference in the mean concentration in the neural and the aneural zones of the muscle. In certain muscles, for example the internal gastrocnemius of the guinea pig, 2 weeks after section of the motor nerve there is a close relationship between the enzymatic concentration in the region of the innervation and that in other muscle regions similar to that found in normal muscle (Couteaux and Nachmansohn, 1939, 1942). In this case the maintenance of an almost normal concentration in the innervated region may be explained to a large extent by an increase in the number of motor end-plates per unit volume of muscle resulting from the atrophy of the muscle fibers (Couteaux and Nachmansohn, 1938). In fact in the muscle deprived of nerve there is indeed a reduction in the cholinesterase activity of the motor end-plate but the major part of this activity neverthe-less remains for a fairly long time after the degeneration of the nerve. It does appear clear that the major part of the cholinesterase in the motor end-plate does not reside in the interior of the nerve ending but is out-side around it.

Taking account of the overall biochemical findings and of progress in the morphological study of the neuromuscular junction it seemed probable a few years later (Couteaux, 1947) that the high cholinesterase activity of the neuromuscular junction was located mainly in the region of the sub-neural apparatus (Fig. 6).

A number of studies which cannot be enumerated here have subse-quently been carried out on the cholinesterase of striated muscle using numerous and diverse biochemical techniques. These have been carried out on homogenates using a wide variety of substrates and of selective inhibitors.

As regards the nonspecific esterases of striated muscle our knowledge has recently been increased by new data. Thus Markert and Hunter (1959) have shown on thirty-two organs and tissues using the method of vertical

21

starch gel electrophoresis (Hunter and Markert, 1957) that the nonspecific esterases form a family comprising a number of enzymes. Using zymograms, as these latter authors, Barron *et al.* (1966, 1968) came to the conclusion that the nonspecific esterases of rat striated muscle comprise a series of eserine-resistant isoenzymes which were sensitive to the action of organophosphorus compounds and particularly that of the compound E600 which inhibits them at a concentration of 10^{-5} M. These enzymes possess the characteristics of nonspecific esterases of type B (aliesterases)

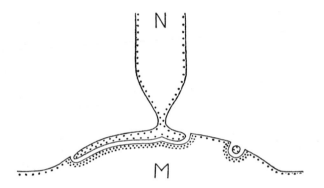

Fig. 6. Diagram showing the distribution of cholinesterase activities at the neuromuscular junction based on results obtained by biochemical and morphological techniques (Couteaux, 1947). *N*, axon; *M*, muscle fibre. The suggested sites of cholinesterase activities are shown as dots, more numerous where the activities are greater.

similar to those defined by Aldridge (1953). Their sensitivity to the action of organophosphorus compounds enables them to be distinguished from nonspecific esterases of type A (arylesterases) as well as those of type C as defined by Bergmann *et al.* (1957).

2.3.1.2 *HISTOCHEMICAL METHODS*

Introduced and controlled at each stage by biochemical determinations, the *in situ* study of cholinesterases and of nonspecific esterases at the neuromuscular junction is one of the questions of enzymatic histochemistry which has been studied in great detail.

The selective inhibitors used by biochemists for the identification of cholinesterases and of nonspecific esterases in homogenates of numerous tissues and notably muscular tissues have permitted histochemists to separate on tissue sections the diverse esterase activities of striated muscle and of the neuromuscular junction and to attempt to localize the site of each.

Amongst the inhibitors of carboxylic esterases of which there exists at the present time a large number belonging to a wide range of chemical substances, a number are very often used in histochemical studies and particularly carried out on striated muscle.

Eserine sulfate or eserine salicylate in a concentration of 10^{-5} M inhibits cholinesterases but does not affect the activity of other esterases.

In order to distinguish acetylcholinesterase from the nonspecific cholinesterases one makes use of compounds which preferentially inhibit either acetylcholinesterase or the nonspecific cholinesterases. Amongst the compounds widely used to inhibit the nonspecific cholinesterases one may mention DFP (di-isopropyl-fluorophosphate) at 10^{-6} M; iso-OMPA (tetra-isopropyl-pyrophosphoramide) at 10^{-6} M and ethopropazine (10-(2-diethylamino-1-propyl) phenothiazine) at 10^{-4} M.

In contrast to the latter compounds the substance 284C51 (1,5-bis(4-allyl-dimethylammonium phenyl) pentane-3-one) and 62C47 (1,5-bis 4-tri-methylammonium phenyl) *n*-pentane-3-one) preferentially inhibit acetylcholinesterase at 10^{-5} M.

When one is dealing with an esterase which is resistant to eserine, that is a nonspecific esterase, the inhibitor most widely used to distinguish esterases of type B and those of type A and C which are resistant to organic phosphates is the compound E600 (diethyl-*p*-nitrophenyl phosphate), which selectively inhibits esterases of type B at a concentration of 10^{-5} M.

Due to the selectivity of these inhibitors it is possible for histochemical studies on cholinesterases and on other carboxylic esterases to use methods which are based on substrates of very unequal specificity. Each method has its own advantages and inconveniences depending on the nature of enzyme. The comparison of the results obtained by all these methods leads to much firmer conclusions, at least when the results are in agreement.

(a) *Localization with the light microscope*

Results obtained using different substrates. The first histochemical method proposed for the localization of cholinesterases was that of Gomori (1948) who used esters of choline and of higher fatty acids principally myristoylcholine as substrate. The principle of this method is briefly as follows: a cobalt salt is added to the incubation medium which contains the substrate; the fatty acid which is liberated by the enzymatic hydrolysis combines with the cobalt and gives a white insoluble precipitate which

23

after reaction with ammonium sulfide gives a black precipitate of cobalt sulfide.

The application of this method to sections obtained after fixation by cold acetone and embedding in paraffin blocks gives very variable results. On frozen sections of the non-fixed diaphragm Denz (1953) was regularly able to obtain staining of the motor end-plate.

As regards the specificity of the method, *in vitro* experiments carried out by Gomori (1952 a, b) on various preparations of cholinesterases have led to the conclusion that the esters used could not be hydrolyzed by some acetylcholinesterases and by certain nonspecific cholinesterases. These latter findings varied, however, according to the ester. It thus appeared that preparations of purified acetylcholinesterases from erythrocytes and from the electric organ could not readily hydrolyze myristoylcholine.

In view of this type of result it was difficult to state with any precision the nature of the enzyme responsible for the staining of the motor end-plate which was observed with this technique.

Denz has studied further the action of acetylcholinesterase on myristoyl-choline using preparations of purified acetylcholinesterase from sheep erythrocytes and from rat brain. He found that these preparations produced an "appreciable hydrolysis" of myristoylcholine and, with the use of selective inhibitors, he established that this hydrolysis was due to acetyl-cholinesterase and not to nonspecific cholinesterases or nonspecific esterases which coexisted in the same preparation. These inhibitors enabled him to conclude that the staining of the motor end-plate obtained with myristoylcholine was also due to the presence of acetylcholinesterase.

The use of acetylthiocholine as a substrate which was introduced into histochemistry by Koelle and Friedenwald (1949) was the start of the impressive progress made since then in the histochemistry of the cholin-esterases.

The main advantage of this substrate is that it is hydrolyzed very rapidly by acetylcholinesterase, indeed at certain pH's more rapidly than acetyl-choline itself. The thiocholine liberated by enzymatic hydrolysis in an incubation medium containing glycin and copper sulfate gives rise to a white precipitate, which may then be converted to a brown precipitate of copper sulfide by ammonium sulfide.

The mechanism of the reactions on which this method is based has not yet been completely elucidated. Malmgren and Sylvén (1955) have carried out a chemical analysis of the initial white precipitate and consider that it consists of cuprothiocholine sulfate. More recent studies, however, lead to the suggestion that its composition is more complex. The hydrolysis of acetylthiocholine appears only to give rise to this precipitate if the incubation medium contains iodine and it seems that iodine is a constituent of the final precipitate (Tsuji, 1968).

Acetylthiocholine is acted on, not only by acetylcholinesterase, but also by the nonspecific cholinesterases. Nevertheless, by a pretreatment of the sections with DFP which preferentially inhibits the nonspecific cholinesterase, Koelle (1950, 1951) was able, using acetylthiocholine as substrate, to demonstrate the separate activity of acetylcholinesterase. In order to localize the nonspecific cholinesterases, he used another ester of thiocholine, butyrylthiocholine, a substrate which is much more rapidly hydrolyzed by nonspecific cholinesterases than by acetylcholinesterase.

When combined with the use of specific inhibitors, the method using esters of thiocholine can reach a high degree of specificity. However, the data on locations is much less rigorous. The latter method may give rise to artefacts due to diffusion which leads to false locations which may be very varied. In the case of striated muscle, this is due to diffusion of the reaction products to neighboring sites rather than diffusion of the enzymes themselves.

Among the factors which determine the diffusion of the reaction products, the pH is certainly the most critical (Couteaux and Taxi, 1951, 1952). In order to avoid this a pH around 5 should be chosen, that is a pH considerably less than that above which a precipitate can no longer be formed with the technique of Koelle and Friedenwald.

The structures stained by diffusion vary according to the pH and the length of incubation. It also depends on whether the tissue has been stained in the fresh condition or after fixation. The optimum pH for the histochemical reaction, that is the pH at which the diffusion artefacts are minimal, varies according to the species and should therefore be determined for each species.

Since the initial work of Koelle and Friedenwald, the thiocholine technique, as applied to cholinesterases of striated muscle, has undergone many modifications. However, these have usually consisted only of changes in the mode of utilization (Koelle, 1950, 1951; Portugalov and Yakovlev, 1951; Couteaux and Taxi, 1952; Coërs, 1953a; Gerebtzoff, 1953, 1959; Holmstedt, 1957b; Lewis, 1961). However, the modifications suggested by Karnovsky and Roots (Karnovsky and Roots, 1964; Karnovsky, 1964) and that of Davis and Koelle (1965) both differ from the original method of Koelle and Friedenwald in the nature of the initial precipitate.

Karnovsky and Roots add to the incubation medium containing the thiocholine ester and $CuSO_4$ some potassium ferricyanide. The sites of

25

cholinesterase appear directly stained by the formation of a brown precipitate of copper ferrocyanide. It seems that the thiocholine liberated by the enzymatic hydrolysis reduces the ferricyanide to ferrocyanide. This combines with Cu^{++} ions to form a brown insoluble precipitate of copper ferrocyanide.

The modification suggested by Davies and Koelle consists of substituting an aurous compound in the incubation medium for the copper sulfate. The authors assumed that under these conditions the first reaction product is aurothiocholine phosphate which is subsequently transformed by the ammonium sulfide into Au_2S. This modification gives with the light microscope results on the motor end-plate comparable to those obtained by the initial technique using copper. However, the image has considerably less contrast and in general the method has little interest except for use with the electron microscope.

The various techniques that have been described using esters of thiocholine as substrate all produce staining of the motor end-plate. From results obtained with the use of selective inhibitors, Denz (1953) concluded that the staining obtained with acetylthiocholine is due to acetylcholinesterase. However, the staining obtained following a long incubation period with butyrylthiocholine indicates the presence of nonspecific cholinesterases. It may be concluded from the studies of Denz and those of Homstedt (1957 a, b), who also used a number of selective inhibitors, that the motor end-plate contains both acetylcholinesterase and nonspecific cholinesterases. However, the concentration of nonspecific cholinesterases at the motor end-plate is relatively less than that of acetylcholinesterase. A number of other authors have reached a similar conclusion, in particular Pécot-Dechavassine, (1961), Barron *et al.* (1967), Eränkö and Teräväinen (1967).

Using beta-naphthyl acetate as substrate Nachlas and Seligman (1949) primarily determined the location of nonspecific esterases. However, both acetylcholinesterase and nonspecific cholinesterases also hydrolyze this substrate (Barrnett and Seligman, 1951). This substrate has also been used to localize cholinesterases (Ravin *et al.*, 1953).

In this technique the naphthol liberated by enzymatic hydrolysis is converted into an insoluble azo dye due to its coupling with a diazonium salt. Gomori (1950) substituted alpha-naphthyl for beta-naphthyl and the former is now most usually used. In the modification proposed by Lehrer and Ornstein (1959) the coupling reaction is carried out with hexazonium pararosanilin.

Using alpha- or beta-naphthyl acetate as substrate and Fast Blue B as a coupling agent Denz (1953) observed in unfixed sections of rat muscle a purple coloration of motor end-plate. However, he did not obtain this effect in paraffin sections of muscle fixed in acetone. In contrast he obtained in both cases a diffused crimson staining throughout the entire extent of the muscle fibers. He showed with the aid of inhibitors that the staining of the motor end-plate obtained when one uses alpha- or beta-naphthyl acetate as substrate is due to acetylcholinesterase. This conclusion added support to the *in vitro* studies he had carried out on the hydrolysis of both the substrates by purified preparations of acetylcholinesterase. The diffuse staining is hardly affected by a 10^{-3} M eserine or by 10^{-5} M E600. This resistance to inhibitors coupled with the observation of a diffuse staining of muscle fibers obtained with the method of Gomori for lipases led Denz to think that this was due to a nonspecific esterase probably of type A which did not have focal concentration in the region of the neuromuscular junction.

The histochemical studies on the distribution of nonspecific esterases in the striated muscle of the rat have recently been taken up again with alpha-naphthyl acetate by two groups (Barron *et al.*, 1967; Eränkö and Teräväinen, 1967) who reached conclusions different from those of Denz. Indeed these authors concluded that there was present both in the striated muscle and in a higher concentration in the motor end-plate a nonspecific esterase which by its resistance to eserine and its sensitivity to the action of organophosphorous compounds (E600) enabled it to be identified as an esterase of type B.

Indoxyl compounds may also be interesting substrates for the detection of muscle esterases. The liberation of indoxyl by enzymatic hydrolysis of indoxyl acetate or of its homologues and its subsequent oxidation gives rise to an insoluble indigo precipitate. Barrnett and Seligman (1951) were the first to develop a method of this type. They chose indoxyl acetate as substrate. Holt and Withers (1952) and subsequently Holt (1954) and Holt and Withers (1958) considerably improved the method by substituting other oxidizing agents for the oxidizing action of the atmosphere and by using other indoxyl derivatives, particularly 5-bromo-4-chloro-indoxyl acetate. This latter compound was the most appropriate for the study of esterases. This conclusion was reached after a systematic comparison of the data obtained with a number of esterases.

Esters of indoxyl are readily hydrolyzed by acetylcholinesterase, by the nonspecific cholinesterases and by the nonspecific esterases. With these substrates it is possible to obtain a staining of the motor end-plate which is comparable to that obtained by the method using esters of choline or with alpha-naphthyl acetate.

The technique using thiolacetic acid (Crevier and Belanger, 1955; Csillik and Sávay, 1958) is not more specific for cholinesterases than are the previous methods since thiolacetic acid can be hydrolyzed by non-specific esterases. The enzymatic hydrolysis of this acid liberates a thiol and in the presence of lead acetate or nitrate the site of the enzyme is indicated by the formation of a precipitate of lead sulfide. This technique also furnishes a staining of the motor end-plate but the identification of the esterases in this case depends entirely on the use of selective inhibitors.

A recent modification of this technique uses an aurous compound also used in the variations of the methods with thiocholine esters mentioned previously. The aurous compound is substituted for the lead salts (Davis and Koelle, 1965; Koelle and Gromadzki, 1966). However, this change which leads to a reduction in the intensity of the staining produces its value only for studies with the electron microscope.

Finally, thiolesters have recently been used as substrates. The thiol liberated by enzymatic activity is coupled with Fast Blue BBN and forms a diazothioether which may be converted into osmium "black", a coordination polymer osmium, by exposing the diazothioether to vapors of OsO_4 (Hanker *et al.*, 1966; Seligman *et al.*, 1966). The hydrolysis of several substrates of this type can thus be visualized by the formation of osmiophilic diazothioethers. A number of these have been used in the study of motor end-plate and in particular 2-naphthyl thiolacetate (NTA), 2-thiolacetoxybenzanilide (TAB) and 2-thiolpropionoxybenzanilide (TPB) (Hanker *et al.*, 1964; Bergman *et al.*, 1968).

Two of these thiolesters (NTA and TAB) are preferentially hydrolyzed by nonspecific cholinesterases and other esterases (Hanker *et al.*, 1964; Seligman *et al.*, 1966).

In spite of these differences the types of staining of the motor end-plate obtained with these three substrates are similar when examined by the light microscope. Only the observations carried out with the electron microscope and which are reported later have enabled to establish a difference between the locations suggested by these preparations.

Discussion

The results which have just been presented clearly establish that a number of substrates (acetylthiocholine, butyrylthiocholine, myristoylcholine, alpha-naphthyl acetate, indoxyl acetate and its homologues, thiolacetic acid, thiolesters) undergo enzymatic hydrolysis at the motor end-plate much more rapidly than they do in other regions of the muscle fiber.

Due to the already high degree of specificity of thiocholine esters and to the selectivity of esterine it has been shown that the enzymes responsible for this hydrolysis are mainly cholinesterases.

The effects obtained on the cholinesterase activities of the motor end-plate by inhibitors which act preferentially on either acetylcholinesterase or the nonspecific cholinesterases as well as the speed with which these hydrolyze acetylthiocholine and butyrylthiocholine respectively makes it very probable that the two types of cholinesterases co-exist at the motor end-plate but that acetylcholinesterase is preponderant.

From recent studies on the nonspecific esterases of striated muscle it appears that esterases of type B also exist at the motor end-plate.

It is now necessary to define the precise sites of the cholinesterases and the nonspecific esterases at the motor end-plate where such a large number of different structures belonging to the nerve ending, the muscle fibery, and the teloglia are juxtaposed.

A precise localization of these enzymes is naturally only possible if the structures of the motor end-plate, some of which are very labile, can be preserved in a satisfactory manner. Fortunately a large proportion of the cholinesterase activity of the neuromuscular junction may still be demonstrated after fixation of the tissue by, for example, formaldehyde (Couteaux and Taxi, 1951; Couteaux, 1951), as well as by other aldehydes such as glutaraldehyde (Sabatini *et al.*, 1963). The fixation of the tissue minimizes the tissue alterations taking place during the histochemical treatments. However, the rate of inactivation of cholinesterase in striated muscle by the fixing agent, for example formaldehyde, may vary considerably from one species to another. Thus it is much more rapid on the muscles of the frog than on the muscles of the mouse. The histochemical recognition of this great difference in the resistance of muscle cholinesterases of different animal species to the action of formaldehyde has been confirmed by biochemical studies carried out on the cholinesterases of other organs (Taxi, 1952). This latter author has shown that the resistance to the action of formaldehyde greatly depends on the type of cholinesterase in question.

These inequalities in the effects of fixation on enzymatic activity necessitate a careful comparison of results obtained in using fresh and fixed tissues.

Using fresh muscle tissue or tissue fixed with formaldehyde, using acetyl-thiocholine as substrate and by choosing a pH of the incubation medium and a duration of incubation such that the diffusion is minimized, it has been demonstrated that the staining of the motor end-plate appears to be limited to the folds of the subneural apparatus (Couteaux and Taxi, 1951,

1952; Couteaux, 1951, 1958; Coërs, 1953 a, b, 1955; Gerebtzoff, 1953; Gerebtzoff *et al.*, 1954) (Fig. 7).

A similar conclusion may be reached using all other substrates the enzymatic hydrolysis of which may be visualized histochemically.

The fact that a selective staining of the subneural apparatus may be obtained by the hydrolysis at the motor end-plate of such diverse substrates as esters of thiocholine, naphthol, indoxyl and thiols constitutes a strong argument in favor of the location of cholinesterases at the subneural apparatus.

Nevertheless, the question remains as to whether the cholinesterase is uniquely located at the folds of the subneural apparatus. Indeed it is not possible with the light microscope to detect the synaptic cleft, a few hundred Ångströms wide, separating the plasma membrane which limits the nerve terminal from the plasma membrane which limits the sarcoplasm. It is therefore impossible to decide using the light microscope whether the axonal plasmalemma in the region of the synoptic cleft is or is not a site for cholinesterase activity distinct from that in the subneural apparatus.

Without recourse to experimentation it would be difficult, in view of the proximity of the pre- and postsynaptic membranes and the possibility that the diffusion of hydrolysis products occurs, to establish to any degree of certainty which of these two is the main site of the cholinesterase activity of the motor end-plate. However, further information on this point is provided by the numerous histochemical observations carried out on denervated motor end-plates. The persistence of significant cholinesterase activities in the region of the motor end-plate of the rat, the guinea pig, and the rabbit after section of the motor nerve and degeneration of the nerve terminals has been indicated in a preliminary note by Sawyer *et al.* (1950) and Kupfer (1951). A similar conclusion was subsequently reached by the more thorough histochemical studies of Coërs (1953c), Snell and MacIntyre (1955, 1956), Sávay and Csillik (1956), Gerebtzoff and Vandersmissen (1956), Schwarzacher (1957) and Bauer *et al.* (1962). These studies have shown that the cholinesterase activities which persist at the motor end-plate after denervation are present as in the normal muscle at the subneural apparatus. Two weeks after section of the motor nerve the general appearance of the subneural apparatus already shows changes; however, it is possible to distinguish the lamellae of this apparatus stained by histochemical methods. These results which are in complete agreement with later biochemical studies demonstrate the location of cholinesterase at postsynaptic subneural sites. It does not, however, exclude the possibility

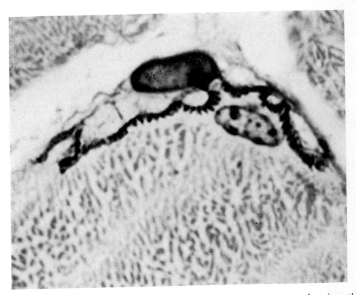

FIG. 7. Hedgehog motor end-plate (Couteaux, 1955), prepared using the Koelle acetylthiocholine method. The section shows the localization of cholinesterases at the subneural apparatus. Nuclei are stained by haematoxylin.

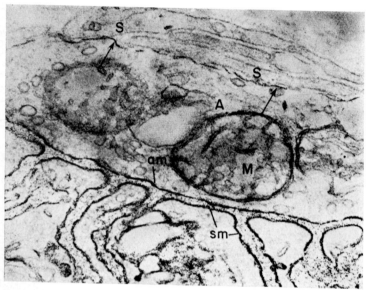

FIG. 8. The localization of AChE activity at a mouse motor end-plate with the electron microscope, using the thiolacetic acid–gold technique after treatment with DFP (3×10^{-7} M). *A*, axon; *M*, mitochondria; *am*, presynaptic axonal membrane; *sm*, sarcoplasmic postsynaptic membrane; *S*, teloglial Schwann cell. The presynaptic and postsynaptic membranes are stained. Moderate staining is also present in the axonal plasma membrane (arrows) facing the teloglial Schwann cell. (After Davis and Koelle, 1967.)

of cholinesterase located at presynaptic sites in the region of the membrane limiting the nerve terminal in the region where it is adjacent to the sub-neural apparatus.

A presynaptic location seems fairly certain at the neuromuscular junction of the hippocampus muscles (Couteaux, 1961). In contrast to the neuromuscular junctions of mammalian and frog fast muscles the plasma-lemma of the muscle fibers does not fold in the subneural region. On the other hand, histochemical studies of these junctions carried out using acetylthiocholine, butyrylthiocholine and alpha-naphthyl acetate (modification of Lehrer and Ornstein) and by using selective inhibitors makes it seem probable that the nerve terminals contain both acetylcholinesterase and nonspecific cholinesterases and that the nonspecific cholinesterases are present in significant quantities.

This presynaptic location is not confined to the terminal ramification of the axon but extends throughout its length. Since the staining of terminals requires approximately the same duration of incubation as that of the other unmyelinated portions of the nerve fibers the cholinesterase activities which reside in the terminals are without doubt nearly equivalent to those of the axon. These activities are thus not primarily located in the nerve terminal but constitute significant level of activity present throughout the motor nerve fiber.

The problem of the cholinesterase content of the postsynaptic membrane of the neuromuscular junction of the hippocampus is comparable to that of the presynaptic location at the neuromuscular junction of other vertebrates as outlined above. The width of the synaptic cleft is of the order of several hundred Ångströms and the presynaptic portions are here very rich in cholinesterases. It is thus impossible to reach a conclusion on preparations studied with the light microscope as to the presence or the absence of a subneural location of cholinesterase activity.

It should be possible by section of the motor nerve and subsequent disappearance of the presynaptic activity to distinguish the presynaptic from the postsynaptic cholinesterase activity in case where there is an important postsynaptic concentration of cholinesterase at the neuro-muscular junction. Unfortunately in the hippocampus section of the motor nerve does not lead to rapid disappearance of cholinesterase activity of the nerve fibers and their endings. This activity persists almost as long as the nerve fibers themselves and although many of the fibers become monili-form or very fragmented they may nevertheless be demonstrated by methods for detecting cholinesterase more than 15 days after nerve section at 20°C. In some cases the degeneration of the nerve terminal appears almost complete at the end of 15 days; the terminal only remains visible due to the fine granules (stained by histochemical treatment) which run along the path of the otherwise vanished nerve terminal; no cholinesterase activity has ever been demonstrated at the adjacent sarcoplasmic membrane. Although not completely conclusive these experiments involving degeneration would thus seem to agree with the hypothesis that a presynaptic location of cholinesterase activity is preponderant at the neuromuscular junction of the hippocampus.

The real demonstration of a subneural location of cholinesterase activity in the hippocampus or of a presynaptic location for those junctions possessing subneural folds will only be possible with an instrument with a higher resolving power than the light microscope. The same is true for the cholinesterase or nonspecific esterase activities residing in structures such as the teloglia which are less readily identified with the light microscope than is the subneural apparatus or which may be masked by other locations.

(b) *Localization with the electron microscope*

Results obtained using different substrates. Those methods which may be used with the light microscope and which have just been described have not all been immediately transposed to the electron microscope. The first requirement which each must satisfy for use with the electron microscope is that the precipitate by virtue of which the enzymatic hydrolysis of the substrate is made visible in the light microscope is itself opaque to electrons. This is not always the case.

Many other conditions must also be satisfied in order that enzymatic histochemistry may afford data useful at the ultrastructural scale.

Primarily it must allow a satisfactory preservation of the ultrastructures and this implies that the tissue must be already fixed before incubation. The fixation of the tissue before incubation must naturally preserve the enzymatic activity which one wishes to localize. This immediately excludes fixatives containing osmium and $KMnO^4$ which in the conditions of time and concentration necessary to achieve good fixation inactivate almost all the cholinesterases and the nonspecific esterases.

Lehrer and Ornstein (1959) were the first to apply to the study of the neuromuscular junction a method of localizing cholinesterases and non-specific esterases which was adapted to the requirements of the electron microscopy. This method, after fixation with formaldehyde, uses alpha-naphthyl acetate as substrate and as coupling agent tetrazoted pararosaniline. When combined with selective inhibitors this method provides electron micrographs where one may observe the subneural location of the azo dye which visualizes the enzymatic hydrolysis. However, the opacity to electrons of this azo dye is unfortunately rather low and other methods have been proposed which allow a better contrast due to a greater opacity of the reaction products. The method with thiolacetic acid where visualization is due to lead salts gives the best contrast one could hope for (Zacks and Blumberg, 1961 a, b; Barrnett, 1962). The modification of this method as proposed by Davis and Koelle (1965, 1967) where an aurous compound $(AuNa_3 (S_2O_3))$ is substituted in the incubation medium for the lead salts gives a finer precipitate of Au_2S which is also very opaque to electrons.

The methods involving esters of thiocholine have also been adapted in various ways to the electron microscope and also give pictures with a high degree of contrast due to the electron opacity of the reaction products.

Since the first attempts to transpose directly to the electron microscopy the technique of Koelle and Friedenwald gave disappointing results, several modifications have been proposed. In the first amongst these (Birks and Brown, 1960; Brown, 1961) silver was substituted for copper but the results obtained by this method on the motor end-plate were not really equivalent to the results subsequently obtained with the electron microscope using the technique of Koelle and Friedenwald (Couteaux, 1963).

We have already seen that with methods using the light microscope Davis and Koelle (1965, 1967) modified the method involving thiocholine esters by substituting gold for copper. They replaced the copper salt by the same aurous compound which they used in the method involving thiolacetic acid by substituting it for the lead salts. After treatment with ammonium sulfide the precipitate is transformed into Au_2S which is opaque to electrons.

Lead, which confers to the reaction products a high degree of electron opacity, has also been substituted for copper (Joó *et al.*, 1965) or used at the same time as copper; in this latter case copper sulfate and lead nitrate are simultaneously introduced into the incubation medium (Kása *et al.*, 1965; Kása and Csillik, 1966).

In addition to the modifications involving the substitution of one metal for another one should also cite the method of Lewis and Shute (1964, 1966) which involves essentially the same techniques as that of Koelle and Friedenwald except that all the details have been adjusted with a view to studies with the electron microscope for the localization of brain cholinesterases. This method, of course, may also be applied to other tissues and in particular the motor end-plates.

Finally there is a last modification to the thiocholine esters method which in principle is very different to those previously described. This is a direct coloring method developed for the light microscope by Karnovsky and Roots (1964) and adapted without difficulty to the electron microscope (Karnovsky, 1964). The ferrocyanide formed at the enzymatic locations is very opaque to electrons and enables even low activities to be detected.

All the methods which have just been outlined utilize as substrate either thiolacetic acid, or esters of thiocholine, and in the electron microscope give a clear picture of the enzymatic locations only because of the presence of a metal in the final reaction product. False localization may often be linked to the use of metallic salts, and particularly heavy metals. Attempts have been made to overcome this whilst preserving the satisfactory electron opacity of the final reaction product. A new method has been made available in this direction by the use of esters, the hydrolysis products of which are osmiophilic (Hanker *et al.*, 1964; Seligman, 1964). The application of this new principle to the histochemical study of the neuromuscular junction has already been referred to in relation to methods involving the light microscope. The three thiolesters which are used as substrates in the light microscope (NTA, TAB, TPB) may also be used with the electron microscope (Bergman *et al.*, 1968). After liberation of a thiol by enzymatic hydrolysis and coupling this method involves the formation of an osmiophilic diazothioether which in the presence of osmium vapors is converted into a precipitate which is very opaque to electrons.

The main limit to this technique for the precise localization with the electron microscope is that the diazothioether appears in the form of droplets which are incomparably less fine than the granules of the precipitate of the metallic compounds involved in the other methods. The recent localization of cytochrome oxydase by a method based on the same principle and the final reaction of which is present in the form of non-droplet deposits (Seligman *et al.*, 1968) leads one to hope that a similar progress may be made in the localization of hydrolases.

In all these methods adapted to the electron microscope which have been reviewed the preservation of the structure is obtained in a satisfactory manner because of a primary fixation before the incubation by aldehydes which allows a substantial portion of enzymatic activity to remain and also due to the complementary fixation by OsO_4 after incubation.

Of the various esters used, only the esters of thiocholine possess any significant degree of specificity in respect to cholinesterases. The inhibition of cholinesterases by low concentrations of eserine enables them to be readily distinguished from nonspecific esterases, particularly thiolesterases,

34

which are able to hydrolyze esters of thiocholine. Thus for the localization of cholinesterases thiocholine esters are of considerable value. Nevertheless, in spite of the considerable amount of work carried out, it does not seem as if the method of Koelle and Friedenwald has been fully elucidated. In particular, the nature of the primary precipitate should still be regarded as ill-defined (Tsuji, 1968). One of the main drawbacks of the thiocholine esters technique is the poor penetration of these esters. This justifies the parallel use of other techniques involving much less specific agents, such as thiolacetic acid, but which have a much greater penetration.

In spite of the great diversity of substrates and processes of visualization employed, the methods utilizing the electron microscope demonstrate that the products of the esterase activities of the motor end-plate accumulate primarily in the primary and secondary synaptic clefts. With some modifications of the methods utilizing thiocholine esters or thiolacetic acid, the accumulation of the precipitate indicating the enzyme activity takes place at the supra- and subsynaptic membranes which delineate these clefts. The location of the precipitate at the membranes can be observed, but inconstantly in the electron micrographs obtained by Kása and Csillik (1966) using thiocholine esters and simultaneously lead and copper salts, equally by Davis and Koelle (1967) with the gold–thiocholine method. The thiolacetic acid–gold technique (Davis and Koelle, 1967) allows this location of the precipitate to be obtained with greater regularity (Fig. 8).

With sections which are perpendicular to the surface of the junction, the pre- and postsynaptic membranes appear with these methods to be more electron-opaque in the region of the junction itself than outside it. Sections cut parallel to these membranes and containing one of them indicate that the special opacity corresponds to the presence of the precipitate the fine granules of which are attached to the membrane surface. Even when the location of precipitate granules at the membranes is particularly pronounced, granules may also be observed in the interior of the synaptic cleft. These, however, are distributed with a much lower density.

These pictures suggest that the enzymatic activities are linked to the membranes themselves and that the granules occasionally seen within the cleft are due to diffusion of the reaction products to a greater or less degree, depending on the method used.

According to Davis and Koelle, the staining of the presynaptic membrane is usually slightly less than that of postsynaptic membrane.

The use of specific inhibitors has led a number of authors to state that enzymes which are located at the pre- and postsynaptic membranes are both acetylcholine esterase and a nonspecific cholin esterase. The slight difference in the intensity of staining of the supra- and subsynaptic membranes which has previously been referred to may be observed equally after treatment with an inhibitor of nonspecific cholinesterases as after an acetylcholinesterase inhibitor.

A prolongation of the incubation period leads to a progressively increasing concentration of the enzymatic hydrolysis products accumulating in the synaptic clefts. These products do not, or only after long incubation periods, cross the pre- and postsynaptic membranes. This is in agreement with the notion that both these enzymes reside in the external portion of the membranes.

Using a modification of the thiocholine ester method introduced by Karnovsky and Roots, Teräväinen (1967) reached the conclusion that acetylcholinesterase and the nonspecific cholinesterases did not reside on the same side of the subsynaptic membrane. Only the nonspecific esterases would be present on the external side of the membrane, whilst acetylcholinesterase would be present on the internal side. It should be pointed out that in order to preserve, in each type of preparation, only one type of cholinesterase, specific or nonspecific, Teräväinen used inhibitors (Iso-OMPA and 284C51) at concentrations higher than those normally used.

In addition to the location at the presynaptic and postsynaptic membranes an additional location of nonspecific cholinesterase has also been demonstrated in the region of the motor end-plate at the teloglial cells. However, it is difficult to state to what extent this teloglial location is due to the plasma membrane or other organites.

According to the experiments of Bergman *et al.* (1968) with the thiolester TPB as substrate there exists between the subneural apparatus and the rest of the muscle fiber a zone rich in nonspecific esterase which constitute a sort of barrier to all diffusion of acetylcholine from the motor end-plate.

Very recently, Csillik and Knyihár (1968) have applied to the study of esterases in the motor end-plate the technique of detecting esterases introduced into electron microscopy by Holt and Hicks (1966). This method depends on the hydrolysis of indoxyl acetate. An azo dye which is strongly osmiophilic is formed by coupling hexazoted pararosaniline with indoxyl liberated by the esterase. With indoxyl acetate and butyrate Csillik and Knyihár obtained at the neuromuscular junction a particularly intense staining of the primary and secondary synaptic clefts.

Discussion

By comparing with the light microscope the histochemical staining obtained on both the normal motor end-plate and the denervated motor end-plate it could already be concluded that there existed a high concentration of cholinesterase at the subneural apparatus. It could also be considered very probable that the location of these cholinesterases was at the postsynaptic membrane.

As regards the presynaptic membrane and because of the small distance which separates it from the postsynaptic membrane and the frequent diffusion of enzymatic hydrolysis products it is not possible with the light microscope only to state the concentration of cholinesterases at this membrane (Couteaux, 1958). In order to solve the problem however, it is not sufficient to have access to an instrument with a higher resolving power. The interpretation of the pictures obtained remains equally difficult in electron microscopy as in light microscopy when the synaptic cleft appears to be filled with the precipitate of the histochemical reaction. The latter was indeed the case with all the electron micrographs studied until the present time with the very recent exception of micrographs obtained using the thiocholine–gold, thiocholine–copper and lead, or thiolacetic acid–gold techniques. It is only with these latter techniques that we have observed that the granules of precipitate visualizing the enzymatic activity are mainly concentrated at the two membranes and are distributed with a much lower density in the space which separates them. These pictures strongly suggest the notion of a location of cholinesterase at the presynaptic membrane as well as at the postsynaptic membrane.

Can one consider the presynaptic location as histochemically established? The frequency of diffusion effects and of the changes observed in the distribution of the primary reaction products makes it necessary to be extremely cautious. Zajicek *et al.* (1954) and Holmstedt (1957) have already emphasized the danger associated with displacements of the precipitate in the technique using esters of thiocholine, and in the conversion of mercaptides into sulfides by treatment with ammonium sulfide. On the other hand, treatment with OsO_4 when carried out after the incubation both in the thiolacetic acid–gold method or in the thiocholine–gold method appears equally capable of causing a modification in the initial distribution of the primary precipitate.

It should be pointed out that without treatment by OsO_4 the precipitate observed by the thiocholine–copper technique is not confined to the membranes but is also distributed in the synaptic cleft (Couteaux, 1963). This is also the case even if one avoids both the treatment with OsO_4 and the treatment with ammonium sulfide (Tsuji, 1968).

It thus seems not impossible, in the conditions of incubation normally carried out, that the enzymatic hydrolysis products can first diffuse into the synaptic cleft from one of the membranes which delineate it and are only secondarily precipitated on the two membranes following chemical treatment.

The treatment which seems to be able to modify the initial distribution of the primary precipitate is not only the action of OsO_4 or of ammonium sulfide but also that of the substances which are used to obtain the best conditions for the polymerization of the embedding medium.

Before it can be considered as established that the "staining" of the presynaptic membrane by the precipitate corresponds to a real enzymatic location, further studies should be carried out.

There seems little doubt of the existence at the neuromuscular junction of concentrations of acetylcholinesterase and of nonspecific cholinesterases and nonspecific esterases greater than the concentrations of these enzymes in other regions of the muscle. However, when the incubation of the sections and the treatment with inhibitors are carried out on sections of muscle of one to some dozen microns in thickness, the conditions in which these diverse locations may be studied are not comparable. One cannot avoid that there exist differences which are sometimes very great between the speeds with which inhibitors and the substances which form the incubation medium reach the enzymatic sites. One can to some extent correct for these differences by allowing the inhibitors to react on the sections for greater or less periods of time before the incubation and by submitting the sections to a prolonged "preincubation" in a medium which is identical to the normal medium but devoid of substrate. It is more difficult, however, to correct for the differences with which the same substrate reaches different enzymatic sites. Under normal conditions of incubation the sites reached more rapidly appear to be more active than they really are in comparison with other sites. In order to correct these "distortions" or at least to disclose them we have been led to make use of an incubation medium in which the concentrations of substrate are greater than the biochemical optimum. This depresses the activity of the first sites reached by a high concentration of substrate. This type of experiment was first attempted with acetylthiocholine iodide. However, the concentrations of substrate necessary to obtain an inhibitory effect were considerably in excess, in the histochemical conditions, on those necessary to obtain the same result with homogenates. This leads to severe difficulties in equilibrating the incubation medium.

Israël and Tsuji (Tsuji, 1968) managed to find a solution to this problem by adding to the preincubation medium acetylcholine in high concentrations. This enabled them to reduce at will the cholinesterase activity and to obtain a more uniform distribution of acetylthiocholine during the incubation.

Methods such as those which have just been outlined can to a certain degree compensate for the irregularities in the penetration of reagents. However, the possibility of carrying out the incubation on ultra-thin sections nevertheless would appear to be conditions under which distribution of the enzymatic activity of the neuromuscular junction may be studied in detail.

At the present time, in the absence of ultra-thin sections the enzymes of which are not inactivated and which may be submitted to histochemical treatment, the thiolacetic acid method, in spite of its lack of specificity, offers the advantage of the use of a reagent the penetration of which across the structures is better than that of choline esters or of ferrocyanide ion. In addition it gives precipitates more stable than those of the other methods and, in particular, less easily displaced by OsO_4.

2.3.1.3. *AUTORADIOGRAPHIC METHODS*

One of the main limitations to enzymatic histochemistry, when this depends on the *in situ* formation of precipitates which are recognizable by their color under the light microscope or their opacity to electrons, is the inaptitude in giving a real quantitative evaluation of enzymatic activities. Autoradiographic methods which are at the present time developing so rapidly will undoubtedly contribute to overcoming this defect particularly in the area of carboxylic esterases.

As early as 1961 Ostrowski and Barnard suggested the utilization of radioactive inhibitors to localize the enzymes sites and to quantitatively evaluate their concentration.

In the first instance this method was applied to the cholinesterases of the motor end-plate using the irreversible enzyme inhibitor di-isopropylflurophosphate (DFP)-^{3}H,-^{32}P,-^{14}C (Ostrowski *et al.*, 1963; Waser and Reller, 1965).

The first attempts were made with the light microscope with DFP (Ostrowski *et al.*, 1963; Barnard and Ostrowski, 1964) but it was subsequently shown by the same group (Rogers *et al.*, 1966) that the quantitative data provided by the studies were wrongly interpreted. This was probably due to misappreciation with unstained preparations of mastocytes of the muscle. These mastocytes, which contain apparently no acetylcholinesterase, are in contrast rich in other esterases. Subsequently taken up by the electron microscope these autoradiographic studies have become particularly fruitful (Salpeter, 1967).

The basis of the technique consists in phosphorylating acetylcholinesterase with ^{3}H-DFP and to quantitatively estimate the distribution of phosphorylated enzyme by electron microscope autoradiography using a layer of emulsion whose sensitivity to tritium has previously been calibrated.

The main problem to be resolved in order to selectively label acetylcholinesterase with ^{3}H-DFP was due to the fact that this inhibitor can phosphorylate other esterases in addition to acetylcholinesterase (see the review of O'Brien, 1960) and although more slowly even other sites which are nonenzymatic (Ashbolt and Rydon, 1957).

The solution of this problem was found by the use of PAM (pyridine–2-aldoxime methiodide) the high selectivity of which as a reactivator of phosphorylated acetylcholinesterase is well established (Wilson and Ginsburg, 1955; Wilson et al., 1958) following treatment of the tissue with nonradioactive DFP which is fixed by all the sites which are available for phosphorylation. The acetylcholinesterase is reactivated by PAM and subsequently rephosphorylated this time with ^{3}H-DFP.

One difficulty, however, remains for the nonspecific linkages which DFP may make with diverse constituents in the tissue. This nonspecific adsorption seems to be responsible for the basic radioactivity which prolonged washings with nonradioactive DFP and buffer fail to completely eliminate. Indeed this level of background radioactivity remains practically the same whether the treatment by ^{3}H-DFP has or has not been preceded by nonradioactive DFP. This effect appears to be due primarily to the lipophilic properties of DFP which explain the reduction in background radioactivity which has been observed by Rogers (Salpeter, 1967) following washing in organic solvents after the unlabeled DFP and buffer washes. This lipophilicity of DFP appears to cause some difficulty in removing all the nonspecific adsorption of DFP to tissue components.

If one takes into account the resolution of the method which under the present conditions can hardly be greater than 800 Ångströms (Bachmann and Salpeter, 1965) it was naturally not possible to demonstrate the location of acetylcholinesterase at the membranes nor even in the synaptic cleft. However, by counting the grains of silver distributed to either side of the primary synaptic cleft it has been possible to reach important conclusions concerning the motor end-plate of the sternomastoid muscle of the mouse (Fig. 9). These conclusions are as follows:

1. Acetylcholinesterase is primarily located in the region of the sub-neural folds (85% of the total quantity of enzyme of the motor end-plate). The number of active sites in this region of the motor end-plate is greater than 20,000 per cubic micron.
2. The resolution of the technique is not sufficient to determine whether there is some acetylcholinesterase in the axon terminal; however, if there is any there the concentration must be less than 10% of that at the subneural folds region.

The type of histogram obtained in enumerating the silver grains at different regions of the motor end-plate and the position of the axon

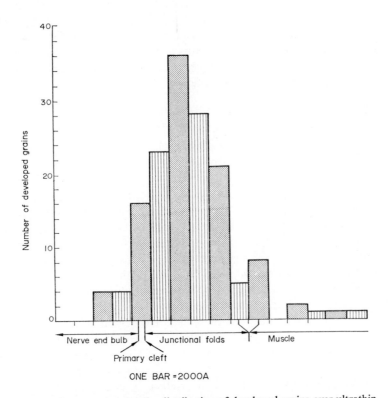

ONE BAR = 2000A

FIG. 9. Histogram showing the distribution of developed grains over ultrathin sections of motor end-plate (sterno-mastoid muscle of the mouse). On the electron microscope autoradiographs the distances were measured from the midpoint of each developed grain to the centre of the primary cleft of the end-plate. (After Salpeter, 1967.)

terminal in the middle of a zone the radioactivity of which is relatively high suggest that the concentration of acetylcholinesterase in this terminal could be less than the already very weak concentration deduced from the number of silver grains it contains.

It should be pointed out that the quantitative results furnished by these autoradiographic studies with the electron microscope were to a certain extent controlled by a comparison of the data with that obtained measuring the global radioactivity of a motor end-plate after treatment with ^{32}P-DFP. These figures were obtained by counting the number of tracks of beta particles by the use of light microscope autoradiography.

In the discussion on the validity of the results obtained by these studies and particularly those results which attribute but a low level of radioactivity to the entire axon terminal one should take into consideration, as has Salpeter, the fact that some substances such as PAM do not readily penetrate into the axon. However, this is not necessarily the same for the axon terminal which is directly accessible to exchange with the extracellular medium by the primary synaptic cleft.

2.3.1.4. *CONCLUSIONS ON THE DISTRIBUTION OF CHOLINESTERASES AND OTHER CARBOXYLIC ESTERASES*

The overall results, biochemical, histochemical, and autoradiographic, obtained with the light microscope and the electron microscope on normal and denervated skeletal muscle show that in most vertebrates and particularly in mammals there exists a location of acetylcholinesterase and of nonspecific cholinesterases at the postsynaptic membrane, at the primary and secondary synaptic clefts of the neuromuscular junction. Furthermore, the activity of this enzyme by unit area of surface of the membrane is considerably higher than in other regions of the postsynaptic membrane.

Amongst the numerous histochemical methods which have been adapted to the electron microscope, some produce micrographs which clearly suggest that there exist a location of acetylcholinesterase and of nonspecific cholinesterases in the junctional region of the presynaptic membrane. However, with the techniques used at the present time it remains conceivable that the "staining" of the presynaptic membrane situated in the immediate neighborhood of a zone of high cholinesterase concentration is due to a diffusion artefact. This staining could indeed correspond to a secondary adsorption on the presynaptic membrane either of enzymatic hydrolysis products, or of the precipitate from the histochemical reaction. This would result from the high activity of the subsynaptic membrane and the diffusion in the primary synaptic cleft.

That there exists a location of cholinesterases in the presynaptic region of the neuromuscular junction can thus not be considered as histochemically established by present-day methods.

Without enabling one to completely reject the location at the presynaptic membrane the results obtained with autoradiographic methods suggest that it has an activity per unit area of surface considerably less than that of the postsynaptic membrane.

Besides the diffusion artefacts which are still insufficiently well controlled there exist numerous other sources of error in the cytochemical localization of carboxylic esterases which reside in the region of the neuromuscular junction. There may also be numerous errors in estimating their relative activity. One of the most important sources of error is due to the great inequality in the penetration of the reagents utilized across the structures which separate them from the enzymatic sites. This is particularly important with regard to substrates and inhibitors which are absolutely essential to distinguish and identify the diverse enzymatic activities. These inconveniences would be considerably reduced if it was possible to expose directly to the action of these reagents ultra-thin sections of the muscle the enzymes of which were not inactivated.

There are difficulties at the present time in estimating the cholinesterase activity of the presynaptic membrane in the case of neuromuscular junctions which are endowed with a significant location of cholinesterases at the postsynaptic membrane. These difficulties should not lead one to forget that the motor nerve fibers of striated muscles and their terminals certainly contain cholinesterases and can on some occasions, for example in the case of the muscles of hippocampus, contain much more enzyme than the subneural region of the muscle fiber.

The best-established location of cholinesterases in the neuromuscular junction is the location at the postsynaptic membrane. However, at the present time there are only very unprecise data available on the site of the cholinesterase activities relative to the membrane structure.

Until quite recently the balance of opinion was that acetylcholinesterase and nonspecific esterases were both linked to the external layer of the membrane. As we have seen above a different opinion based on the histochemical results has recently been proposed. According to this a nonspecific cholinesterase is situated on the external side of the membrane and the acetylcholinesterase is located on the internal side.

The micropharmacological studies of Pécot-Dechavassine (1968) on the frog neuromuscular junction suggests that acetylcholinesterase and nonspecific cholinesterases may have different locations relative to the subsynaptic membrane. It is known that eserine when acting on frog muscle homogenates inhibits acetylcholinesterase and nonspecific cholinesterases at very similar concentrations. On the other hand, butyrylcholine as well as acetylcholine when applied iontophoretically to the neuromuscular junction is able to depolarize the subsynaptic membrane. Pécot-Dechavassine has shown that eserine when acting *in situ* potentiates the depolarization produced by butyrylcholine, but not that produced by acetylcholine. It seems that acetylcholinesterase is less accessible to eserine than nonspecific cholinesterases and this may imply a different location of the two enzymes relative to the receptors.

Sites of cholinesterases other than those of the pre- and postsynaptic membranes have also been described histochemically at the neuromuscular junction. One of the most well established amongst these is the location of a nonspecific cholinesterase in the teloglial cells.

Although the nonspecific esterases of the neuromuscular junction have for a long time been neglected or even completely unknown it would seem that they may take an important place in further biochemical and cytochemical studies relative to carboxylic esterases at the neuromuscular junction.

Extensive studies on the nature and distribution of these esterases have been carried out simultaneously by a number of teams and it is likely that this will shed light on their functional significance.

2.3.2. DISTRIBUTION OF CHOLINE ACETYLTRANSFERASE AND OF ACETYLCHOLINE

The choline acetyltransferase (ChAT-E.C. 2.3.1.6, acetyl-CoA: choline *O*-acetyltransferase) and acetylcholine (ACh) content of nerve and muscle has been the subject of numerous studies for a long time. The first studies from which one can draw accurate indications of their distribution in the neuromuscular junction are those of Hebb *et al.* (1964) on the rat diaphragm and those of Israël and Gautron (1969) on the rat diaphragm and sternomastoid muscle.

(a) Distribution of choline acetyltransferase

The quantity of ACh formed during 1 hour of incubation at 39°C in homogenates of muscle has been determined in the studies of Hebb *et al.* These authors used as test for ACh the rectus abdominis muscle of the frog and the dorsal muscle of the leech. The determinations were carried out both on the phrenic nerve on the one hand and on the diaphragm on the other. Each diaphragm was divided into two sections. One, the neural, contained the intramuscular branches of the phrenic nerve and almost all the motor end-plates. The other portion therefore contained only a small number of motor end-plates and could be considered as almost aneural.

The quantity of ACh formed by a rat phrenic nerve homogenate per hour and per gram was on average 1610 mcg. The total activity of the muscle varied between 60 mcg and 166 mcg of ACh/hr/g and the activity of the aneural portion of the muscle varied between 6 and 46 mcg of ACh/hr/g. It is possible that these figures may be slightly superior to that of "pure" muscle since the separation between the innervated and non-innervated zone was not absolutely complete.

The ChAT activity of the neural portion which corresponded to approximately 40% of the total muscle represented about 87.8% of the total muscle activity.

If the nerve fibers situated in the interior of the neural portion of the diaphragm had a ChAT activity per unit weight similar to that in the phrenic nerve it is possible to calculate, as has been done by Hebb *et al.*, that the intramuscular branches of the nerve can contain only between one-quarter ($\frac{1}{4}$) and one-half ($\frac{1}{2}$) of the activity found in the muscle. One is thus led to form two hypotheses. One of these is that the nerve fibers have a ChAT activity higher in their intramuscular portion than within the phrenic nerve. This hypothesis is supported by the fact that an increase of the activity in the 2 to 3 cm proximal to the section has been observed following section of the nerve (Hebb and Waites, 1956; Hebb and Silver, 1961; Hebb, 1962). The nerve fibers of the central end of the cut nerve undergo changes which would make them comparable to the terminal portions of normal nerve fibers (Hebb and Silver, 1961).

One can supply another explanation for the high concentration of the neural portion in ChAT by supposing that the enzyme is present in a high concentration at neuromuscular junctions.

In order to establish how this activity at the neuromuscular junction is distributed between the presynaptic and postsynaptic portions, experiments were to be carried out to study the variation in activity of the neural and aneural portions after section of nerve. These experiments are similar to those carried out with cholinesterases.

Hebb *et al.* have shown that 41 days after section of the phrenic nerve the activity of the neural and aneural portions fell to about 4% of the normal values. However, the time after denervation was too long to enable one to exclude by this experiment the possibility of a concentration of ChAT in the subsynaptic portion of the normal neuromuscular junction.

The studies of Israël and Gautron (1968) have provided data on the distribution of ChAT in striated muscle and particularly at the neuromuscular junction. These data complete the results of Hebb *et al.* The former authors carried out estimations of ChAT using a radiochemical technique where radioactive acetyl-CoA was synthesized from ^{14}C labeled acetate and where the concentration of radioactive acetylcholine formed was measured with a scintillation counter. The results obtained with the use of this method on the normal rat diaphragm are similar to those of Hebb *et al.* (1964). They have also carried out estimations on the sternomastoid muscle of the rat which offers certain advantages over the diaphragm. Thus the former muscle may readily provide large areas completely devoid of motor end-plates. The intramuscular portion of the motor nerve is less long and its reimplantation in muscle after section may readily be carried out. By following on this denervated muscle and on the symmetrical normal muscle the variations in the ratio between the activity of the denervated neural portion and the normal neural portion, Israël and Gautron found that 48 hours after section of the nerve the activity of the denervated neural portion had already fallen to less than 20% of the normal activity of this portion and ultimately reached values which were between the limits of the normal variation in the activity of the aneural portion.

The rapidity with which, after section of the motor nerve, the difference in activity which normally exists between the neural and aneural portions is abolished make it seem very probable that this difference is entirely or almost entirely due to the enzymatic activity of the presynaptic portion of the neural zone and that the disappearance of the activity is directly correlated to the degeneration of the axons. In contrast with the ChAT activity which declines so rapidly, the cholinesterase activity of the neural zone remains in the same muscle almost unchanged 72 and 92 hours after section of the motor nerve.

Experiments involving reimplantation of the motor nerve which has previously been sectioned have enabled a reinnervation of the sternomastoid muscle some 20 days later. This was accompanied by an almost complete restoration of the proportions of ChAT activity in the neural and aneural portions.

In conclusion, the experiments involving denervation have made it possible to demonstrate that the difference in ChAT activity observed between the neural and aneural portions may be entirely attributed or almost entirely attributed to the motor nerve fibers and their terminals.

It remains to be established by other methods, and principally those requiring the preparation by centrifugation of fractions containing only the motor nerve terminals ("synaptosomes"), whether the high activity residing in the nervous elements of the neural portion of the muscle is due to a concentration of ChAT distributed throughout the intramuscular portion of the motor innervation, or due to an extremely high concentration of the enzyme in the nerve endings only.

Knowing the close relationship which exists between the electric organs and striated muscle it was of interest to compare the ChAT activity of these two organs.

In the experiments of Bull *et al.* (1969), carried out by using techniques similar to those used for muscle by Hebb *et al.* (1964), the ChAT activity of the electric organ of torpedo was found to vary between 2600 and 3200 mcg of ACh/hr/g at 39°C. This activity was 1200 mcg of ACh/hr/g at 21°C. Using a radiochemical method applied to muscle Israël and Gautron (1969) obtained on this organ at 18°C figures ranging between 500 and 600 mcg ACh/hr/g. This activity rose to 800 mcg ACh/hr/g in particularly small specimens.

Section of the electric nerves results in a lowering of enzymatic activity in the organ, but the effect is here considerably more delayed than in the case of striated muscle (Israël, personal communication). Both morphological and electrophysiological observations suggest that the degeneration of the nerve terminals in the electric organ of torpedo is also much slower than the degeneration of motor nerve terminals in striated muscle. Clear-cut conclusions from these experiments on the distribution of ChAT in this type of organ can thus not be drawn.

(b) *Distribution of acetylcholine*

Only the distribution of "bound" acetylcholine will be discussed here, that is the acetylcholine which is shown to be active on biological preparations only after physical or chemical treatment of the tissue. This acetylcholine is protected in the tissue from the action of esterases and may be estimated after extraction.

Hebb *et al.* (1964) have studied the distribution of ACh in parallel with that of ChAT in the rat phrenic nerve and in the neural and aneural portions of the diaphragm.

In the phrenic nerve the ACh content was on average 2250 ng/g. That of the total muscle varied between 126 and 291 ng/g (average: 181.7 ng/g). This concentration of ACh in the diaphragm is many times higher than that which has been found in some other skeletal muscles (Chang and Gaddum, 1933; Bhatnagar and MacIntosh, 1960; Hebb, 1962; Israël and Gautron, 1969).

The particularly high concentration of ACh in the diaphragm is at least partially explained by the fact that the intramuscular portion of most motor nerve fibers is much longer in the diaphragm than in other striated muscles studied. Thereby the ratio between the weight of the nerve fibers and the weight of the muscle fibers is probably increased.

The ACh content found by Hebb *et al.* for the aneural portion of the diaphragm is on average 19.4 ng/g. The ACh content of "pure" muscle might indeed be even less if the separation between the neural and aneural portions was complete.

The neural portion which corresponds to approximately 40% of the weight of the diaphragm contains on average 89.7% of the total ACh content of the muscle.

Israël and Gautron obtained similar figures for the ratio in the ACh content of the neural and aneural portions of the sternomastoid muscle of the rat.

In their experiments on the denervated diaphragm Hebb *et al.* found that 20 days after section of the phrenic nerve the ACh content of the neural and aneural portions fell to approximately 20% of the normal values. After 6 weeks the content in the neural portion fell to 10% and was practically indeterminable in the aneural portion.

It may be concluded from the overall results previously discussed that the distribution of ACh is parallel with that of ChAT. Furthermore, the difference in the content of the neural and aneural portions is entirely or almost entirely due to the high ACh concentration in the motor nerve fibers and in their terminals, that is in the presynaptic portion.

If one takes into consideration, as for ChAT, the total volume of the nerve elements of the neural portion of the muscle one finds that the quantity of ACh in the presynaptic portion corresponds to a ACh concentration considerably higher than that in the phrenic nerve. The question thus arises whether, as for ChAT, the ACh is in a higher concentration in all the intramuscular portion of the motor nerve fibers than in the nerve trunk or whether only the nerve terminals are extremely rich in ACh.

As yet to our knowledge there is no data on the concentration of ACh in the motor nerve terminals of striated muscle. However, recent studies on ACh content of various fractions of the electric organ of torpedo has supplied some interesting data on this point.

It has been known for a long time that the ACh content of the electric organ of torpedo is extremely high (Feldberg *et al.*, 1940; Feldberg and Fessard, 1942). More recent studies have fully confirmed these first observations (Sheridan *et al.*, 1966; Morris *et al.*, 1966; Bull *et al.*, 1969). In particular Bull *et al.* have shown that ACh content of the electric organ of torpedo estimated following various extraction procedures varied between 65 and 165 mcg/g of fresh tissue.

Israël *et al.* (1968) have carried out fractionation experiments on this organ using various media. After a first centrifugation the supernatant containing more than 60% of the ACh content of the homogenate was put on a density gradient. In this manner a synaptic vesicles fraction was isolated. This fraction contained more than 80% of the ACh content of the initial fraction.

These experiments demonstrate that the greatest portion of the bound acetylcholine in the electric organ is associated with vesicles lying in the nerve terminals.

It seems probable that this is also the case for the greatest portion of the bound acetylcholine of the neuromuscular junction.

REFERENCES

ALDRIDGE, W. N. (1953) Serum esterases. I. Two types of esterases (A and B) hydrolysing *p*-nitrophenyl acetate, propionate and butyrate, and a method for their determination. *Biochem. J.* **53**: 110.

ANDERSSON-CEDERGREN, E. (1959) Ultrastructure of motor end-plate and sarcoplasmic components of mouse skeletal muscle fiber. *J. Ultrastr. Res.*, suppl. **1**: 5–181.

ASHBOLT, R. F. and RYDON, H. N. (1957) The action of diisopropyl phosphorofluoridate and other anticholinesterases on amino acids. *Biochem. J.* **66**: 237–42.

BACHMANN, L. and SALPETER, M. M. (1965) Autoradiography with the electron microscope. A quantitative evaluation. *Lab. Invest.* **14**: 1041–53.

BARNARD E. A. and OSTROWSKI, K. (1964) Autoradiographic methods in enzyme cytochemistry. II. Studies on some properties of acetylcholinesterase in its sites at the motor end-plate. *Exp. Cell. Res.* **36**: 28–42.

BARRNETT, R. J. (1962) The fine structural localization of acetylcholinesterase at the myoneural junction. *J. Cell Biol.* **12**: 247.

BARRNETT, R. J. and SELIGMAN, A. M. (1951) Histochemical demonstration of esterases by production of indigo. *Science* **114**: 579–80.

BARRON, K. D., BERNSOHN, J. and HESS, A. R. (1966) Esterases and proteins of normal and atrophic feline muscle. *J. Histochem. Cytochem.* **14**: 1–24.

BARRON, K. D., BERNSOHN, J. and ORDINARIO, A. T. (1967) Proteins non specific and cholinesterases of rat gastrocnemius and effects of tenotomy and denervation. *J. Histochem. Cytochem.* **15**: 782–3.

BARRON, K. D., ORDINARIO, A. T., BERNSOHN, J., HESS, A. R. and HEDRICK, M. T. (1968) Cholinesterases and nonspecific esterases of developing and adult (normal and atrophic) rat gastrocnemius. I. Chemical assay and electrophoresis. *J. Histochem. Cytochem.* **16**: 346–61.

BAUER, W. C., BLUMBERG, J. M. and ZACKS, S. I. (1962) Short and long term ultra-structure changes in denervated mouse motor end-plates. In: *Proc. IV Int. Congress of Neuropathology, Munich*, 1962, pp. 16–18. Georg Thieme Verlag, Stuttgart.

BENEDETTI, E. L. and EMMELOT, P. (1966) On the fine structure of cellular membranes. In: *VIth Int. Conf. Electron Microsc., Kyoto*, Vol. II, pp. 399–400. Ryozi Uyeda-Maruzen Co., Tokyo.

BENEDETTI, E. L. and EMMELOT, P. (1967) Studies on plasma membranes. IV. The ultra-structural localization and content of sialic acid in plasma membranes isolated from rat liver and hepatoma. *J. Cell Sci.* **2**: 499–512.

BENNETT, H. S. (1963) Morphological aspects of extracellular polysaccharides. *J. Histochem. Cytochem.* **11**: 14–23.

BERGMANN, F., SEGAL, R. and RIMON, S. (1957) A new type of esterase in hog kidney extract. *Biochem. J.* **67**: 481.

BERGMAN, R. A., UENO, H., MORIZONO, Y., HANKER, J. S. and SELIGMAN, A. M. (1968) Ultrastructural demonstration of acetylcholinesterase activity of motor endplates via osmiophilic diazothioethers. *Histochemie* **11**: 1–12.

BHATNAGAR, S. P. and MACINTOSH, F. C. (1960) Acetylcholine content of striated muscle. *Proc. Canad. Fed. Biol. Soc.* **3**: 12–13.

BIRKS, R. I. and BROWN, L. M. (1960) A method for locating cholinesterase of a mammalian myoneural junction. *J. Physiol. (Lond.)* **152**: 5–7.

BIRKS, R., HUXLEY, H. E. and KATZ, B. (1960) The fine structure of the neuromuscular junction of the frog. *J. Physiol. (Lond.)* **150**: 134–44.

BIRKS, R., KATZ, B. and MILEDI, R. (1959) Dissociation of the "surface membrane complex" in atrophic muscle fibres. *Nature (Lond.)* **184**:1507–8.

BROWN, L. M. (1961) A thiocholine method for locating cholinesterase activity by electron microscopy. Histochemistry of cholinesterase. Symposium, Basel, 1960. *Bibl. Anat.* **2**: 21–33.

BROWN, G. L., DALE, H. H. and FELDBERG, W. (1936) Reactions of the normal mammalian muscle to acetylcholine and eserine. *J. Physiol.* **87**: 394–424.

BRZIN, M. and MAJCEN-TKACEN, Z. (1963) Cholinesterase content of normal and denervated endplates and muscle fibres. *J. Cell Biol.* **19**: 349–58.

BRZIN, M. and ZAJICEK, J. (1958) Quantitative determination of cholinesterase activity in individual end-plates of normal and denervated gastrocnemius. *Nature (Lond.)* **181**: 626.

BUCKLEY, G. A. and NOWELL, P. T. (1966) Micro-calorimetric determination of cholinesterase activity of motor end-plates in the rat diaphragm. *J. Pharm. Pharmac.* **18**: suppl. 146S-150S.

BULL, G., HEBB, C and MORRIS, D. (1969) Synthesis of acetylcholine in the electric organ of torpedo. *Comp. Biochem. Physiol.* **28**: 11–28.

CHANG, H. C. and GADDUM, J. H. (1933) Choline esters in tissue extracts. *J. Physiol.* **79**: 255–85.

COËRS, C. (1953a) La détection histochimique de la cholinestérase au niveau de la jonction neuro-musculaire. *Rev. Belge Pathol. Méd. Exp.* **22**: 306–14.

COËRS, C. (1953b) Contribution à l'étude de la jonction neuromusculaire. Données nouvelles concernant la structure de l'arborisation terminale et de l'appareil sous-neural chez l'homme. *Arch. Biol. (Paris)* **64**: 133–47.

COËRS, C. (1953c) Etude chimique des variations de l'activité cholinestérasique au niveau de la jonction neuro-musculaire après section nerveuse. *Bull. Acad. Roy. Belg., Cl. Sci.* **39**: 447–50.

COËRS, C. (1955) Les variations structurelles normales et pathologiques de la jonction neuromusculaire. *Acta Neurol. Belg.* **55**: 741–866.

COËRS, C. (1967) Structure and organization of the myoneural junction. *Inter. Rev. Cytol.* **22**: 239–67.

COËRS, C. and WOOLF, A. L. (1959) *The Innervation of Muscle: a Biopsy Study*. Charles C. Thomas, Springfield, Illinois.

COUTEAUX, R. (1946) Sur les gouttières synaptiques du muscle strié. *C.R. Soc. Biol., Paris* **140**: 270–1.

COUTEAUX, R. (1947) Contribution à l'étude de la synapse myoneurale. *Rev. Canad. Biol.* **6**: 563–711.

COUTEAUX, R. (1951) Remarques sur les méthodes actuelles de détection histochimique des activités cholinestérasiques. *Arch. Int. Physiol.* **59**: 52–63.

COUTEAUX, R. (1958) Morphological and cytochemical observations on the post-synaptic membrane at motor end-plates and ganglionic synapses. *Exp. Cell Res. Suppl.* **5**: 294–322.

COUTEAUX, R. (1960) Motor end-plate structure. In: *Muscle*, Vol. I, pp. 337–80. Bourne (ed.). Academic Press, New York.

COUTEAUX, R. (1961) Remarques sur la distribution des activités cholinestérasiques dans les muscles striés de l'Hippocampe. Fasc. 2. Histochemie der cholinesterase. *Bibl. Anat.*, pp. 207–19.

COUTEAUX, R. (1963) The differentiation of synaptic areas. *Proc. Roy. Soc. Biol.* **158**: 457–80.

COUTEAUX, R. and NACHMANSOHN, D. (1938) Cholinesterase at the end-plates of voluntary muscle after nerve degeneration. *Nature* **142**: 1481.

COUTEAUX, R. and NACHMANSOHN, D. (1939) La cholinestérase des plaques motrices après section du nerf moteur. *Bull. Soc. Chim. Biol.* **21**: 1054–5.

COUTEAUX, R. and NACHMANSOHN, D. (1940) Changes of cholinesterase at the end-plates of voluntary muscle following section of sciatic nerve. *Proc. Soc. Exp. Biol. N.Y.* **43**: 177–81.

COUTEAUX, R. and NACHMANSOHN, D. (1942) La cholinestérase des plaques motrices après section du nerf moteur. *Bull. Biol. France et Belg.* **76**: 14–57.

COUTEAUX, R. and PÉCOT-DECHAVASSINE, M. (1968) Particularités structurales du sarcoplasme sous-neural. *C.R. Acad. Sci. Paris* **266**: 8–10.

COUTEAUX, R. and TAXI, J. (1951) Recherches histochimiques sur les cholinestérases synaptiques. *Compt. Rend. Assoc. Anat.*, 38e *Réunion* (*Nancy*), pp. 1030–1.

COUTEAUX, R. and TAXI, J. (1952) Recherches histochimiques sur la distribution des activités cholinestérasiques au niveau de la synapse myoneurale. *Arch. Anat. Microscop. Morphol. Exptl.* **41**: 352–92.

CREVIER, M. and BÉLANGER, L. F. (1955) Simple method for histochemical detection of esterase activity. *Science* **122**: 256–557.

CSILLIK, B. (1965) *Functional Structure of the Postsynaptic Membrane in the Myoneural Junction*. Akadémiai Kiado, Budapest. 154 pp.

CSILLIK, B., JOÓ, F., KÁSA, P. and SÁVAY, G. (1966) Pb-Thiocholine techniques for the electron histochemical localization of acetylcholinesterase. *Acta Histochem.* **25**: 58–70.

CSILLIK, B. and KNYIHÁR, E. (1968) On the effect of motor nerve degeneration on the fine-structural localization of esterases in the mammalian motor end-plate. *J. Cell. Sci.* **3**: 529–38.

CSILLIK, B. and SÁVAY, Gy. (1958) Die Regeneration der subneuralen Apparate der motorischen Endplatten. *Acta Neuroveg.*, Wien **19**: 41–52.

DALE, H. H., FELDBERG, W. and VOGT, M. (1936) Release of acetylcholine at voluntary motor nerve endings. *J. Physiol.* **86**: 353–80.

DAVIS, R. and KOELLE, G. B. (1965) Electron microscopic localization of acetylcholinesterase (AChE) at the motor endplate by the gold–thiolacetic acid and gold–thiocholine methods. *J. Histochem. Cytochem.* **13**: 703 (Abstr.).

DAVIS, R. and KOELLE, G. B. (1967) Electron microscopic localization of acetylcholinesterase and nonspecific cholinesterase at the neuromuscular junction by the gold–thiocholine and gold–thiolacetic acid methods. *J. Cell Biol.* **34**: 157–71.

DENZ, F. A. (1953) On the histochemistry of the myoneural junction. *Brit. J. Exptl. Pathol.* **34**: 329–39.

ERÄNKÖ, O. and TERÄVÄINEN, H. (1967) Distribution of esterases in the myoneural junction of the striated muscle of the rat. *J. Histochem. Cytochem.* **15**: 399–403.

FELDBERG, W. and FESSARD, A. (1942) The cholinergic nature of the nerves of the electric organ of the torpedo (*Torpedo marmorata*). *J. Physiol. (Lond.)* **101**: 200–15.

FELDBERG, W., FESSARD, A. and NACHMANSOHN, D. (1940) The cholinergic nature of the nervous supply of the electric organ of the torpedo (*Torpedo marmorata*). *J. Physiol. (Lond.)* **97**: 3P–6P.

FENG, T. P. and TING, Y. C. (1938) Studies on the neuromuscular junction. XI. A note on the local concentration of cholinesterase at motor nerve endings. *Chin. J. Physiol.* **13**: 141–4.

GASIC, G. J. and BERWICK, L. (1963) Hale stain for sialic-acid-containing mucins. Adaptation to electron microscopy. *J. Cell Biol.* **19**: 223–8.

GEREBTZOFF, M. A. (1953) Recherches histochimiques sur les acetylcholine et cholin-estérases. *Acta Anat. (Basel)* **19**: 366–79.

GEREBTZOFF, M. A. (1959) *Cholinesterases.* Pergamon Press, London. 195 pp.

GEREBTZOFF, M. A., PHILIPOT, E. and DALLEMAGNE, M. J. (1954) Recherches histo-chimiques sur les acétylcholine et choline estérases. 2. Activité enzymatique dans les muscles lents et rapides des mammifères et des oiseaux. *Acta Anat.* **20**: 234–57.

GEREBTZOFF, M. A. and VANDERSMISSEN, L. (1956) Etude de la relation spatiale entre acétylcholinestérase et récepteur de l'acétylcholine. *Ann. Histochim.* **1**: 221–9.

GIACOBINI, E. and HOLMSTEDT, B. (1960) Cholinesterase in muscles. A histochemical and microgasometric study. *Acta Pharmacol. (Kobenhavn)* **17**: 94–105.

GOLDSTEIN, D. J. (1959) Some histochemical observations of human striated muscle. *Anat. Rec.* **134**: 217–32.

GOMORI, G. (1948) Histochemical demonstration of sites of cholinesterase activity. *Proc. Soc. Exp. Biol. Med.* **68**: 354–8.

GOMORI, G. (1952a) *Microscopic Histochemistry.* University of Chicago Press, Chicago, Ill. 273 pp.

GOMORI, G. (1952b) The histochemistry of esterases. *Int. Rev. Cytol.* **1**: 323–35.

HANKER, J. S., KATZOFF, L., ROSEN, H. R., SELIGMAN, M. L., UENO, H. and SELIGMAN, A. M. (1966) Design and synthesis of thiolesters for histochemical demonstration of esterase and lipase via the formation of osmiophilic diazothioethers. *J. Med. Chem.* **9**: 288.

HANKER, J. S., SEAMAN, A. R., WEISS, L. P., BERGMAN, R. A. and SELIGMAN, A. M. (1964) New cytochemical principles for light and electron microscopy. *Science* **146**: 1039.

HARVEN, E. DE and COËRS, C. (1959) Electron microscopy study of the human neuro-muscular junction. *J. Biophys. Biochem. Cytol.* **6**: 7–10.

HEBB, C. O. (1962) Acetylcholine content of the rabbit plantaris muscle after denerva-tion. *J. Physiol. (Lond.)* **163**: 294–306.

HEBB, C., KRNJEVIĆ, K. and SILVER, A. (1964) Acetylcholine and choline acetyltrans-ferase in the diaphragm of the rat. *J. Physiol. (Lond.)* **171**: 504–13.

HEBB, C. O. and SILVER, A. (1961) Gradient of choline acetylase activity. *Nature (Lond.)* **189**: 123–5.

HEBB, C. O. and WAITES, G. M. H. (1956) Choline acetylase in antero- and retro-grade degeneration of cholinergic nerves. *J. Physiol. (Lond.),* **132**: 667–71.

HOLMSTEDT, B. (1957a) A modification of the thiocholine method for the determination of cholinesterase. I. Biochemical evaluation of selective inhibitors. *Acta Physiol. Scand.* **40**: 322–30.

HOLMSTEDT, B. (1957b) A modification of the thiocholine method for the determination of cholinesterase. II. Histochemical application. *Acta Physiol. Scand.* **40**: 331–7.

HOLT, S. J. (1954) A new approach to the cytochemical localization of enzymes. *Proc. Roy. Soc. (Biol.)* **142**: 160–9.

HOLT, S. J. and HICKS, R. M. (1966) The importance of osmiophilia in the production of stable azoindoxyl complexes of high contrast for combined enzyme cytochemistry and electron microscopy. *J. Cell Biol.* **29**: 361–6.

HOLT, S. J. and WITHERS, R. F. J. (1952) Cytochemical localization of esterases using indoxyl derivatives. *Nature (Lond.)* **170**: 1012–14.

HOLT, S. J. and WITHERS, R. F. J. (1958) Studies in enzyme cytochemistry. V. An appraisal of indigogenic reactions for esterase localization. *Proc. Roy. Soc. (Biol.)* **148**: 520–32.

HUNTER, R. L. and MARKERT, C. L. (1957) Histochemical demonstration of enzymes separated by zone electrophoresis in starch gels. *Science* **125**: 1294–5.

ISRAËL, M. and GAUTRON, J. (1969) Cellular and subcellular localization of acetylcholine in electric organs. *Symposia of the International Society for Cell Biology*, 6 (Paris, Sept. 1968) (in the press).

ISRAËL, M., GAUTRON, J. and LESBATS, B. (1968) Isolement des vésicules synaptiques de l'organe électrique de la Torpille et localisation de l acétylcholine à leur niveau. *C.R. Acad. Sci. (Paris)* **266**: 273–5.

JOÓ, F., SÁVAY, G. and CSILLIK, B. (1965) A new modification of the Koelle–Friedenwald method for the histochemical demonstration of cholinesterase activity. *Acta Histochem.* **22**: 40–45.

KARNOVSKY, M. J. (1964) The localization of cholinesterase activity in rat cardiac muscle by electron miscroscopy. *J. Cell Biol.* **23**: 217–32.

KARNOVSKY, M. J. and ROOTS, L. (1964) A "direct-coloring" thiocholine method for cholinesterases. *J. Histochem. Cytochem.* **12**: 219.

KÁSA, P. and CSILLIK, B. (1966) Electron microscopic localization of cholinesterase by a copper–lead thiocholine technique. *J. Neurochem.* **13**: 1345–9.

KOELLE, G. B. (1950) The histochemical differentiation of types of cholinesterase and their localizations in tissues of the cat. *J. Pharmacol. Exp. Ther.* **100**: 158–79.

KOELLE, G. B. (1951) The elimination of enzymatic diffusion artifacts in the histochemical localization of cholinesterases and a survey of their cellular distributions. *J. Pharmacol. Exp. Ther.* **103**: 153–71.

KOELLE, G. B. and FRIEDENWALD, J. S. (1949) A histochemical method for localizing cholinesterase activity. *Proc. Soc. Exp. Biol. (N. Y.)* **70**: 617–22.

KOELLE, G. B. and GROMADZKI, C. G. (1966) Comparison of the gold–thiocholine and gold–thiolacetic acid methods for the histochemical localization of acetylcholinesterase and cholinesterases. *J. Histochem. Cytochem.* **14**: 443–54.

KUPFER, C. (1951) Histochemistry of muscle cholinesterase after motor nerve section. *J. Cell. Physiol.* **38**: 469–73.

LEBLOND, C. P., GLEGG, R. E. and EIDINGER, D. (1957) Presence of carbohydrates with free 1,2-glycol groups in sites stained by the periodic acid-Schiff technique. *J. Histochem. Cytochem.* **5**: 445–58.

LEHRER, G. M. and ORNSTEIN, L. (1959) A diazo coupling method for the electronmicroscopic localization of cholinesterase. *J. Biophys. Biochem. Cytol.* **6**: 399–406.

LEWIS, P. R. (1961) The effect of varying the conditions in the Koelle technique. *Bibl. Anat.* **2**: 11–20.

LEWIS, P. R. and SHUTE, C. C. D. (1964) Demonstration of cholinesterase activity with the electron microscope. *J. Physiol. (Lond.)*, **175**: 5 P (Abstr.).

LEWIS, P. R. and SHUTE, C. C. D. (1966) The distribution of cholinesterase in cholinergic neurons demonstrated with the electron microscope. *J. Cell Sci.* **1**: 381–90.

53

LUFT, J. H. (1966) Ruthenium red staining of the striated muscle cell membrane and the myotendinal junction. In: *VIth Int. Conf. Electron Microsc., Kyoto*, Vol. II, pp. 65–66. Ryozi Uyeda-Maruzen Co., Tokyo.

MCMANUS, J. F. A. (1946) Histological demonstration of mucin after periodic acid. *Nature (Lond.)* **158**: 202.

MALMGREN, H. and SYLVÉN, B. (1955) On the chemistry of the thiocholine method of Koelle. *J. Histochem. Cytochem.* **3**: 441–5.

MARINOZZI, V. (1967) Réaction de l'acide phosphotungstique avec la mucine et les glycoprotéines des plasmamembranes. *J. Microscopie* **6**: 68a–69a.

MARINOZZI, V. (1968) Phosphotungstic acid (PTA) as a stain for polysaccharides and glycoproteins in electron microscopy. In: *Electron Microscopy*, Vol. II, pp. 55–56 (*Fourth European Regional Conference, Roma, Sept. 1968*). D. S. Bocciarelli (ed.). Tipografia Poliglotta Vaticana.

MARKERT, C. L. and HUNTER, R. L. (1959) The distribution of esterases in mouse tissues. *J. Histochem. Cytochem.* **7**: 42–49.

MARNAY, A. and NACHMANSOHN, D. (1937) Sur la répartition de la cholinesterase dans le muscle couturier de la Grenouille. *C.R. Soc. Biol.* **125**: 41–43.

MARNAY, A. and NACHMANSOHN, D. (1938) Cholinesterase in voluntary muscle. *J. Physiol. (Lond.)* **92**: 37–47.

MORRIS, D., BULL, G. and HEBB, C. (1966) Acetylcholine in the electric organ of torpedo. *Nature (Lond.)* **207**: 1295.

NACHLAS, M. M. and SELIGMAN, A. M. (1949) Comparative distribution of esterase in tissues of five mammals by histochemical technique. *Anat. Rec.* **105**: 677–95.

NAKAMURA, T., NAMBA, T. and EBANKS, P. H. (1966) Demonstration of motor endplate by binding of divalent metal ions with subneural apparatus. *Fed. Proc.* **25**: 718.

NAMBA, T. and GROB, D. (1967) Cholinergic receptors in skeletal muscle: isolation and properties of muscle ribonucleoprotein with affinity for *d*-tubocurarine and acetylcholine, and binding activity of the subneural apparatus of motor end plates with divalent metal ions. *Ann. N.Y. Acad. Sci.* **144**: 772–802.

NAMBA, T. and GROB, D. (1968) Cholinesterase activity of the motor endplate in isolated muscle membrane. *J. Neurochem.* **15**: 1445–54.

NOËL, R. (1957) Télosomes et manchon périéloneuritique. *Acta Anat.* **30**: 530–41.

O'BRIEN, R. D. (1960) *Toxic Phosphorus Esters*. Academic Press, New York.

OSTROWSKI, K. and BARNARD, E. A. (1961) Application of isotopically-labelled specific inhibitors as a method in enzyme cytochemistry. *Exp. Cell Res.* **25**: 465–8.

OSTROWSKI, K., BARNARD, E. A., STOCKA, Z. and DARZYNKIEWICZ, Z. (1963) Autoradiographic methods in enzyme cytochemistry. I. Localisation of acetylcholinesterase activity using a ^{3}H-labelled irreversible inhibitor. *Exp. Cell Res.* **31**: 89–99.

PALADE, G. E. and PALAY, S. L. (1954) Electron microscope observations of interneuronal and neuromuscular synapses. *Anat. Rec.* **118**: 335.

PEASE, D. C. (1966) Polysaccharides associated with the exterior surface of epithelial cells: kidney, intestine, brain. *J. Ultrastruct. Res.* **15**: 555–88.

PÉCOT-DECHAVASSINE, M. (1961) Etude biochimique, pharmacologique et histochimique des cholinestérases des muscles striés chez les Poissons, les Batraciens et les Mammifères. *Arch. Anat. Micro., Morph. Exp.* **51**: 341–438.

PÉCOT-DECHAVASSINE, M. (1968) Différence dans l'action de l'ésérine sur les dépolarisations de la membrane musculaire par l'acétylcholine et la butyrylcholine. *C.R. Acad. Sci. (Paris)* **266**: 1149–52.

PLATTNER, F. and HINTNER, H. (1930) Die Spaltung von Acetylcholin durch Organextrakte und Körperflüssigkeiten. *Pflüger's Arch.* **225**: 19–25.

PORTUGALOV, V. V. and YAKOVLEV, V. A. (1951) Lokalizacija kholinesterazi v. poperetshnopolosatich mishcach. *Dokl. Akad. Nauk SSSR* **78**: 1021.

RAMBOURG, A. (1967) Détection des glycoprotéines en microscopie électronique: coloration de la surface cellulaire et de l'appareil de Golgi par un mélange acide chromique-phosphotungstique. *C.R. Acad. Sci. (Paris)* **265**: 1426–8.

RAMBOURG, A. (1968) Détection des glycoprotéines en microscopie électronique par l'acide phosphotungstique à bas pH. In: *Electron Microscopy*, Vol. II, pp. 57–58. *(Fourth European Regional Conference, Roma, Sept.* 1968). D. S. Bocciarelli (ed.). Tipografia Poliglotta Vaticana.

RAMBOURG, A. and LEBLOND, C. P. (1967) Electron microscope observations on the carbohydrate-rich cell coat present at the surface of cells in the rat. *J. Cell Biol.* **32**: 27–53.

RAMBOURG, A., NEUTRA, M. and LEBLOND, C. P. (1966) Presence of a "cell coat" rich in carbohydrate at the surface of cells in the rat. *Anat. Rec.* **154**: 41.

RAVIN, H. A., ZACKS, S. J. and SELIGMAN, A. M. (1953) The histochemical localization of acetylcholinesterase in nervous system. *J. Pharmacol. Exp. Ther.* **107**: 37.

REGER, J. F. (1954) Electron microscopy of the motor end-plate in intercostal muscle of the rat. *Anat. Rec.* **118**: 344.

REGER, J. F. (1958) The fine structure of neuromuscular synapses of gastrocnemii from mouse and frog. *Anat. Rec.* **130**: 7–14.

ROBERTSON, J. D. (1954). Electron microscope observations on a reptilian myoneural junction. *Anat. Rec.* **118**: 346.

ROBERTSON, J. D. (1956a) Some features of the ultrastructure of reptilian skeletal muscle. *J. Biophys. Biochem. Cytol.* **2**: 369–80.

ROBERTSON, J. D. (1956b) The ultrastructure of reptilian myoneural junction. *J. Biophys. Biochem. Cytol.* **2**: 381–94.

ROBERTSON, J. D. (1960) Electron microscopy of the motor endplate and the neuromuscular spindle. *Amer. J. Phys. Med.* **39**: 1–43.

ROGERS, A. W., DARZYNKIEVICZ, Z., BARNARD, E. A. and SALPETER, M. M. (1966) Number and location of acetylcholinesterase molecules at motor endplates of the mouse. *Nature (Lond.)* **210**: 1003–6.

SABATINI, D. D., BENSCH, K. G. and BARRNETT, R. J. (1963) Cytochemistry and electron microscopy. The preservation of cellular ultrastructure and enzymatic activity by aldehyde fixation. *J. Cell Biol.* **17**: 19–58.

SALPETER, M. M. (1967) Electron microscope radioautography as a quantitative tool in enzyme cytochemistry. I. The distribution of acetylcholinesterase at motor end plates of a vertebrate twitch muscle. *J. Cell Biol.* **32**: 379–89.

SÁVAY, G. and CSILLIK, B. (1956) The effect of denervation of the cholinesterase activity of motor end-plates. *Acta Morph. Acad. Sci. Hung.* **6**: 289–97.

SÁVAY, G. and CSILLIK, B. (1958) Lead reactive substances in myoneural synapses. *Nature* **181**: 1137–8.

SAWYER, C. H., DAVENPORT, C. and ALEXANDER, L. M. (1950) Sites of cholinesterase activity in neuromuscular and ganglionic transmission. *Anat. Rec.* **106**: 287–8.

SCHIEBLER, T. H. (1953) Herzstudie. I. Mitteilung-Histochemische Untersuchung der Purkinjefasern von Säugern. *Z. Zellforsch.* **39**: 152–67.

SCHWARZACHER, H. G. (1957) Der histochemisch nachweisbare Cholinesterasegehalt in Muskelendplatten nach Durchschneidung des motorischen Nerven. *Acta Anat. (Basel)* **31**: 507–21.

SELIGMAN, A. M. (1964) Some recent trends and advances in enzyme histochemistry. In: *Proc. 2nd Int. Congr. for Histo- and Cytochemistry*, p. 9. Springer-Verlag, Berlin.

SELIGMAN, A. M., KARNOVSKY, M. J., WASSERKRUG, H. L. and HANKER, J. S. (1968) Non droplet ultrastructural demonstration of cytochrome oxidase activity with a polymerizing osmiophilic reagent, diaminobenzidine (DAB). *J. Cell Biol.* **38**: 1–14.

SELIGMAN, A. M., UENO, H., WASSERKRUG, H. and HANKER, J. S. (1966) Esterase method for light and electron microscopy via the formation of osmiophilic diazothioethers. *Ann. Histochem.* **11**: 115.

SHERIDAN, M. N., WHITTAKER, V. P. and ISRAËL, M. (1966) The subcellular fractionation of the electric organ of torpedo. *Z. Zellforsch.* **74**: 291–307.

SNELL, R. S. and McINTYRE, N. (1955) Effect of denervation on the histochemical appearance of cholinesterase at the myoneural junction. *Nature* **176**: 884–5.

SNELL, R. S. and McINTYRE, N. (1956) Changes in the histochemical appearance of cholinesterase at the motor endplate following denervation. *Brit. J. Exp. Path.* **37**: 44–48.

TAXI, J. (1952) Action du formol sur l'activité de diverses préparations de cholinestérases. *J. Physiol. (Paris)* **44**: 595–9.

TERÄVÄINEN, H. (1967) Electron microscopic localization of cholinesterases in the rat myoneural junction. *Histochemie* **10**: 266–71.

TSUJI, S. (1968) Sur la localisation des cholinestérases à l'aide d'iodures d'esters de thiocholine. *C.R. Acad. Sci. (Paris)* **267**: 801–3.

WASER, P. G. and RELLER, J. (1965) Bestimmung der Zahl activer Zentren der Acetylcholinesterase in motorischen Endplatten. *Experientia* **21**: 402.

WILSON, I. B. and GINSBURG, S. (1955) A powerful reactivator of alkylphosphate-inhibited acetylcholinesterase. *Biochem. Biophys. Acta* **18**: 168–70.

WILSON, I. B., GINSBURG, S. and QUAN, C. (1958) Molecular complementariness as basis for reactivation of alkyl phosphiate-inhibited enzyme. *Arch. Biochem. Biophysics* **77**: 286–96.

ZACKS, S. I. (1964) *The Motor Endplate*, pp. 321. W. B. Saunders Co., Philadelphia.

ZACKS, S. I. and BLUMBERG, J. M. (1961a) The histochemical localization of acetylcholinesterase in the fine structure of neuromuscular junctions of mouse and human intercostal muscle. *J. Histochem. Cytochem.* **9**: 317–24.

ZACKS, S. I. and BLUMBERG, J. M. (1961b) Observations on the fine structure and cytochemistry of mouse and human intercostal neuromuscular junctions. *J. Biophys. Biochem. Cytol.* **10**: 517–28.

ZAJICEK, J., SYLVÉN, B. and DATTA, N. (1954) Attempts to demonstrate acetylcholinesterase activity in blood and bone-marrow cells by a modified thiocholine technique. *J. Histochem. Cytochem.* **2**: 115.

CHAPTER 3

PHYSIOLOGICAL AND BIOCHEMICAL ASPECTS OF THE NORMAL NEUROMUSCULAR JUNCTION

J. I. Hubbard

Evanston, Ill.

3.1. HISTORICAL INTRODUCTION

The first demonstration of the nerve muscle junction as a distinct entity was made by Claude Bernard (1856) using the South American Indian arrow poison, curare, as his analytical tool. Curarized muscle, he found, contracted in the normal way when stimulated directly, but did not contract when its nerve was stimulated. The nerve, however, appeared to conduct impulses towards the region of the nerve muscle junction. Bernard deduced a block of transmission at the motor nerve in its most distal part where contact was made with the muscle. Later experimenters found, however, that another drug, nicotine, excited the contraction of skeletal muscle and this contraction was prevented, even in denervated preparations, by treatment with curare (Heidenhain, 1883; Langley, 1905, 1908; Edmunds and Roth, 1908). The site of drug action was thus the muscle.

Elliott (1905) had suggested, in connection with the contraction of smooth muscle caused by adrenaline, that this drug reacted with a special receptor substance in the muscle. Langley applied these ideas to skeletal muscle, and in a series of skilful quantitative experiments showed that the receptor substance for curare and nicotine was localized beneath the terminations of motor nerves on skeletal muscle (Langley, 1905, 1907, 1909, 1914). It followed from these experiments that since curare blocked the action of nerve impulses, the nerve impulse too caused muscle contraction by affecting the receptor substance. Langley (1905, 1909), following Elliott's (1904) suggestion of sympathetic nerve action by liberation of adrenaline, felt that motor nerves affected the receptor substance by releasing a chemical. A few years later Loewi (1921) demonstrated that nerve endings could release chemical mediators. He found that upon stimulation of the vagal nerve supply to the frog heart a chemical, later shown to be acetylcholine (ACh), was released which inhibited another isolated frog heart when added to the perfusate. A second example of what came to be called chemical transmission followed when stimulation of sympathetic nerves was shown to release an adrenaline-like substance which accelerated the heart (Cannon and Bacq, 1931; Cannon and Rosenblueth, 1933).

In a long series of investigations Dale and his colleagues extended the scope of chemical transmission from the peripheral synapses of the autonomic nervous system to the nerve–muscle junction. The transmitter was again ACh. Amongst the many stimulating contributions of the Dale school a few highlights may be mentioned. These include the first discovery of ACh in the animal body (Dale and Dudley, 1929); the demonstration of ACh release from the motor nerve terminal in response to nerve stimulation (Dale *et al.*, 1936); and the mimicking of nerve stimulation of muscle by close intra-arterial injection of ACh (Brown *et al.*, 1936). Dale and his colleagues explained these observations by supposing that nerve impulses released ACh. The ACh acted on a specialized region of the muscle to release a propagated wave of excitation in the muscle fiber which was in turn followed by contraction.

Fresh light was thrown on ACh action when Gopfert and Schaefer (1938) found that nerve stimulation of curarized muscle set up a local electrical potential which could be recorded with leads placed over the nerve–muscle junction. This potential, which consisted of a quick negative deflection and a slower return to the initial potential level, became known as the end-plate potential (e.p.p.). Pharmacological evidence, such as the progressive reduction of e.p.p. amplitudes with increasing curare concentrations and the prolongation of e.p.p. time courses by substances preventing ACh destruction, indicated that e.p.p.s were set up by a reaction of the ACh released from nerve terminals with muscle receptors. The e.p.p. in turn, if its amplitude exceeded a certain critical level, triggered the generation of muscle action potentials (Eccles *et al.*, 1941, 1942; Eccles and MacFarlane, 1949). Final proof of the chemical hypothesis was afforded by the use of intracellular recording. An accurate quantitative measure of the e.p.p. made possible the measurement of total charge displacement during neuromuscular transmission (Fatt and Katz, 1951). This charge could not possibly be provided by the action potential in nerve terminals, but could easily be accounted for by the ACh hypothesis.

More recent research has been marked by an increasing knowledge of

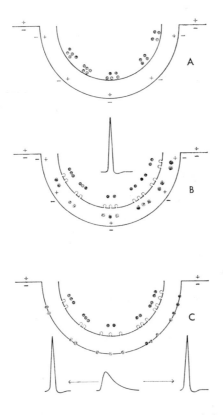

F<small>IG</small>. 1. A schematic presentation of neuromuscular transmission. A, B, C show a nerve terminal lying in a groove in the muscle membrane. The packets of acetylcholine (ACh) in the terminals are indicated by circles. The polarization of the muscle membrane is indicated by the + and − signs. A shows the resting junction, B the terminal invaded by a nerve impulse with a number of packets of ACh released into the synaptic cleft. In C the ACh has combined with receptors in the muscle membrane and set up the end-plate potential shown below. The end-plate potential in turn (arrows) set up the muscle action potentials indicated to the right and left of the end-plate potential.

the physicochemical basis of the transmitter process. In physical terms neuromuscular junctions in vertebrates are transducing elements in which electrical activity, in the form of action potentials in nerve terminals, is translated into the release of ACh (Fig. 1). ACh diffuses across the narrow synaptic cleft to react with receptors in the outer surface of the muscle membrane, causing this area to become permeable to ions (Fig. 1, B).

The resultant flow of ionic current across this localized area of membrane generates a nonpropagated electrical potential. If this potential, the e.p.p., is large enough, an action potential is initiated in the surrounding muscle membrane, and the transducing cycle is complete (Fig. 1, C). Muscular contraction is triggered in turn by the depolarizing effect of muscle action potentials propagating along the muscle fiber in all directions from the junctional region.

TERMINOLOGY

The neuromuscular junction is a functional junction between nerve and muscle cells. It may be termed therefore (widening the meaning of a term introduced by Sherrington (1897) for such connections between neurones) a synapse. Like all synapses it consists of two elements—presynaptic and postsynaptic. The term presynaptic will be used to denote a specialized terminal portion of the motor nerve, distinguished by its position in relation to the muscle membrane and, as electron microscopy has revealed, by its content of abundant mitochondria and, adjacent to the terminal membrane, a multitude of synaptic vesicles.

The term postsynaptic usually denotes not only the area of the muscle in relation to the nerve terminal, but also the whole muscle cell. It is convenient, however, both for descriptive purposes and in pharmacological and physiological investigation, to divide the muscle membrane into an area of membrane directly under the nerve terminal which is specialized for reaction with ACh, the subsynaptic membrane, and the rest of the membrane, the postsynaptic membrane.

3.2. PRESYNAPTIC PHYSIOLOGY

3.2.1. THE BIOSYNTHESIS OF ACh

The ability to synthesize ACh is a property of motor nerves which is most evident in their terminal portion. Essentially the process involves the acetylation of choline (Fig. 2). There are at least two steps in this reaction, the first being the generation of the high-energy compound acetyl coenzyme A (acetyl-CoA) by reactions between ATP, CoA and free acetate involving the formation of the intermediate adenyl-acetate (Berg, 1956 a, b):

(i) acetate $+$ ATP $\rightarrow$ adenyl-acetate $+$ P–P
(ii) adenyl-acetate $+$ CoA $\rightleftharpoons$ acetyl-CoA $+$ adenylic acid

The second and specific step is the transfer of the acetyl group from

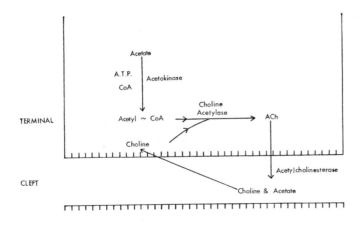

Summary of ACh Metabolism

FIG. 2. A schematic summary of the metabolism of ACh. In the terminal, the high-energy compound acetyl-CoA is formed from ATP, coenzyme A and acetate under the influence of the enzyme acetokinase. Acetyl-CoA is combined with choline by the enzyme choline acetylase to form ACh. The ACh is liberated into the synaptic cleft and broken down to choline and acetate fragments by the enzyme acetylcholinesterase (AChE). The choline is then reabsorbed by the nerve terminal. The ACh metabolism is thus dependent on a supply of energy (ATP) and the circulation of choline.

acetyl-CoA to choline. This reaction, catalyzed by the enzyme choline acetylase (ChAc), is illustrated in Fig. 3 (Nachmansohn, 1963).

CHOLINE ACETYLASE

This enzyme, now termed choline acetyltransferase (Korey *et al.*, 1951), was first isolated in a cell-free form by Nachmansohn and Machado (1943). It is found in the spinal cord, in high concentration in ventral roots and in lesser concentration in nerve trunks such as the sciatic and phrenic nerves (Hebb, 1963). In rat diaphragm muscle careful investigation has shown that most of the ChAc activity is concentrated in the part of the muscle containing the phrenic nerve and the majority of the nerve endings (Hebb *et al.*, 1964). The calculations of these authors suggest that, if the intramuscular nerve fibers contained as much ChAc as does the phrenic nerve, most of the ChAc activity must be concentrated in the nerve endings. Furthermore, the amount of ChAc activity in the endings, provided that the enzyme was as efficient *in vivo* as *in vitro*, would be enough to synthesize ACh at about three times the observed maximal rates of release during prolonged stimulation.

The ChAc found in nerve terminals is probably produced in moto-neurons. The initial evidence for central production and peripheral accumulation was the observation that the enzyme was most concentrated in ventral roots and the peripheral portions of motor nerves, with intermediate concentrations in the regions between (Feldberg and Vogt, 1948). Later it was found that ligaturing of the cervical sympathetic or sciatic nerves led to accumulation of ChAc above the ligature and its disappearance below the ligature (Hebb and Waites, 1956; Hebb and Silver, 1963).

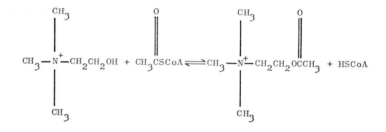

Fig. 3. The formation of ACh. Choline and acetyl-coenzyme A are combined under the influence of choline acetyltransferase to form ACh + coenzyme A. The full formula of coenzyme A is not shown. The S atom indicates that there is a sulfide link between enzyme and acetate.

3.2.2. ACh RELEASE

The evidence that motor nerve terminals release ACh upon nerve stimulation is direct and unequivocal. It rests on the collection of ACh from nerve-stimulated muscle preparations by methods which have been increasingly refined. In the earliest experiments mixed nerves to perfused muscles were stimulated and substances incompletely identified as ACh were found in the venous effluent (e.g. Brinkman and Ruiter, 1924, 1925). In later experiments, which were corner-stones of the chemical theory of transmission, Dale *et al.* (1936) showed clearly that motor nerve stimulation alone lead to the appearance of ACh in the venous effluent from dog, cat and frog muscle perfused intra-arterially *in vivo*. Emmelin and MacIntosh (1956) with improved perfusion techniques found that about 5×10^{-12} g of ACh was released by a maximal nerve impulse in the cat tibialis anticus, the stimulus rate being 20–25/sec. These experiments have more recently been supplemented by experiments with isolated nerve–muscle preparations placed in a suitable bathing medium containing an anticholinesterase (Straughan, 1960; Krnjević and Mitchell, 1961). In the rat diaphragm the amount of ACh released per nerve impulse is very similar to the amount released in cat tibialis anticus, being 3.5×10^{-12} g/impulse at a stimulus rate of 6/sec (Straughan, 1960). By lowering the stimulus rate still further (to 2/sec) Krnjević and Mitchell (1961) were able to collect 1.76×10^{-11} g (0.12 pmole)/impulse. If it is assumed that there are 10,000 synapses in the rat diaphragm (Krnjević and Miledi, 1958b) the output at each synapse would be 1.76×10^{-15} g $(10^{-17}$ mole)/impulse.

With these sensitive techniques a spontaneous release of ACh from diaphragm muscle has been detected (Brooks, 1954; Straughan, 1960; Krnjević and Mitchell, 1961). The amount is about one-twentieth to one-thirtieth of the amount released during stimulation. Part of this release can be accounted for by the spontaneous release of ACh recorded as miniature end-plate potentials (q.v.), but a portion is apparently of non-nervous origin for it can still be detected after denervation of muscle (McIntyre, 1959; Straughan, 1960; Krnjević and Mitchell, 1961; Mitchell and Silver, 1963). This release from denervated preparations is increased by stimulation of the muscle, and it has been claimed that this is inconsistent with the assumed presynaptic origin of ACh (McIntyre, 1959; Hayes and Riker, 1963). It appears most probable that the release in denervated preparations arises from the ChAc activity of remnants of the nerve, such as Schwann cells, for after denervation the release falls in parallel with degeneration of the nerve and only arises from the middle region of the muscle which normally contains the nerve branches (Mitchell and Silver, 1963; Krnjević and Straughan, 1964). Certainly Hebb *et al.* (1964) found that denervated diaphragm muscle has residual ChAc activity which is more than enough to supply ACh for the spontaneous release, although only 3–6% of the amount of ChAc found in innervated muscle.

A further and often more convenient method of assessing ACh release is to measure the depolarization of the postsynaptic membrane produced by ACh which can be recorded by either an intracellular or an extracellular electrode in close proximity to the synaptic region. This type of experiment has lead to a very important and unifying hypothesis—the quantal hypothesis.

3.2.3. THE QUANTAL HYPOTHESIS

In 1950 Fatt and Katz, while recording intracellularly from the frog

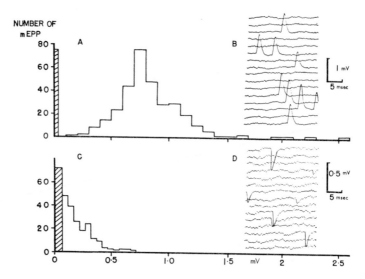

Fig. 4. Miniature end-plate potentials (m.e.p.p.s). A, B show the amplitude distribution and sample intracellular records of m.e.p.p.s from a neuromuscular synapse in the rat diaphragm. Note in A the presence of a few m.e.p.p.s with amplitudes much greater than the mean. C, D show the amplitude distribution and sample records from the same synapse, on extracellular recording. The skew distribution of m.e.p.p. amplitudes (C) arises because an extracellular electrode records only from some fraction of the end-plate area. The majority of recorded potentials are thus small and just above the noise level (hatched bar in A and C). The width of the cells in the histograms was 100 μV in A and 50 μV in C. The records (B, D) are composite and do not give an accurate representation of m.e.p.p. frequency. The temperature was 25°C. The records have been retouched (Hubbard and Schmidt, 1963).

neuromuscular synapse, detected small potentials of fairly uniform amplitude appearing apparently at random intervals (Fig. 4, A, B). Their observation was fundamental to the quantal hypothesis for these small potentials, termed by Fatt and Katz (1950) miniature endplate potentials (m.e.p.p.s), are the basic units of the release mechanism. They have since been recorded from the postsynaptic cell at all the vertebrate and invertebrate neuromuscular synapses explored (Boyd and Martin, 1956a; Brooks, 1956; Liley, 1956a; Burke, 1957; Takeuchi, 1959; Elmqvist *et al.*, 1960; Ginsborg, 1960a; Dudel and Kuffler, 1961; Burnstock and Holman, 1962a; Usherwood, 1963).

The first investigators (Fatt and Katz, 1950, 1952) found that these potentials were produced by multimolecular packets or quanta of ACh, for the potentials were smoothly graded in amplitude and time course by drugs such as tubocurarine and prostigmine. This would not be expected if single molecules of ACh were involved. Further, externally applied ACh produced only a smoothly graded depolarization with no increase in frequency of m.e.p.p.s (Fatt and Katz, 1952; Hubbard *et al.*, 1965). If the m.e.p.p.s were produced by individual ACh molecules then the application of ACh in solution should greatly increase the discharge frequency. The effect of ACh thus again suggests that the m.e.p.p.s were produced by multimolecular ACh packets. Recent estimates of the number of ACh molecules involved in the production of a single m.e.p.p. range between 10^4 and 10^5 (Krnjević and Mitchell, 1961; Elmqvist and Quastel, 1965a).

The origin of the quanta of ACh is necessarily from the nerve terminal for m.e.p.p.s cease to be detectable after degeneration of the terminal (Fatt and Katz, 1952; Liley, 1956a). A further telling point is that the frequency of m.e.p.p.s can be markedly altered by polarizing currents applied to the nerve terminal, while polarizing currents applied to the postsynaptic membrane are without effect on their frequency (del Castillo and Katz, 1954d; Liley, 1956c).

The quantal size is not absolutely fixed but the variation is small (Fig. 4, A). Multiples occur, but rarely (Liley, 1957). It appears that the quantal size is not only uniform at each junction in a muscle but is similar at all junctions in a given preparation. The apparent variation in amplitude of focally recorded m.e.p.p.s from different muscle fibers can be almost entirely attributed to the variation of the diameter of fibers. Fiber diameter affects the input resistance of the fiber and thus the amplitude of the recorded potential (Katz and Thesleff, 1957a). The only known presynaptic factors which affect quantal size are drugs which affect ACh synthesis, e.g. hemicholinium (see Presynaptic ACh stores) and the disease myasthenia gravis. In both cases quantal size is reduced (Elmqvist and Quastel, 1965a; Elmqvist *et al.*, 1964).

While the m.e.p.p. amplitude reflects a standard quantum of ACh, the m.e.p.p. frequency at any particular synapse appears very variable in time (Fig. 4, B). In the resting state it was established that the succession of m.e.p.p.s was random (Fatt and Katz, 1952). The evidence for this conclusion was that when the intervals between successive potentials were measured, the distribution of intervals fitted a simple exponential curve. Similar results have been obtained at all other neuromuscular synapses investigated in this way. Recently it has been shown that of the various possible types of random processes, the one involved is the Poisson process (Gage and Hubbard, 1965). Thus the probability of finding any particular

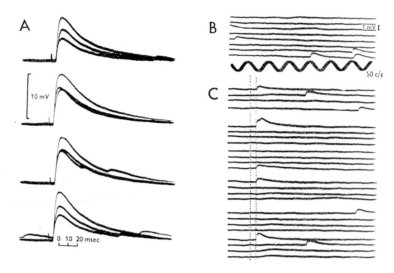

FIG. 5. The effect of increasing the Mg concentration upon the quantal content of e.p.p.s. A shows fluctuation of e.p.p. response at a single frog neuro-muscular synapse, treated with 10 mM Mg (Ca concentration was normal: 1.8 mM; prostigmine 10^{-6}). Intracellular recording. In each record, three superimposed responses are seen. Note the scattered spontaneous miniature potentials. B shows a frog neuromuscular synapse treated with reduced Ca (0.9 mM) and 14 mM Mg concentration. The top part shows a few spontaneous potentials (traces separated by 1 mV steps). C (below the 50 c/sec time signal) shows responses to single nerve impulses. Stimulus artefact and response latency are indicated by a pair of dotted vertical lines. The proportion of failures was very high: there are only five responses to twenty-four impulses (reproduced from Del Castillo and Katz, 1954b).

number of m.e.p.p.s in any unit time interval (e.g. oscilloscope sweep) is given by the function

$$\text{Probability } (n = k) = e^{-\lambda}\ \lambda^k/k! \qquad (1)$$

where λ is the mean frequency of m.e.p.p.s per unit time interval; λ is the important parameter of a Poisson distribution. It can be shown that the mean of such a distribution is equal to λ and that the variance of such a distribution is also equal to λ (Feller, 1950).

The establishment of m.e.p.p. frequency as a Poisson process has the important corollary that the release of quanta giving rise to m.e.p.p.s must by definition be independent events, involving a large number of potentially releasable quanta each with a low probability of release. It

66

will be appreciated that the mean frequency (λ) must be given by the product of this probability (p) and the number of potentially releasable units (n), i.e.

$$\lambda = np. \tag{2}$$

The importance of this unit potential, produced by a standard quantum of ACh, lies in the fact that the e.p.p. produced by nerve stimulation can be fractionated into units identical in all respects with m.e.p.p.s. The means of fractionation is to raise the magnesium or lower the calcium concentration of the solution bathing the synaptic region (Fig. 5). By these methods the e.p.p.s can be reduced in a stepwise manner until single units are obtained on nerve stimulation. With a further reduction of the calcium concentration or raising of the magnesium concentration the responses to stimulation are intermittent so that there are occasional failures (Fig. 5, C).

It was the achievement of del Castillo and Katz (1954 a, b) to show that when the e.p.p. had been reduced to small numbers of constituent units the number of such units in a long series of responses was distributed according to the Poisson distribution. To do this an estimate had to be obtained of the mean number of units (m) in responses, in this case the mean of the number of units or quanta in all e.p.p.s rather than the mean frequency as in the m.e.p.p. example.

Obviously the simplest way to obtain such an estimate would be to divide the mean e.p.p. amplitude ($\bar{v}$) by the mean m.e.p.p. amplitude ($\bar{v}_1$) thus obtaining an estimate (m_1) of the average number of constituent units, that is the average quantal content

$$m_1 = \bar{v}/\bar{v}_1. \tag{3}$$

Alternatively, if after raising the magnesium concentration of the bathing medium there were a large number of nerve stimuli to which there was no release of transmitter (Fig. 5, C) then m may be estimated from the Poisson function with $n = 0$, for as the probability of $n = k$ is given by

$$n_k = e^{-m} m^k/k! \tag{4}$$

which is as (1) but substituting m for λ, then if $k = 0$

$$n_0 = e^{-m} m^0/0! = e^{-m} \tag{5}$$

and for N trials

$$n_0 = Ne^{-m}. \tag{6}$$

It is therefore only necessary to count the total number of trials (N) and the number of these trials in which no quantum was released (n_0); m may then be directly estimated from (6) by

$$m = \log_e N/n_0. \tag{7}$$

It is found that the relative numbers of failures, unit responses, and responses containing two or more quanta, are found to agree satisfactorily with the Poisson law. Moreover, when the depression is less extreme, the quantum content as judged by the proportion of failures always agrees closely with the quantum content as judged from the ratio of e.p.p. amplitude to m.e.p.p. amplitude. This type of analysis while first successfully carried out at vertebrate neuromuscular junctions (del Castillo and Katz, 1954b; Liley, 1956b; Boyd and Martin, 1956b) has been extended to crustacean neuromuscular junctions where ACh is not the transmitter (Dudel and Kuffler, 1961).

It is difficult to carry out these tests when the quantal content of e.p.p.s is larger than about 3. A further method is available, however, which can be used for e.p.p.s of any quantal content. This is the variance method, based on the fundamental property of a Poisson distribution that the variance and mean are identical. The standard deviation (σ) is then equal to the square root of the mean (i.e. $(m)^{\frac{1}{2}}$). It is more convenient to work with the coefficient of variation ($CV = \sigma/m = 1/(m)^{\frac{1}{2}}$ for a Poisson distribution) rather than the standard deviation. In a series of synaptic potentials, the quantal contents of the individual potentials should be distributed according to the Poisson distribution with $CV = 1/m^{\frac{1}{2}}$. The coefficient of variation of the amplitude of the e.p.p.s should be similarly distributed, except that allowance must be made for the small variation of amplitude of the individual quantal components (Fig. 4, A). This will increase the value of the observed CV by a fraction $1 + (cv)^2$, where cv is the coefficient of variation of the unit potential amplitude (Blackman, Ginsborg and Ray, 1963; Martin and Pilar, 1964). Then

$$CV/1 + (cv)^2 = 1/m^{\frac{1}{2}}. \tag{8}$$

It has been found (reviewed by Martin, 1966) that in practice $[1+(cv)^2]^{\frac{1}{2}} = 1.05$ and can be ignored; thus

$$m = 1/(CV)^2. \tag{9}$$

This method cannot be used for values of $m > 10$, without a preliminary correction of e.p.p. amplitudes to allow for the nonlinear addition of the individual quantal units. The nonlinearity arises because each quantum of transmitter produces a conductance change in the postsynaptic membrane (see Sect. 3.3.2), and the amount of potential change produced by each quantum decreases as the number of quanta released (i.e. total membraine depolarization) increases. Individual e.p.p. amplitudes (v) must be corrected to allow for this (Martin, 1955). If the membrane potential is E, and the equilibrium potential for the synaptic potentials is Ve, then the corrected e.p.p. amplitude $v^1(mV)$ is given by

$$v^1 = v[(E - Ve)/(E - Ve - v)]. \tag{10}$$

With this method it has been demonstrated that nerve impulses release between 100–300 quanta in curarized amphibian and mammalian muscle (Martin, 1955; Liley, 1956b; Boyd and Martin, 1956a; Takeuchi and Takeuchi, 1959; Elmqvist and Quastel, 1965b). Martin (1955) has also shown that the quantal content of e.p.p.s is not altered by the presence of d-tubocurarine, therefore presumably the normal quantal content of responses is approximately of this order.

PROBABILITY OF RELEASE

As in the case of spontaneous release, quantal content can be considered in terms of n, the number of releasable units, and p, the probability of release. When compared with spontaneous release n is presumably the same, but p is enormously increased over a small but finite time interval. Katz and Miledi (1965d) have given a graphic illustration of this process by recording the latency of e.p.p.s at 4.5°C using a frog preparation (Fig. 6). This graph may be regarded as illustrating the probability of quantal release at successive intervals of time after the stimulus. It can be seen that this probability reaches a maximum and then declines slowly. At the frog nerve terminal at 20°C the complete sequence takes some 3–4 msec (Katz and Miledi, 1965b). The parameter p is not, therefore, constant over the period of release. However, if the number of quanta released during successive short intervals after a nerve impulse were compared in successive trials, the number in each interval would be expected to follow the Poisson law. Since the sum of any number of Poisson variates is also a Poisson variate, it would be expected that the number of quanta released during any defined interval following a nerve impulse should follow the Poisson law, as indeed experiment shows (Martin, 1955; Elmqvist and Quastel, 1965b).

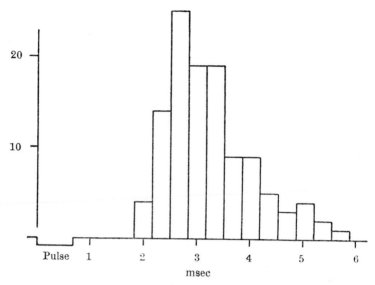

Fig. 6. Time course of the probability of ACh release after depolarization of motor nerve terminals. The histogram indicates the latency distribution of e.p.p.s evoked by constant current pulses of 0.68 msec duration (pulse) applied to nerve terminals in a frog sartorius muscle *in vitro*. The bathing solution contained tetrodotoxin (4×10^{-6} g/ml) so that the depolarization of terminals released ACh presumably without entry of sodium ions into the terminals. Temperature 4.5°C. Ordinate: number of observed responses. Abscissa: time interval between the start of the depolarizing pulse and the start of e.p.p.s (Katz and Miledi, 1965d).

3.2.4. ACh STORES

As would be expected from the Poisson character of release the amount of ACh thought to be contained in motor nerve terminals (1.8×10^{10} molecules, Krnjević and Mitchell, 1961) is large compared with the amount of ACh thought to be contained in a single quantum (10^4–10^5 molecules, Krnjević and Mitchell, 1961; Elmqvist and Quastel, 1965a). The investigation of the perturbations of quantal release caused by stimulation has shown, however, that not all this ACh is immediately available for release by nerve impulses. This difficulty has been resolved by postulating ACh stores, the contents of which differ in their availability for release.

IMMEDIATELY AVAILABLE ACh

The basic observation which has lead to the concept of immediately

70

available ACh was that after 1 e.p.p. has been elicited by nerve stimulation in a curarized preparation, further stimuli elicit e.p.p.s which are smaller in amplitude (because of a smaller quantal content) for periods up to 10 seconds (Liley and North, 1953; Lundberg and Quilisch, 1953; Takeuchi, 1958; Thies, 1965). The size of this depression of the second response is directly correlated with the number of quanta released by the first impulse (Otsuka *et al.*, 1962). If, for instance, this number is drastically reduced, e.g. by increasing the MgCl$_2$ content of the bathing medium, then the depression disappears and the second response may now have a larger quantal content than the first for intervals of up to 200 msec. Conversely, if the quantal content of the first e.p.p. is increased by, for example, increasing the CaCl$_2$ concentration of the bathing medium, this depression is increased in magnitude but not in duration (Lundberg and Quilisch, 1953; Thies, 1965). A simple explanation of these findings is that the release of a large number of quanta entails the depletion of some factor needed for subsequent e.p.p.s. In all probability this is simply the emptying of a store of 300–1000 immediately available performed quanta of ACh (Elmqvist and Quastel, 1965b).

This apparent contradiction of the Poisson character of release is most plausibly explained if the process generating the Poisson distribution is not the actual release of quanta, but lies one step behind. This would arise directly if only a small fraction of a pool of quanta in the nerve terminal were at any moment available for release, either because of a particularly favorable location or because of some kind of activation. If the other quanta each had at any moment a low probability of becoming immediately available for liberation, then there would be a Poisson distributed entry of quanta into the "immediately available store" and the number in this store would fluctuate according to the Poisson law, no matter what the probability of the quanta leaving (Quastel and Vere-Jones, unpublished calculations; Vere-Jones, 1966).

MOBILIZATION

If nerve impulses are repeated at rates greater than 0.1/sec, the amplitude of the e.p.p.s so elicited declines progressively and eventually reaches a plateau after four to eight impulses (Fig. 7). The progressive decline in amplitude of the first few e.p.p.s (early tetanic rundown) is due to a progressive fall in quantal content ascribed to a progressive depletion by the repeated stimuli of the "immediately available store". It is presumed that the quantal content of the e.p.p.s does not fall to zero because the "immediately available store" is sustained by a "repletion" or "mobilization"

71

process. Presumably depletion of the immediately available store is the actual stimulus for mobilization into it and it seems that the frequency of stimulation is also important (Liley and North, 1953; Elmqvist and Quastel, 1965b).

As yet, there has been very little investigation of the mobilization process despite its great physiological importance in permitting the sustained

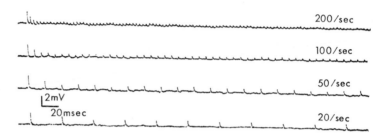

FIG. 7. The effects of repetitive stimulation upon end-plate potential (e.p.p.) amplitude in a curarized rat diaphragm preparation. Note that the e.p.p. amplitude is largest at the beginning of stimulation and falls during stimulation to a plateau level. The level of this plateau is greater the lower the frequency of stimulation. Even in this plateau phase e.p.p.s show some variation in amplitude, due to the Poisson character of release. This variability enables quantal content to be determined by the "variance" method. The illustrations are of intracellular records all from the same synapse at the indicated frequency of stimulation. The temperature of the bathing Krebs–Ringer solution was 37°C and the curare concentration 2×10^{-6} g/ml (Hubbard, unpublished observations).

release of ACh. The application of a hyperpolarizing current to nerve terminals is the only process which has been shown to affect it (Hubbard and Willis, 1962).

With prolonged tetani, at frequencies of more than about 5/sec, e.p.p. quantal contents and therefore e.p.p. amplitudes do not remain at their initial level, but fall slowly and progressively, to be maintained eventually at a level which is much lower than that found at first (del Castillo and Katz, 1954c; Brooks and Thies, 1962; Elmqvist and Quastel, 1965b). If this fall is also ascribed to depletion of a presynaptic store, it is possible to arrive at a figure for a "mobilization store". Elmqvist and Quastel (1965b) found this store was about 50–100 times larger than the immediately available store. The anatomical substrate of the mobilization store is unknown, certainly it appears to be only a fraction of the total amount of ACh normally stored in a nerve terminal.

PRESYNAPTIC ACh STORE

It has recently become possible to estimate the size of the presynaptic store at individual neuro-muscular junctions, using the drug hemicholinium No. 3 (αα-dimethyl ethanolamine 4,4'-biacetophenone, HC3). HC3 blocks ACh synthesis in intact nervous tissue but not in homogenates. Apparently the drug does not interfere with ChAc action directly but in some way affects choline metabolism (MacIntosh *et al.*, 1956; Schueler, 1960; MacIntosh, 1961). At mammalian neuromuscular synapses *in vitro* it has been found that e.p.p.s and m.e.p.p.s run down in amplitude to apparent extinction when stimulation is prolonged in the presence of 10^{-5} g/ml of HC3 (Elmqvist *et al.*, 1964; Elmqvist and Quastel, 1965a).

If it is assumed that HC3 completely blocks synthesis, the amount of ACh in a nerve terminal can be determined as the amount released after synthesis is blocked by HC3. This amount can be determined as the sum of all e.p.p.s elicited at a synapse by prolonged repetitive stimulation until such time as the e.p.p.s vanish. Alternatively, m.e.p.p.s released by raising the potassium concentration of the bathing medium can be recorded. By plotting the size of e.p.p.s or m.e.p.p.s against the sum of all foregoing e.p.p.s or m.e.p.p.s, and by extrapolating the resulting curve to zero e.p.p. or m.e.p.p. amplitude, it is possible to obtain an estimate of total releasable transmitter. Usually the result is expressed in terms of the initial quantum size because it is then independent of differences of postsynaptic sensitivity due to, for instance, muscle fiber dimensions or membrane potential (Katz and Thesleff, 1957a), or the presence of postsynaptically depressing substances such as Mg^{2+}, K^+, tubocurarine or HC3. Furthermore, it appears that the store estimates are quite independent of how rapidly the nerve terminals are emptied (Elmqvist and Quastel, 1965a).

In the rat diaphragm the store was found to be 270,000 ± 70,000 quanta (mean of fourteen determinations ± S.D.). Similar results were obtained at the human neuromuscular synapse (Elmqvist *et al.*, 1964; Elmqvist and Quastel, 1965a). The amount of ACh in a nerve terminal in the rat diaphragm has been estimated at 1.8×10^{10} molecules (Krnjević and Mitchell, 1961) so that each quantum in the store would contain about 76,000 molecules.

3.2.5. THE NATURE OF THE RELEASE MECHANISM

The quantal nature of the release mechanism is an inherent property of the presynaptic terminals. The alternative possibility that the fractionation of release occurs because the nerve impulse fails to invade fine terminals of the motor nerve can be dismissed. In the first place, while elevation of the $MgCl_2$ concentration of the bathing medium increases the threshold for invasion of the terminals by a nerve impulse (Hubbard *et al.*, 1965), increasing the $CaCl_2$ which would further raise the invasion threshold (Katz and Miledi, 1965c) reverses the Mg-induced fractionation of release (del Castillo and Katz, 1954a; Boyd and Martin, 1956b). Secondly, direct evidence bearing on this point was obtained by Dudel and Kuffler (1961) who recorded extracellularly from individual terminal branches on the crayfish muscle. Both spontaneous and nerve-induced responses were as expected for a Poisson process, yet only one terminal was involved. Finally, Katz and Miledi (1965c) have shown that changing the $CaCl_2$ concentration in the region of a single branch of the terminals of a frog motor nerve affects transmitter release without any alteration of the action potential recorded extracellularly from the nerve terminal.

Therefore it seems that in the nerve terminal there is a process spontaneously liberating quanta of ACh at a low rate which is momentarily and enormously accelerated by nerve impulses. There are thus two problems involved:

1. The nature of the release mechanism, and
2. The nature of the coupling between the nerve impulse and the release mechanism.

THE VESICLE HYPOTHESIS

This hypothesis (del Castillo and Katz, 1955b) states that ACh is contained within the 500 Å diameter vesicles which are clustered on the presynaptic side of neuromuscular synapses (Robertson, 1956; Birks *et al.*, 1960a). The content of one vesicle presumably corresponds to a quantum of ACh, registered as a m.e.p.p. by the postsynaptic membrane. The evidence for this hypothesis comes from several sources. Firstly, upon degeneration or regeneration of nerve terminals, m.e.p.p.s and vesicles disappear or appear at about the same time (Fatt and Katz, 1952; Liley, 1956a; Birks *et al.*, 1960b; Miledi, 1960c). Secondly, synaptic vesicles take up and retain ferritin particles indicating that they communicate with the extracellular fluid at some time (S. Page, quoted by Katz and Miledi, 1965e; Birks, 1966). Thirdly, the amount of ACh per quantum is estimated to be about 70,000–80,000 molecules (Elmqvist and Quastel, 1965a), which is of the order of the total amount of ACh (62,000 molecules) which could be accommodated in a vesicle of 500 Å (Canepa, 1964). Finally, there have been experimental attempts to influence vesicle numbers. At the frog neuromuscular synapse, increased ACh release by exposing preparations to hyperosmotic or high potassium containing solutions was not associated with detectable effects on vesicle numbers (Birks *et al.*, 1960a; Birks, 1966). However, at other synapses similar experiments have apparently been successful. For instance, the rate of spontaneous release of transmitter is reduced at synapses in the vas deferens of the guinea pig after reserpine treatment (Burnstock and Holman, 1962b) which deplete tissues of cate-cholamines (Burn and Rand, 1959) and nerve terminals of presumed adren-ergic vesicles (Pelligrino de Iraldi and de Robertis, 1961). Reported altera-tions in vesicle number and diameter in rod and cone synapses after light adaptation of rabbit retina (de Robertis and Franchi, 1956) have, however, not been confirmed when repeated with adequate controls (Mountford, 1963). Reports of changes in vesicle numbers in nerve endings in the adrenal medulla after splanchnic nerve stimulation (de Robertis and Ferreira, 1957; de Robertis, 1958) await confirmation. At human neuro-muscular synapses *in vitro* stimulation of nerves did not produce any de-tectable changes in the appearance of vesicles (Woolf, 1966).

The site of formation of the vesicles found in motor nerve terminals is not known with certainty. On the one hand Breemen *et al.* (1958) suggest that the vesicles are formed in the perikaryon of motoneurons and move with the axoplasm down to the terminals. On the other hand, there are a number of physiological observations consistent with production of the vesicles in the terminals, perhaps by budding off from the terminal membrane. In favor of central production Breemen *et al.* (1958) report the presence of vesicle profiles in frog nerves above the terminal, and the accumulation of vesicles above a ligature on the frog sciatic nerve. In favor of peripheral production there is the ability of rat diaphragm preparations to continue release of quanta of ACh measured as m.e.p.p.s at a rate of over 100/sec for a period of at least 8 hours *in vitro* (Hubbard and Landau, unpublished observations). There are only about 3×10^5 vesicles in the nerve terminals at this junction (Hubbard, unpublished observations), therefore replacement of vesicles would seem mandatory. Similar evidence has been reported by de Robertis (1964) for presumed adrenergic vesicles.

THE ROLE OF CALCIUM

Although the vesicle hypothesis provides an explanation for the quantal release of ACh, the actual release process remains obscure. It seems clear that calcium ions are involved, for, without calcium, release of ACh ceases (del Castillo and Stark, 1952; Jenkinson, 1957; Elmqvist and Feld-

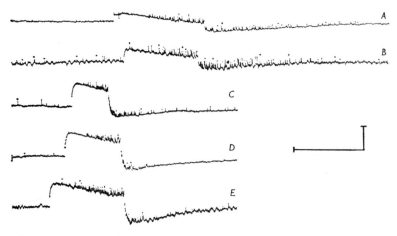

Fig. 8. The calcium step in ACh release. Intracellular records of m.e.p.p.s before, during (elevated baseline) and after the passage of 7.0×10^{-5} Å through a micropipette containing 0.2 M CaCl$_2$ and positioned at the subsynaptic region of a neuromuscular synapse in a rat diaphragm *in vitro*. The diaphragm had been incubated for 3 hours at 32°C in the following solutions: A, calcium-free with 20 mM KCl; B and C, calcium-free with ethylenediamine tetra-acetic acid (EDTA) 1 mM and 20 mM KCl; D and E, calcium-free with EDTA 1 mM and ouabain 160 mg/ml. Time calibration: A, 250 msec, B–E, 500 msec. Voltage 2 mV in all records. Membrane potentials (mV): A, 38; B, 52; C, 52; D, 44; E, 40 (Elmqvist and Feldman, 1965a).

man, 1965a). The critical concentration necessary for release at individual junctions lies between 10^{-3} and 10^{-4} M (Elmqvist and Feldman, 1965a). As shown in Fig. 8, if the calcium concentration at a calcium depressed junction is suddenly increased by microelectrophoretic administration, m.e.p.p.s can again be detected after an invariable latency of about 250 msec (Elmqvist and Feldman, 1965a). This striking latency gives some indication that complex reactions are involved in the release mechanism. It is well established that m.e.p.p. frequency and the quantal content of e.p.p.s varies with extracellular calcium concentration in both amphibian and mammalian preparations (Boyd and Martin, 1956a; Hubbard, 1961; Mambrini and Benoit, 1964; Elmqvist and Quastel, 1965b). The form of the relationship between the calcium concentration and m.e.p.p. frequency indicates that calcium ions form complexes, presumably with membrane components which appear to be associated with the ability of nerve impulses to release ACh (Gage and Quastel, 1966; Hubbard *et al.*, 1967).

Other ways of increasing the spontaneous release of ACh are known which do not appear to involve the calcium mechanism so directly. These include changes in extracellular osmotic pressure, stretching of the nerve terminals, mechanical damage to the terminals and hypoxia (Fatt and Katz, 1952; Hutter and Trautwein, 1956; Liley, 1956a; Furshpan, 1956; Hubbard and Løyning, 1966). Extensive *in vitro* investigations indicate that m.e.p.p. frequency is logarithmically proportional to extracellular osmotic pressure over a very wide range of osmotic pressures (Hubbard, Jones and Landau, 1968).

EXCITATION-RELEASE COUPLING

Recent investigations make it certain that vertebrate motor nerve terminals do not differ substantially from the parent nerve in their electrical properties. Contrary to earlier beliefs nerve impulses are conducted along the nerve terminals, and nerve impulses can be set up in the terminals as in the parent fibre by depolarizing current pulses (Hubbard and Schmidt, 1963; Katz and Miledi, 1965 a, b; Braun and Schmidt, 1966). The belief that the depolarization brought about by the nerve impulse begins the coupling process has been strengthened by experiments in which nerve terminals have been depolarized by application of electric currents or by raising the extracellular potassium ion concentration.

THE EFFECT OF POLARIZING CURRENTS

When polarizing currents are applied to nerve terminals the m.e.p.p. frequency is a logarithmic function of the applied current strength, being increased by depolarizing and decreased by hyperpolarizing currents (del Castillo and Katz, 1954d; Liley, 1956c). This effect is markedly reduced if the extracellular Ca concentration is lowered.

THE ROLE OF POTASSIUM IONS

Further light on the release process has come from *in vitro* experiments in which m.e.p.p. frequency has been examined in various extracellular $[K^+]$ (Fig. 9, A). It is found that the frequency of m.e.p.p.s is related logarithmically to the logarithm of the extracellular $[K^+]$ at levels above 10^{-2} M (Liley, 1956c). Presumably potassium ions act by lowering the membrane potential of the terminals, and the potential should be a logarithmic function of the extracellular $[K^+]$ (Katz, 1962). This enormous effect illustrated in Fig. 9 is related to the calcium mechanism by the requirement that a minimum concentration of calcium ions be present before the potassium mechanism operates (Liley, 1956c). The importance of this

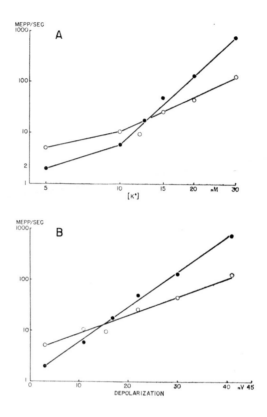

FIG. 9. The relationship between m.e.p.p. frequency and $[K^+]$. In A the open circles indicate the mean m.e.p.p. frequency in a rat diaphragm preparation 2–7 minutes after increasing $[K^+]$ from 5 mM to the indicated value. Each point is the mean of two or more diaphragms in each of which the frequency was determined at 14–25 synapses during the 5-minute period. The filled circles show the relationship between mean m.e.p.p. frequency and $[K^+]$ after 20 minutes at 38°C, found by Liley (1956c). B, the relationship between m.e.p.p. frequency and potassium-induced depolarization. In this figure, the data of Fig. 4, A is replotted converting $[K^+]$ to the assumed membrane depolarization, using the Nernst equation (Katz, 1962). Open and filled circles as in Fig. 4, A. Ordinate: m.e.p.p. frequency (logarithmic scale). Abscissa: membrane depolarization in millivolts. It will be noted that the m.e.p.p. frequency recorded 2–7 minutes after raising the $[K^+]$ is much lower than the frequency found after 20 minutes. It is thought that these lower values (open circles) more accurately reflect the depolarization of terminals and give a better quantitative indication of the relationship between nerve terminal depolarization and ACh release (Hubbard, Jones and Landau, 1967).

observation lies in the relationship between the magnitude of terminal depolarization and the release of transmitter. Liley (1956c) suggested that extrapolation of the relationship between depolarization and release, to the level of depolarization expected from a nerve impulse, could explain the observed release of ACh by nerve impulses. Later re-examination of the effect of potassium ions has shown that the effect on frequency was not as rapid as would be expected if it was mediated solely through terminal depolarization. For instance, Gage and Quastel (1965) found that when 20 mM KCl was added to the bathing solution of a rat diaphragm preparation, m.e.p.p. frequency continued to increase for over 2 hours. These prolonged effects are at present unexplained.

The action of increased magnesium or sodium ion concentrations, which inhibit the ACh release produced by nerve impulses or by increased extracellular [K^+] concentrations, is apparently a competitive inhibition of Ca (Jenkinson, 1957; Hubbard, 1961; Birks and Cohen, 1965; Kelly, 1965; Gage and Quastel, 1966). The possibility that the entry of sodium ions during the nerve impulse played a role in the release process (Birks, 1963; Birks and Cohen, 1965) appears excluded by experiments using the Puffer fish poison, tetrodotoxin. This poison is known to block the initial depolarizing component of action potentials in nerve and muscle fibres, presumably by preventing the normal sodium ion influx (Nakamura *et al.*, 1965; Narahashi *et al.*, 1964; Narahashi *et al.*, 1960). However, tetrodotoxin does not affect either the m.e.p.p. frequency or the ability (Fig. 6) to release ACh from nerve terminals by depolarizing pulses (Elmqvist and Feldman, 1965b; Katz and Miledi, 1965d).

3.2.6. RELEASE HYPOTHESES

The common ground of present release hypotheses (Fig. 10) is that the synaptic vesicles are in Brownian motion and that ACh, presumably within the vesicles, is released when the vesicles interact with the nerve terminal membrane. The hypotheses differ however in the role assigned to nerve terminal polarization. According to Bass and Moore (1966), terminal depolarization removes a charge and hydration barrier normally preventing impingement of charged hydrated vesicles with the terminal membrane (Fig. 10, A). However, according to del Castillo and Katz (1957d), depolarization increases the number of membrane receptors available for combination with presumably uncharged vesicles (Fig. 10, B), it being assumed that combination inevitably leads to release of ACh.

It has been suggested that calcium complexes move through membranes

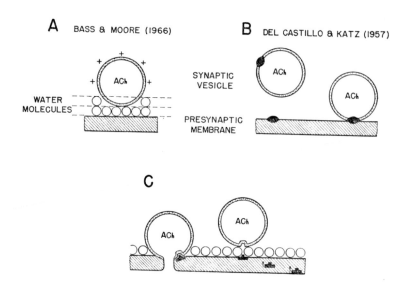

FIG. 10. Release models. In these models synaptic vesicles, shown as circles, are assumed to contain ACh and to be in Brownian motion. Release of ACh occurs when the vesicle interacts with the presynaptic membrane. In A (Bass and Moore, 1966) a charge and hydration barrier is thought to prevent impinging of vesicle and membrane. Spontaneous release occurs only if vesicles have above average kinetic energies. Depolarization removes the charge barrier. In B (Del Castillo and Katz, 1957d) release occurs when specific sites on vesicle and membrane interact. Depolarization is thought to increase the number of sites. In C calcium complexes are indicated moving through the membrane to form receptors which interact with vesicles to cause release. Depolarization is thought to increase the rate of movement of complexes (Hubbard, Jones and Landau, 1967).

(Luttgau and Niedergerke, 1958) to form the vesicle receptors (Gage and Quastel, 1966). Figure 10, C shows one possible mechanism, it being presumed, as in the del Castillo and Katz theory (Fig. 10, B), that release occurs upon combination of complex and vesicle. Depolarization presumably increases the rate of movement of complexes. Several possible mechanisms have been described. For instance, conformational changes occur in cell membranes during the generation of action potentials (see, for example, Schmidt and Davison, 1965). Speculatively, depolarization may therefore facilitate movement of complex either by inducing membrane pores and/or by providing an electrical gradient favoring the movement of an appropriately charged complex. Osmotic pressure alterations may

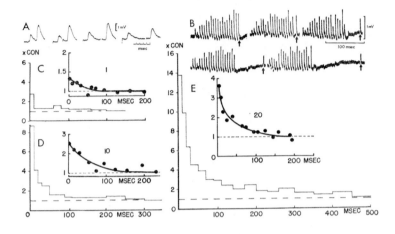

FIG. 11. Potentiation of e.p.p amplitudes and m.e.p.p. frequency after one to twenty nerve impulses in a Mg-poisoned preparation. A shows potentiation of an e.p.p. elicited by the second of paired stimuli in a Mg-paralysed preparation. In C (inset) the amplitude of this second potentiated e.p.p. is plotted as a multiple of the first e.p.p. for intervals up to 200 msec; each point represents the average of ten to fifteen trials at each interval. Also shown in C is the probability of m.e.p.p. occurrence at intervals up to 250 msec after an impulse. This graph was constructed from data obtained in over 200 trials in which m.e.p.p.s were counted in a 500-msec period before a single impulse and in 10-msec periods thereafter. From the total count before stimulation (270) the average number of m.e.p.p.s to be expected in any period after stimulation could be calculated (assuming stimulation had no effect). In fact there was always an excess of m.e.p.p.s in the first 200-msec period after stimulation, the greater part of this excess falling in periods immediately after stimulation. In the graph this has been shown by lines placed to indicate m.e.p.p. numbers as a multiple of the number expected in that interval. The intervals are shown by the line lengths, which represent 10 msec immediately after the stimulus, then 20 msec and at later periods 50 msec. In some places the lines are confluent, the numbers of m.e.p.p.s in adjacent periods being then the same (Hubbard, 1963). B shows e.p.p.s in response to twenty stimuli at 200/sec, and to a testing stimulus (arrow) at various intervals after the short tetanus. In the graphs inset in D and E the amplitude of the e.p.p. response to a testing stimulus is plotted after 10 (D) and 20 (E) impulses at 200/sec, for intervals up to 200 msec. Each point represents the average e.p.p. amplitude determined from ten to fifteen trials at each interval and expressed as a multiple of the average e.p.p. amplitude in the absence of stimulation. The main graphs in D and E show the increased probability of m.e.p.p. occurrence after the same number and frequency of stimuli, calculated as in C; B, D, E were all obtained from the same junction. The temperature was 36°C and the Mg concentration 11 mm/l (Hubbard, 1963).

81

affect ACh release by stripping away water molecule layers thus reducing the energy barrier separating vesicle and membrane receptor (Fig. 10, A, C). Alternatively, or additionally, alterations in membrane structure may be brought about by dehydration.

3.2.7. REPETITIVE ACTIVATION

At the neuromuscular synapse, as at many other synapses (Hughes, 1958), repetitive nerve impulses initiate processes increasing (potentiating) the release of transmitter by subsequent impulses. These potentiating processes are of particular interest for the light their study throws on the processes responsible for sustaining ACh release. These processes occur concurrently with the depletion of quanta of ACh due to release (see ACh stores), and the observed quantal content of e.p.p.s can be considered as a balance between potentiating and depleting processes.

To demonstrate the potentiating processes it is most convenient to avoid depletion by reducing the average quantal content of responses to a very low value. This is most easily done by raising the $MgCl_2$ and/or lowering the $CaCl_2$ content of the bathing medium. Under these circumstances it is easy to show (Fig. 11, A, C) that after a single impulse, e.p.p.s elicited by a second impulse will on average be larger in amplitude for a period of 100–200 msec, and over this period the probability of occurrence of m.e.p.p.s is likewise increased (Fig. 11, C). The presynaptic nature of this potentiation is strikingly indicated by the finding that no ACh need be liberated by the first impulse for the potentiation of e.p.p. amplitude and m.e.p.p. frequency to be demonstrable (del Castillo and Katz, 1954b; Hubbard, 1963; Braun *et al.*, 1966).

During repetitive stimulation it appears that the potentiating influence is additive, for, beginning at frequencies of 5–10/sec which correspond to an interval of 200–100 msec between impulses, successive e.p.p.s show a progressive increase in amplitude (Fig. 11, B) to a virtual plateau of response characteristic of that frequency (Fig. 12, A, C). Close investigation indicates that no steady level is finally attained, for even after 6000 impulses del Castillo and Katz (1954c) found e.p.p. amplitudes still continuing to increase. During the period of progressive e.p.p. amplitude potentiation, m.e.p.p. frequency is likewise increased (Fig. 12, B).

After repetitive stimulation, as after single stimuli, single impulses elicit larger e.p.p.s than in the absence of the conditioning stimulus. Two forms of post-tetanic potentiation have been detected (Hubbard, 1963). The first form corresponds to the running down of the potentiation of e.p.p. amplitude and m.e.p.p. frequency developed during the tetanus (Fig. 13, A, 5 msec). The second (Fig. 13, A, 2 sec; C) develops after a delay which is longer the greater the duration and frequency of stimulation, and is more prolonged. Both the duration of this form of potentiation and the delay at its beginning are determined by the frequency and strength of stimulation. A duration of 4–8 minutes would not be unusual (Feng, 1941; Liley and North, 1953; Hubbard, 1963; Braun *et al.*, 1966).

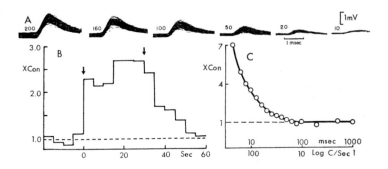

FIG. 12. The effect of stimulation frequency upon the amplitude of e.p.p.s and frequency of m.e.p.p.s during repetitive stimulation. A shows records of e.p.p. responses made by superposing faint traces during repetative stimulation in a Mg-paralysed preparation. In C the average e.p.p. amplitude measured from these and other records in the same experiment is plotted as a multiple of the e.p.p. amplitude during stimulation at a frequency of 1/sec (interrupted line). In these experiments e.p.p. amplitudes during stimulation at frequencies above 10–12.5/sec were always greater than the control amplitude. B shows m.e.p.p. frequency over 5-second periods before, during and after a tetanus of 1500 impulses at 50/sec. The frequency is shown as a multiple of the mean frequency for 20 seconds before stimulation (interrupted line); arrows mark the beginning and end of the tetanus (Hubbard, 1963).

If the quantal content of e.p.p.s is large, as in curarized preparations, traces of the potentiating processes can still be seen during and after repetitive stimulation, but generally the potentiating influences are lost in the depression of response caused by depletion (Hubbard, 1963). An exception is the late posttetanic potentiation which can be demonstrated irrespective of the quantal content of responses.

It is well established that all forms of potentiation are presynaptic in origin, for all are due to an increase in the quantal content of responses (Hutter, 1952; del Castillo and Katz, 1954c; Liley and North, 1953; Liley, 1956b).

83

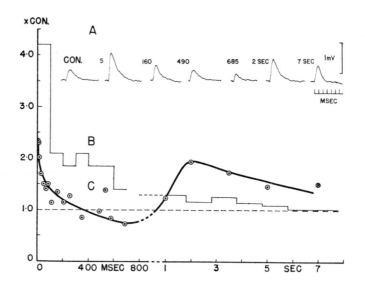

FIG. 13. Early and late post-tetanic potentiation. The effect of fifty impulses at a frequency of 200/sec upon e.p.p. amplitude and m.e.p.p. frequency in a Mg-paralysed preparation. A shows records of testing e.p.p.s elicited at the indicated interval (msec or second) after the tetanus. The records were selected to illustrate the average amplitude found in four to six trials at each interval. In the graph C this average amplitude is plotted as a multiple of the control e.p.p. amplitude found in the absence of tetanic stimulation. This control amplitude was measured repeatedly after two to three intervals had been assessed and was remarkably constant throughout the experiment. In this and other experiments the amplitude of testing e.p.p.s was potentiated at intervals up to 400 msec after the tetanus, was depressed at longer intervals up to 1 second, and thereafter potentiated again. Also shown (B) is the probability of m.e.p.p. occurrence after fifty impulses at 200/sec, as a multiple of the control probability. This probability was calculated as in Fig. 11, C, but for 100-msec periods for the first 700 msec after the tetanus and thereafter for 1-second periods. The control m.e.p.p. probability and e.p.p. amplitude are shown by the same interrupted line. Note the break in the abscissal scale between 800 msec and 1 second and the similar breaks in the graphs. The e.p.p. and m.e.p.p. results are not from the same junction, but are representative of seven experiments in which e.p.p. amplitudes were successfully measured and four experiments in which m.e.p.p. frequency was assessed. The Mg concentration was 11 mM/l, and the temperature 37°C for all these experiments (Hubbard, 1963).

Quantal content can be considered as a product of probability of release and the number of releasable units (see Probability of release, p. 69). It appears that the increased quantal content of responses after single stimuli and at the beginning of a tetanic train, as well as the late and long-lasting posttetanic potentiation must be ascribed to an increased probability of release by the impulse (Liley and North, 1953; Elmqvist and Quastel, 1965b). The mechanism producing this increase is obscure.

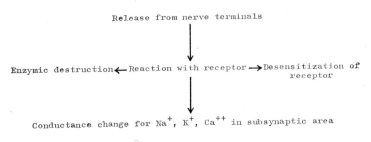

FIG. 14. The effects and fate of ACh.

Testing of current theories indicates that none is completely satisfactory (Gage and Hubbard, 1966 a, b). It appears most probable that some component of the excitation-release coupling process, perhaps the calcium step, is more easily activated after previous use (Katz and Miledi, 1965c).

3.3. SUBSYNAPTIC MEMBRANE

In the subsynaptic membrane lie the receptors for ACh, and an enzyme acetylcholinesterase (AChE) which terminates ACh action by destroying it. The known effects and fate of ACh are summarized in Fig. 14.

3.3.1. THE ACh RECEPTOR

EFFECT OF ACh

The existence of a receptor for curare and nicotine at the neuromuscular synapse was first demonstrated by Langley (1907) when he showed that nicotine caused a contraction of frog muscle if it was applied in the region

85

of innervation, and that this action was blocked by curare. ACh is similarly only effective in producing contraction when applied in the synaptic region (Buchtal and Lindhart, 1937). Kuffler (1943), using single frog muscle fibers, was able to demonstrate that ACh and nicotine application produced an extracellularly recorded depolarization in the synaptic region which was opposed by curare. None of these drugs was effective

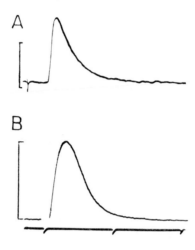

Fig. 15. Comparison of potentials set up by nerve stimulation (A) and microelectrophoresis of ACh (B). A shows an intracellularly recorded e.p.p. evoked by nerve stimulation at a synapse in a rat diaphragm muscle *in vitro*. The muscle was paralysed by the addition of 15 mM/l. $MgCl_2$ to the bathing solution. B shows an intracellularly evoked ACh potential evoked in another rat diaphragm muscle by a 1-msec pulse of current (3.5×10^{-8} Å) applied through an external micropipette containing 4 M acetylcholine chloride. In both cases the temperature was 24–25°C. The voltage scale is 5 mV in A and 10 mV in B and the time scale which has 10-msec calibration applies to A and B. There is a remarkable similarity in the time courses of the potentials evoked by the nerve (A) and by ACh (B) (Krnjević and Miledi, 1958a).

elsewhere in the muscle. If the depolarization exceeded a threshold value, muscle action potentials were set up and muscle contraction followed. Refinement and generalization of these experiments has become possible following the introduction of the microelectrode technique. A minute amount of ACh can now be applied electrophoretically in the close vicinity of single synapses in the whole muscle, and the subsequent depolarization recorded with an intracellular electrode. It is found that ACh administered with brief pulses of current can produce a large transient depolarization, and initiate a muscle action potential (Nastuk, 1951; del Castillo and Katz, 1955a, 1957a). Applying ACh to synapses in the rat diaphragm Krnjević and Miledi (1958a) were able to produce potentials which had almost as fast a time course as e.p.p.s (Fig. 15). Only about 2.8×10^{-15} g/ACh was required to set up such potentials, which is of the same order as the amount of ACh released at a synapse by an impulse (Krnjević and Mitchell, 1961).

RECEPTOR POSITION AND NATURE

The receptors are obviously located on the outside of the membrane for ACh is ineffective if applied intracellularly in a dose which was effective when applied from the extracellular position (del Castillo and Katz, 1955a). By autoradiographic means the presumed ACh receptor sites (identified by binding of ^{14}C muscarone or ^{14}C decamethonium) have been distinguished from the curare receptors (identified by binding of ^{14}C curarine or ^{14}C toxiferin) and the active centers of cholinesterase molecules (identified by binding with ^{32}P or ^{14}C diisopropyl phosphofluoridate). The three receptors, although different, form a closely related topographical unit (Waser, 1967). Earlier experiments also suggested that the ACh receptor and AChE were topographically distinct (Waser, 1960). For instance, in the electroplax, block of electrical activity can be achieved with essentially unaltered AChE activity (Altimirano *et al.*, 1955).

The effects of ACh are customarily classified as either muscarinic or nicotinic, according to whether the ACh action resembles that of muscarine and is blocked by atropine, or resembles nicotine and is blocked by curare. At the neuromuscular synapse ACh action is clearly nicotinic, being mimicked by nicotine (Kuffler, 1943) and blocked by curare but not atropine (Brown *et al.*, 1936) in similar concentrations.

The physical nature of the receptor is still obscure. Claims that the receptor had been isolated in a protein fraction from electroplax tissues (Ehrenpreis, 1960) have later been abandoned with the demonstration that the fraction was not homogeneous (Beychok, 1965) and did not have the pharmacological specificity required (Ehrenpreis, 1961). Some workers in this field still consider that acetylcholinesterases may be the receptor (Ehrenpreis, 1967).

RECEPTOR AREA AND DENSITY

ACh receptors are found in greatest density in the subsynaptic region but also occur outside the synapse on the surrounding muscle membrane.

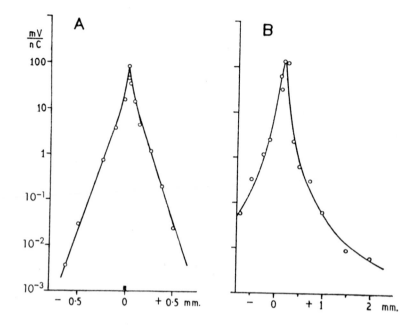

Fɪɢ. 16. ACh receptor distribution along a rat diaphragm muscle fiber (A) and a frog sartorius muscle fiber (B), tested by microelectrophoresis of ACh. The abscissae shows distance in millimeters from a recording electrode inserted near the synapse. The ordinates indicate sensitivity to ACh expressed in arbitrary units (ratio of depolarization in millivolts to number of coulombs of electric charge (nC) passing through the micropipette to release ACh). The approximate diameter of a synapse in diaphragm muscle fibers is indicated by the square on the horizontal axis in A (Miledi, 1962b).

Waser (1967) has estimated that the subsynaptic receptors are capable of combining with $50-70 \times 10^6$ molecules of ACh while the capacity of the extrasynaptic receptors is greater ($1.6-1.9 \times 10^9$ molecules). The sub- and extrasynaptic receptors are pharmacologically alike (del Castillo and Katz, 1957b; Goldsmith, 1963) but not identical.

The receptor area depends on the state of muscle innervation. Fetal muscle and muscles deprived of their nerve supply or poisoned with botulinum toxin have ACh receptors uniformly distributed over the membrane. After birth, and upon reinnervation of denervated or botulinum toxin poisoned muscle, the receptor area shrinks to a focus (Fig. 16) with the maximum density inside an area of $\frac{1}{2}$ mm (rat, Fig. 16, A) to

2 mm (frog, Fig. 16, B) diameter around the subsynaptic region (Ginetzin-sky and Shamarina, 1942; Axelsson and Thesleff, 1959; Miledi, 1960a, b, c; Thesleff, 1960; Diamond and Miledi, 1962).

In many frog sartorius muscles and in tortoise retractor capitis muscle there is a low ACh sensitivity in areas remote from the synapse (Katz and Miledi, 1964; Levine, 1966). The possibility thus arises that the inability to detect extrasynaptic ACh sensitivity in some frog sartori and in mammalian innervated muscle merely reflects a subthreshold density of receptors. The muscle membrane would then be in all cases a composite of electrically and chemically (ACh) excitable elements (Levine, 1966). The proportion of ACh excitable elements would then depend on local factors and the state of innervation. The finding that fibrillation potentials in denervated muscle arise at the denervated synaptic region indicates, however, that this region has some special properties (Belmar and Eyza-guirre, 1966).

3.3.2. THE ACh-RECEPTOR COMBINATION

When ACh is applied to the synapse either by nerve stimulation or artificially, a depolarization of the area is recorded (Gopfert and Schaefer, 1938; Kuffler, 1943). It is clear that this depolarization is not due to the influx of ACh cations (Fatt, 1950) for direct measurements of the electric charge displacement show that there is a much larger ionic flux than could be accounted for in this way (Fatt and Katz, 1951). Measurements of the interaction of e.p.p.s and spike potentials indicate that ACh causes an increased conductance of the muscle membrane (Fatt and Katz, 1951) by briefly and suddenly causing a localized increase in its permeability to ions (Fatt and Katz, 1951; del Castillo and Katz, 1954e). Further investigation of this increased conductance at the frog neuromuscular synapse indicates that the permeability increase does not involve all ions but specifically Na, K and to a small extent Ca ions (Takeuchi and Takeuchi, 1960; N. Takeuchi, 1963a, b). It seems likely that the Na and K ions move through the membrane in separate channels (Maeno, 1966).

The conductance increase at the synapse, unlike that associated with the nerve impulse, does not depend on an alteration of membrane potential for its initiation (Fatt and Katz, 1951; Takeuchi and Takeuchi, 1960). The most striking demonstration of this point was provided by del Castillo and Katz (1955b) who immersed frog sartorius muscles in isotonic K_2SO_4. Despite the depolarization of the fibers and the absence of Na and Cl ions in the bathing solution it was still possible to detect the spontaneous release of ACh (m.e.p.p.s) by measurement of the small fall each quantum produced in the membrane resistance.

SYNAPTIC CURRENT

The current (Isyn) which flows as a result of the membrane conductance change *is*, however, dependent on membrane potential. This arises because for each ion species the driving force is the difference between the membrane potential (E) and the equilibrium potential (V_v) of that ion. Thus considering the frog neuromuscular synapse and neglecting the effect of calcium (Takeuchi and Takeuchi, 1960):

$$I_{syn} = \Delta g_{Na} (E - V_{Na}) + \Delta g_K (E - V_K) \qquad (11)$$

where Δg_{Na} is the sodium conductance change,
   Δg_K is the potassium conductance change.

The net fluxes of Na and K are in opposite directions because the concentration of K is high inside the cell, while the higher Na concentration is external. The electrochemical gradient is higher for Na than for K because of the greater displacement of Na from its equilibrium potential; hence the ratio of fluxes (Na/K) in normal frog Ringer at room temperature is 1.29 in keeping with the net inward current depolarizing the membrane. For analysis, it is convenient to rearrange equation (11) into the form

$$I_{syn} = (\Delta g_{Na} + \Delta g_K) \left(\frac{E - \Delta g_{Na} V_{Na} + \Delta g_K V_K}{\Delta g_{Na} + \Delta g_K} \right). \qquad (12)$$

The composite term subtracted from E is, in fact, the equilibrium potential V_e, the potential at which there is no net flux, therefore

$$I_{syn} = \Delta G (E - V_e) \qquad (13)$$

where $\Delta G = \Delta g_{Na} + \Delta g_K$ is the net conductance change. V_e for frog muscle is about 15 mV inside negative (del Castillo and Katz, 1954e; Burke and Ginsborg, 1956b; Takeuchi and Takeuchi, 1960). An important link in the chain of evidence pointing to ACh as the transmitter substance at the neuromuscular synapse was the demonstration that ACh potentials and e.p.p.s have the same equilibrium potential and involve the same ionic shifts (Takeuchi, 1963b).

EFFECTS OF Ca^{++} AND Mg^{++}

At the frog neuromuscular synapse, and in all probability at many other synapses, an increase in extracellular $[Ca^{++}]$ or $[Mg^{++}]$ raises the equilibrium potential, probably by decreasing sodium conductance (Takeuchi, 1963b). It may be noted, however, that unless there is a concomitant lowering of the extracellular sodium concentration, the effects are not large in the range of calcium and magnesium concentrations normally used to block neuromuscular transmission. In conformity with this finding, magnesium ions in excess decrease the magnitude of the depolarization produced by bath-applied ACh, and also the magnitude of m.e.p.p.s. However, in the presence of *d*-tubocurarine, magnesium ions enhance the ACh effect instead of further depressing it (del Castillo and Engbaek, 1954; del Castillo and Katz, 1954a). Calcium ions in excess likewise decrease the amplitude of m.e.p.p.s (Fatt and Katz, 1952; Mambrini and Benoit, 1964) and diminish the depolarization produced by electrophoretic pulses of ACh (Mambrini and Benoit, 1964).

THE NATURE OF THE ACh RECEPTOR COMBINATION

Most of our information about the nature of this reaction has come from studies of the mode of action of drugs which combine with ACh receptors. These drugs fall into two classes depending upon whether or not the conductance change which normally follows the ACh receptor combination is inhibited. As Thesleff and Quastel (1965) have pointed out, this classification must be considered to a large extent artificial, for there is a considerable overlap in the mode of action of any one drug in different circumstances. One interpretation of this variability is that the ACh receptor combination is a two-step reaction, an intermediate inactive compound being formed, which is then changed to an active depolarizing form (del Castillo and Katz, 1957c). Substrates of the receptor, other than ACh, would be predominantly competitive inhibitors of ACh or depolarizers like ACh, depending on the rate constants of the two steps.

The mode of action of the receptor at the molecular level is quite unknown. A suggested mechanism (Nachmansohn, 1959) is based on the well-established difference in enzymic activity of both AChE and ChAc towards substrates with tertiary and quaternary nitrogen derivatives. Activity is generally accelerated by the presence of the fourth alkyl group— thus the enzymes react much faster with ACh and choline respectively than with their tertiary analogs dimethylethyl acetate and dimethylethanolamine (Wilson and Cabib, 1956; Berman *et al.*, 1953; Berman-Reisberg, 1957). However, the addition of this fourth group does not alter the binding forces of the enzyme substrate complex (Wilson, 1952). There is some evidence that, as the quaternary nitrogen group is structurally almost spherical, an enzyme could only have simultaneous contact with all the

91

methyl groups by enveloping the reactant, i.e. a change of configuration of the protein occurs in the formation of the complex (Berman *et al.*, 1953; Wilson and Cabib, 1956). Such a structural change in the receptor, if it is a protein, could well explain the membrane permeability change which follows combination with ACh.

3.3.3. TERMINATION OF ACh ACTION

It has been calculated that at many synapses, diffusion alone would remove the transmitter from the vicinity of the receptor in a time sufficient to account for the observed decay of transmitter action (Ogston, 1955; Eccles and Jaeger, 1958). At vertebrate neuromuscular synapses, diffusion is supplemented by an enzyme (AChE), which is present in very high concentration in the subsynaptic membrane in very close proximity to the ACh receptor (Waser, 1960, 1967), and which probably binds ACh in a very similar manner to the receptor. As might be expected, therefore, many drugs reacting with the ACh receptor also inhibit AChE and vice versa. The type of receptor combination varies with the structure of the drug and both predominantly depolarizing and non-depolarizing effects have been reported in association with anticholinesterase actions.

THE ACh–AChE COMBINATION

AChE, a hydrolytic enzyme, is one of the fastest enzymes known. At a single neuromuscular synapse 0.2×10^{-6} mg (1.6×10^{9} molecules) of ACh may be hydrolyzed in a millisecond (Marnay and Nachmansohn, 1938; Nachmansohn, 1939). AChE action has been closely studied by Wilson and his colleagues, and it appears that during the reaction an ACh enzyme complex is formed (Fig. 17). An important part of the stability of this complex is thought to be due to an ionic bond formed between the positive charge of ACh and a negatively charged region of the enzyme surface (Wilson and Bergmann, 1950 a, b; Wilson, 1952). At another site two further bonds are formed, a covalent bond between a basic group in the enzyme (Fig. 17, B) and the carbonyl carbon of the ACh molecule and a hydrogen bond between acidic groups in the enzyme and one of the ACh oxygen atoms (Fig. 17, A). This latter site may be termed an esteratic site since the ester linkage is broken during the later steps of the reaction. The mechanism of hydrolysis proposed by Wilson *et al.* (1950) involves two consecutive steps following the formation of the enzyme substrate complex. In the first step the enzyme is acetylated with elimination of choline, and in the final step the acetyl-enzyme reacts with water to form acetic acid and regenerate the enzyme. The choline in all probability is reabsorbed by the presynaptic element. In human neuromuscular and cat ganglionic synapses, *in vitro*, addition of choline to the bathing fluid improves ACh output, so this may be an important function of AChE (Birks and MacIntosh, 1961; Elmqvist and Quastel, 1965a).

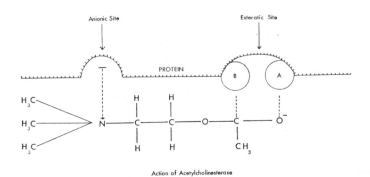

Fig. 17. The ACh–AChE combination. The diagram indicates the covalent and hydrogen bonds between two active groups (A, B) of the enzyme and its substrate, ACh, at an esteratic site and the ionic bonding between the positive charge of ACh and a negatively charged region (anionic site) of the enzyme (Wilson and Bergmann, 1950b).

ORIGIN AND DISTRIBUTION OF AChE

The first appearance of AChE in muscle generally precedes innervation (Karczmar, 1963), and is associated with the appearance of the specialized muscle nuclei in the subsynaptic area (Kupfer and Koelle, 1951). The muscle origin of AChE is supported by the experiments in which muscles were tenotomized, or atrophied as a consequence of spinal cord section (Gwynn and Vrbova, 1966). In both cases, despite intact innervation, profound alterations occurred in the histochemical appearance of AChE in the subsynaptic structures. The motor nerve clearly has some regulatory influence over AChE, however, for the amount of AChE in the subsynaptic region falls on denervation to 40–50% of normal and rises coincident with reinnervation (Csillik, 1965; Guth *et al.*, 1964; Guth and Brown, 1965). Furthermore, AChE appears at synapses formed after implantation of nerves into aneural or denervated muscle (Miledi, 1962a; Guth and Zalewski, 1963).

At the synapse AChE is concentrated on the subsynaptic folds, activity here being 15,000 to 30,000 times greater than in the surrounding region (Marnay and Nachmansohn, 1938; Feng and Ting, 1938). A high concentration is also found at the musculocutaneous junction (Couteaux, 1958). Recent investigations, in which autoradiography and electron microscopy were combined, have confirmed the predominantly subsynaptic location of AChE (Rogers *et al.*, 1966). A small concentration of AChE is associated with the nerve terminal, perhaps derived from the AChE found in motor nerves and neurons (Koelle, 1963).

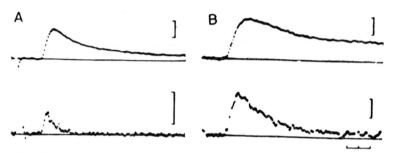

FIG. 18. AChE inhibition. A shows e.p.p. (above) and end-plate current (below) recorded from a curarized frog sartorius preparation. B shows the e.p.p. and end-plate current from the same synapse in the presence of curare and 1×10^{-5} g/ml physostigmine. Note the increased amplitude and prolonged time course of the e.p.p. in the presence of the anticholinesterase and the associated great increase in end-plate current caused by the prolongation of ACh action. Voltage scale: 2 mV. Current scale: 1×10^{-7} Å. Time scale: 2 msec. Temperature: 18°C (Takeuchi and Takeuchi, 1959).

AChE is not the only esterase found in the subsynaptic region. For instance, butyryl cholinesterase, which hydrolyzes butyryl thiocholine at a faster rate than acetyl thiocholine, is also present (Denz, 1953). Recent calculations based on autoradiographic techniques at the light and electron microscope level suggest indeed that the AChE concentration is only 35% of the total esterase concentration in the subsynaptic area. Interestingly, the calculated number of active sites of AChE ($1-4 \times 10^7$/ synapse, Rogers *et al.*, 1966; Waser, 1966) is of the same order as the maximum number of ACh molecules thought to be released by a nerve impulse (6×10^6/synapse, Krnjević and Mitchell, 1961).

AChE INHIBITION

When AChE is inhibited by anticholinesterases such as physostigmine e.p.p.s are found to be increased in amplitude and to have a prolonged time course (Eccles *et al.*, 1941, 1942; Eccles and MacFarlane, 1949; Fatt and Katz, 1951). The mode of anticholinesterase action has been elegantly demonstrated by Takeuchi and Takeuchi (1959) using the voltage clamp technique (Fig. 18). In the presence of the anticholinesterase the end plate current set up by ACh is greatly increased in amplitude and prolonged in time course (Fig. 18, cf. A and B). Presumably the end-plate current reflects the occupation of receptor sites by ACh. Figure 18, B, thus indicates that in the presence of physostigmine ACh survives much longer than normally.

3.3.4. DESENSITIZATION OF RECEPTORS

Early investigators of ACh action found that although the application of ACh to the synaptic region of muscle caused contraction, later applications were ineffective (e.g. Buchtal and Lindhart, 1937). An explanation for this effect was found by Fatt (1950) who reported that at the frog synapse the depolarization produced by high doses of ACh was not well maintained and could not be restored by addition of further ACh. Investigations by Thesleff and his colleagues using microphoretic application of ACh indicate that this refractoriness of ACh receptors, termed desensitization, develops at both amphibian and mammalian neuromuscular synapses (Thesleff, 1955 a, b; Katz and Thesleff, 1957b; Axelsson and Thesleff, 1958). The degree and speed of onset of desensitization was graded and increased with the concentration of ACh applied, but the rate of recovery was constant. Increasing the calcium concentration of the bathing solution also increases the speed of onset of desensitization and this action is antagonized by increasing the bathing sodium concentration (Manthey, 1966, quoted by Nastuk, 1966).

With mammalian muscle ACh applied electrophoretically for 1–2 msec did not have a desensitizing effect although amounts of ACh producing a depolarization as little as that of a m.e.p.p. did desensitize if maintained for longer periods (3–6 msec). It was therefore suggested that desensitization might develop during normal synaptic activity (Axelsson and Thesleff, 1958). In conformity with this idea Thesleff (1959) reported some desensitization at the mammalian synapse after a short train of e.p.p.s. The preparation he used, however, paralysed as it was by immersion in a solution with a high NaCl content, is prone to spontaneous movement. Otsuka *et al.* (1962) who repeated Thesleff's experiment, found this movement was the most probable cause of the reported effect, and also observed that the depression of e.p.p. amplitude after a brief train of stimuli was increased by raising the $CaCl_2$ concentration of the bathing medium but unaltered by the presence of an anticholinesterase. This implies that the depression depended on the amount of ACh released, not the amount reaching the receptors. Moreover, it has been directly demonstrated that the depression of e.p.p.s produced by prolonged stimulation as well as the depression found after a single conditioning stimulus is due to a presynaptic cause—a reduction in quantal content (del Castillo and Katz, 1954c; Thies, 1965).

3.4   POSTSYNAPTIC MEMBRANE

Muscle cells resemble cables being usually 10–100 μ in diameter and a few millimeters to several centimeters in length. They consist of sections—sarcomeres—each 2–3 μ long arranged in series. Each fiber has a surface membrane which is continuous with an internal system of tubules—the transverse tubular system. The surface area of this internal system is 5–7 times that of the surface membrane (Peachey, 1965). A second system of internal tubules—the sarcoplasmic reticulum, is in contact with, but is not continuous with, the transverse tubular system.

In cats, chickens and frogs two types of muscle fiber can be distinguished by their innervation, response to stimulation and ACh, membrane properties and fibrillar structure. One is the common twitch fiber, singly or sparcely innervated with compact nerve endings of the "en plaque" type, responding to stimulation by a propagated action potential and twitch and having regular, distinct and punctate myofibrils. The other is the so-called slow fiber, multiply innervated with endings of the "en grappe" type, responding to stimulation with a contracture (a reversible, prolonged, nonpropagated contraction) and generally unable to produce action potentials. The myofibrils of this type are large, irregular and poorly defined. In cats slow fibers are found only in the extraocular muscles (Hess and Pilar, 1964), but in chickens and frogs the slow system is more widespread (Kuffler and Vaughan Williams, 1953 a, b; Burke and Ginsborg, 1956 a, b; Ginsborg, 1960 a, b). All of the muscles which contain slow fibers have twitch fibers in addition.

3.4.1.   THE GENERATION OF THE e.p.p.

In both twitch and slow muscle fibers the e.p.p. is generated by the rapid displacement of electrical charge (depolarization) under the influence of ACh. This active phase terminates as ACh is removed by AChE and diffusion, and the time course of the e.p.p. is then determined by the passive spreading of charge along and across the muscle fiber membrane (Eccles *et al.*, 1941; Kuffler, 1942; Katz, 1948). To appreciate the evidence for these concepts it is necessary to know something of the electrical properties of muscle membranes. It is conventional to represent excitable tissues such as muscle by a battery, in series with a resistance (or conductance) and shunted by a capacitor (Fig. 19, A). The battery represents the potential difference (some 70–90 mV outside positive) which muscle cells maintain across their membrane. In 1902 Bernstein proposed that this potential was a potassium diffusion potential, and accordingly its magnitude would

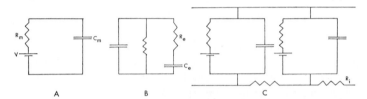

Fɪɢ. 19. Electrical models of the muscle fiber membrane. A shows the conventional electrical representation of a muscle fiber. *V* represents the membrane potential, C_m the membrane capacitance and R_m the membrane resistance (or conductance). B indicates a modification of A to include the capacitance (C_e) and the resistivity (R_e) of the transverse tubules, the walls of which are continuous with the surface membrane. C indicates the cable property of muscle. Because of the length of muscle cells the membrane must be considered as a series of resistive and capacitive elements connected by the internal resistance (R_i) of the myoplasm.

be determined by the intracellular (K_i^+) and extracellular (K_o^+) potassium ion concentrations, the exact relationship being given by the Nernst equation for potassium ions:

$$E_k = RT/FZ_k \quad \log_e [K_i^+]/[K_o^+]$$

where E_k is the equilibrium potential for potassium,
R the universal gas constant (8.2 joules per mol degree),
T the absolute temperature,
F the Faraday number (number of coulombs for mol of charge, 96,500)
Z the valence (for $K^+ = 1$).

At 37°C the equation simplifies to

$$E_K = 61 \quad \log_{10} [K_i^+]/[K_o^+].$$

The most important evidence supporting the Bernstein hypothesis is that the membrane potential varies in the predicted way when the potassium concentration ratio is varied. In summary, in skeletal muscle when $[K_o^+]$ is greater than 10 mM, the membrane potential is close to that of a potassium electrode. At lower concentrations it deviates in the manner expected from a slight permeability to sodium (Hodgkin and Horowicz, 1959).

The resistance (conductance) of Fig. 19, A, represents largely the ability of potassium and chloride ions to cross the muscle membrane. It has been found that in frog muscle potassium permeability depends greatly on the direction of net potassium movement. The membrane permeability for inward movement of potassium ions is much greater (up to $100\times$) than the permeability to outward movement of potassium ions (Hodgkin and Horowicz, 1959; Adrian, 1960; Adrian and Freygang, 1962). Muscle cells are also permeable to chloride ions (Boyle and Conway, 1941). In frog muscle in the resting state, the chloride ion permeability is two-thirds of the total membrane permeability (Hodgkin and Horowicz, 1959; Hutter and Noble, 1960). This chloride permeability remains at a constant value over a wide range of extracellular potassium and chloride concentrations (Hodgkin and Horowicz, 1959), and at any given resting potential the intracellular and extracellular chloride concentrations can reach equilibrium.

Muscle cell membranes are also found to have a large capacitative element, for while measurements of cell membrane capacitance (C_m) are generally of the order of 1 μF/cm^2 (e.g. the squid giant axon, Curtis and Cole, 1938), vertebrate muscle membranes have capacitances of 2–8 μF/cm^2 (Katz, 1948; Fatt and Katz, 1951; Boyd and Martin, 1956b, 1959; Elmqvist *et al.*, 1960). Recent investigations suggest that this discrepancy arises because of the infoldings of the muscle fiber surface membrane in the channels of the transverse tubular system. Falk and Fatt (1964, 1965) suggest that the membrane capacitance is best described in two parts C_m and C_e, with a resistance R_e in series with C_e (Fig. 19, B). The location of the second impedance element is thought to be the channels of the transverse tubules, C_e representing the capacitance across the walls of the channels leading from the surface while R_e represents the resistivity of the channel interior.

Electrically the properties of muscle fibres may be represented by a coaxial cable (Fig. 19, C) consisting of a series of reactive elements. When a charge is applied to such a network it is found that the resultant potential takes some time to reach the steady state. Two useful membrane constants are used to define this property. They are (1) time constant (τ), which is

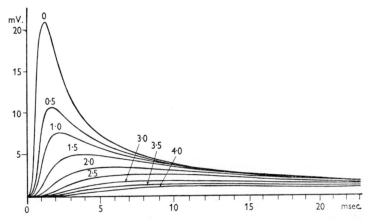

FIG. 20. E.p.p.s at differing distances from the site of e.p.p. generation. The figure shows superimposed tracings of e.p.p.s intracellularly recorded from a frog sartorius muscle fiber at the indicated distance (mm × 0.97) from the subsynaptic focus. The common point of the records is the stimulus artefact. The preparation was paralysed by the addition of d-tubocurarine chloride to the bathing medium. Note the decline in peak amplitude of e.p.p.s and the slowing of the time to rise to the peak which is found with increasing distance from the focus (Fatt and Katz, 1951).

the time (msec) for an applied potential to rise or fall to $1/e$ of its final or initial steady value. Values range from 34.5 msec for the frog sartorius muscle (Fatt and Katz, 1951) to 4.8 msec for the cat tenuissimus muscle (Boyd and Martin, 1959), and (2) length constant (λ), the distance (mm) from the point of application of an applied potential at which its amplitude is $1/e$ of the amplitude at the site of application. Values for amphibian muscle (2.4 mm, Fatt and Katz, 1951) are slightly greater than in human (2.2 mm, Elmqvist *et al.*, 1960) or feline muscle (1.10 mm, Boyd and Martin, 1959).

Quantitative evidence for the generation of e.p.p.s by an ACh-triggered active process and the later passive recharging of the membrane was obtained by Fatt and Katz (1951) and Takeuchi and Takeuchi (1959) using curarized frog nerve-muscle preparations. Fatt and Katz (1951) measured e.p.p.s at varying distances from the synapse (Fig. 20), thus gaining a quantitative measure of the time course and spread of displacement of charge. It was found that the charge was built up to a maximum in about 2 msec and afterward decayed exponentially with a time constant of about 25 msec. This value corresponds to the time constant found from

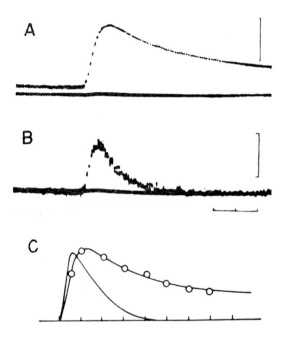

FIG. 21. The charge displacement during ACh action. A, e.p.p. recorded intracellularly from a frog sartorius muscle fiber paralysed by addition of 3×10^{-6} g/ml d-tubocurarine Cl to the bathing medium. B, end-plate current (I syn) recorded from the same synapse using a feedback circuit. The lower beam shows the membrane potential recorded simultaneously with the current. Voltage scale: 5 mV. Current scale: 1×10^{-7} Å. Temperature 17°C. C, superimposed tracings of e.p.p. and end-plate current recorded from same synapse. Circles indicate potential change calculated from end-plate current, assuming membrane time constant to be 25 msec and effective resistance 320 kΩ, peak amplitude of e.p.p. being 8.9 mV and that of end-plate current 1.4×10^{-7} Å. Time in msec (Takeuchi and Takeuchi, 1959).

observation of the potentials produced by application of square pulses to the membrane. Furthermore, the rise time of e.p.p.s at different distances from the focus (Fig. 20) agreed very well with the rise time predicted from cable theory (Hodgkin and Rushton, 1946). Takeuchi and Takeuchi (1959) elegantly confirmed earlier ideas by directly measuring the charge displacement during ACh action. This was done by applying a voltage clamp to the subsynaptic area of frog muscle fibres. The current which had to be supplied to the clamping system to keep the membrane potential stable during ACh action (Fig. 21, B) gave a measure of charge displacement from which an excellent facsimile of the e.p.p. could be recovered (Fig. 21, C, open circles) by applying the cable equations of Hodgkin and Rushton (1946) with the appropriate membrane constants.

In slow muscle fibers the e.p.p. (also known as the small fiber junctional potential—s.j.p.) has a hyperpolarizing phase succeeding the decline of the depolarizing phase. This is attributable to the properties of the slow fiber membrane for a similar hyperpolarization is found after electrical depolarizing pulses are applied to such membranes (Kuffler and Vaughan Williams, 1953a; Burke and Ginsborg, 1956a; Hess and Pilar, 1964).

3.4.2. GENERATION OF MUSCLE ACTION POTENTIALS

In twitch muscle fibers, if the e.p.p. amplitude exceeds 10–20 mV at mammalian neuromuscular junctions (Boyd and Martin, 1956b; Liley, 1956a) or 40–50 mV at amphibian and reptilian junctions (Fatt and Katz, 1951; Jenerick and Gerard, 1953; Nastuk, 1953; Levine, 1966) the electrically excitable mechanism found in the postsynaptic membrane will be triggered (Fig. 22, A, B, C).

The electrically excitable mechanism in muscle appears identical with that described for the squid axon by Hodgkin and Huxley, that is, upon reduction of the membrane potential, i.e. depolarization, to a threshold level characteristic of the particular cell there is a sudden increase in the membrane conductance for sodium ions. This drives the membrane potential toward the sodium equilibrium potential and is accompanied by a slower rising increase in potassium conductance. The sodium conductance charge is self-limiting, and the membrane potential then returns toward the potassium equilibrium potential, under the influence of a maintained potassium conductance increase (Nastuk and Hodgkin, 1950; Hodgkin and Huxley, 1952 a, b; Noble, 1966). The active area, being at a lower potential than surrounding areas, will draw current from them so that they will in turn be depolarized to the critical level setting off the explosive conductance change. The action potential thus propagates in all directions from the original focus by local circuit action, its velocity of propagation being determined by the length constant of the membrane for this determines the distance over which local circuit action is effective.

Action potentials set up by brief pulses of current have the same form wherever in the muscle cell the pulse is applied or the action potential is recorded. Action potentials set up by nerve stimulation in amphibians and reptiles have a different form, however, if recorded in the synaptic area (Fig. 23, N). There is a prominent step formed by superposition of

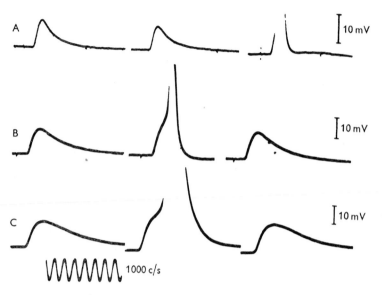

FIG. 22. Generation of muscle action potentials in cat tenuissimus muscle fibers *in vitro*. Three successive end-plate responses recorded intracellularly from each of three fibers at a critical level of block, showing action potentials rising from the peak of e.p.p.s. A, 1.5 × 10⁻⁶ (w/v) tubocurarine chloride, 37°C. B, 5 × 10⁻⁶ (w/v) tubocurarine chloride; 10⁻⁷ (w/v) prostigmine, 37°C. C, magnesium and calcium increased to 28.1 and 10.1 mM respectively, 21°C. Thresholds are approximately 10 mV (A), 14 mV (B) and 18 mV (C). Note the prolongation of the e.p.p. time course in B due to the presence of the anticholinesterase, prostigmine, and the increased threshold in C, probably due to the raised calcium and magnesium concentration of the bathing medium (Boyd and Martin, 1956b).

spike and end-plate potentials, and the overshoot of the spike potential, normally about 35 mV, is only 20 mV, i.e. the spike is smaller in amplitude. The spike also rises faster than the normal spike, and shows a pronounced hump on its declining phase. There is no doubt that these characteristics are due to the simultaneous activation of both the electrically excitable and ACh receptor mechanisms, for this particular spike shape is only found if action potential and e.p.p. coexist in the synaptic area.

The increased rate of rise of the spike is explained by the presence of two parallel mechanisms increasing sodium conductance—the ACh receptor mechanism and the electrically activated mechanism. The reduced spike amplitude arises because the equilibrium potential for ACH action is about 15 mV (inside negative) whereas the spike potential normally has

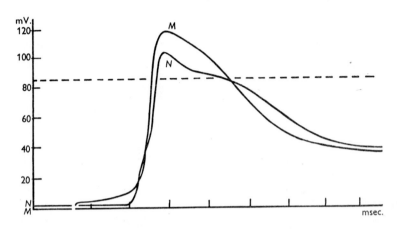

FIG. 23. Muscle action potentials in the synaptic region. M and N are tracings of action potentials recorded intracellularly from the synaptic region of the frog sartorius muscle fiber. M was generated by a direct stimulus, N by nerve stimulation. Note the hump on the rising phase of N, its lesser amplitude when compared with M and the hump on its declining phase. All these features are explained by the coincidence of e.p.p. and action potential (Fatt and Katz, 1951).

an overshoot making the inside of the muscle about 35 mV positive to the outside. The spike amplitude is thus reduced slightly by the simultaneous ACh action while persistance of ACh action causes a hump to appear on the declining phase of the spike (Fatt and Katz, 1951; Nastuk, 1953; del Castillo and Katz, 1955a; Levine, 1966).

In mammalian muscle the spike in the subsynaptic region differs less markedly in shape from the spike recorded elsewhere. There is often no detectable transition between e.p.p. and spike potential, and the spike, while it rises more rapidly and has a decreased overshoot, does not show a hump on its declining phase. Instead the repolarization phase of the spike appears prolonged (Boyd and Martin, 1956b; Muscholl, 1957). These differences from amphibian muscle arise because mammalian fibers have a lower threshold and smaller time and length constant than amphibian fibers (Boyd and Martin, 1959). At the threshold level (about 10 mV) the transition between e.p.p. and spike potential does not involve an appreciable change in the rate of rise of potential, while the short time and length constants mean that mammalian e.p.p.s have a short time course and are rapidly attenuated with increasing distance from the synapse. Spikes with e.p.p. humps (Fig. 23) are thus not observed, the tail of the e.p.p. appearing instead as an apparent negative after potential (Muscholl, 1957).

Slow muscle fibers apparently lack the membrane potential linked sodium conductance system, but contraction is ensured by the presence of multiple innervation. The whole muscle membrane is depolarized at once by the almost simultaneous e.p.p.s (Kuffler and Vaughan Williams, 1953b).

3.4.3. EXCITATION-CONTRACTION COUPLING

Depolarization of the muscle membrane, either by action potentials as in twitch fibers, or by widely distributed e.p.p.s as in slow fibers, is the first step in the series of processes leading to muscle contraction. Important evidence for the effect of depolarization came from the experiments of Huxley and Taylor (1958) in which depolarizing pulses applied to single muscle fibers elicited contraction only if the site of stimulation corresponded to the distribution of the transverse tubular system (Fig. 24, T). The contraction was graded with the strength of stimulation suggesting that a graded depolarization was transmitted down the tubules. It has since been shown that the tubular system is functionally open to the extracellular milieu, for particles of ferritin and fluorescent dyes are taken up by the tubules (Huxley, 1964; Page, 1964; Endo, 1966). With the adoption of glutaraldehyde fixation it has been possible to obtain electron micrographs of fish and frog muscle showing openings of the tubular system on the muscle surface (Franzini-Armstrong and Porter, 1964).

While the intermediate steps in the coupling mechanism are not known exactly, it seems likely that the final result of depolarization of the tubular system is release of calcium ions from the specialized terminal cisternae of the sarcoplasmic reticulum to activate the myofibrils. As Fig. 24 shows these cisternae (Fig. 24, C) are adjacent to the walls of the transverse tubules (Fig. 24, T), the complex being termed a triad. Direct evidence for this hypothesis has come from experiments with fragments of the coupling system. For instance, Costantin and Podolsky (1966) showed that after removal of the outer membrane muscle fibers would contract locally wherever calcium was applied. Electrical stimulation was, however, still only effective at discrete regions, presumably where the triads were intact. Lee and his colleagues (Lee *et al.*, 1966) found that fragments of sarcoplasmic reticulum isolated from skeletal muscle took up calcium actively from the bathing media, released the calcium on electrical stimulation and took it up again when stimulation ceased. Autoradiographic techniques show that labeled calcium is deposited mainly in the region of

Myofibrils

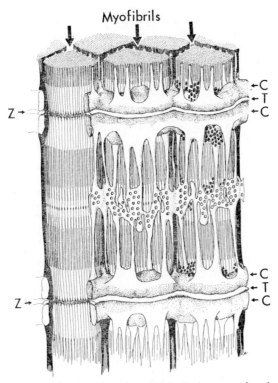

FIG. 24. Three-dimensional reconstruction of the sarcoplasmic reticulum associated with several myofibrils of frog sartorius muscle. Z, Z line. T indicates the opening of the transverse tubular system known to communicate with the external milieu. C indicates the transverse cisternae of the sarcoplasmic reticulum which are thought to store calcium and release it on stimulation thus initiating contraction (Peachey, 1965).

the triads in resting muscle and mainly in the myofibrils in contracted muscle (Winegrad, 1965 a, b). It seems probable that the cisternae store calcium at rest, release it upon activation and pump it back again when activation ends (Hasselbach, 1964). Diffusion of calcium into the myofibrils presumably activates the contractile process, and the uptake of calcium by the cisternae of the sarcoplasmic reticulum causes relaxation.

REFERENCES

ADRIAN, R. H. (1960) Potassium chloride movement and the membrane potential frog muscle. *J. Physiol.* **151**: 154–85.

ADRIAN, R. H. and FREYGANG, W. H. (1962) The potassium and chloride conductance of frog muscle membrane. *J. Physiol.* **163**: 61–103.

ALTAMIRANO, M., SCHLEYER, W. L., COATES, C. W. and NACHMANSOHN, D. (1955) Electrical activity in electric tissue. I. The difference between tertiary and quaternary nitrogen compounds in relation to their chemical and electrical activities. *Biochim. Biophys. Acta* **16**: 268–82.

AXELSSON, J. and THESLEFF, S. (1958) The "desensitizing" effect of acetylcholine and the mammalian motor end-plate. *Acta Physiol. Scand.* **43**: 15–26.

AXELSSON, J. and THESLEFF, S. (1959) A study of supersensitivity in denervated mammalian skeletal muscle. *J. Physiol.* **147**: 178–93.

BASS, L. and MOORE, W. J. (1966) Electrokinetic mechanism of miniature postsynaptic potentials. *Proc. Nat. Acad. Sci. U.S.A.* **55**: 1214–17.

BELMAR, J. and EYZAGUIRRE, C. (1966) Pacemaker site of fibrillation potentials in denervated mammalian muscle. *J. Neurophysiol.* **29**: 425–41.

BERG, P. (1956a) Acyl adenylates: an enzymic mechanism of acetate activation. *J. Biol. Chem.* **222**: 991–1013.

BERG, P. (1956b) Acyl adenylates: the synthesis and properties of adenyl acetate. *J. Biol. Chem.* **222**: 1015–23.

BERMAN-REISBERG, R. (1957) Properties and biological significance of choline acetylase. *Yale J. Biol. Med.* **29**: 403–35.

BERMAN, R., WILSON I. B. and NACHMANSOHN, D. (1953) Choline acetylase specificity in relation to biological function. *Biochim. Biophys. Acta* **12**: 315–24.

BERNARD, C. (1856) Analyse physiologique des propriétés des systèmes musculaire et nerveux au moyen du curare. *C.R. Acad. Sci. (Paris)* **43**: 825–29.

BERNSTEIN, T. (1902) Untersuchungen zur Thermodynamik der bioelektrischen Strome, Erster Theil. *Pflug. Arch. Ges. Physiol.* **92**: 521–62.

BEYCHOK, S. (1965) On the problem of isolation of the specific acetylcholine receptor. *Biochem Pharmacol.* **14**: 1249–55.

BIRKS, R. I. (1963) The role of sodium ions in the metabolism of acetylcholine. *Canad. J. Biochem. Physiol.* **41**: 2573–97.

BIRKS, R. I. (1966) The fine structure of motor nerve endings at frog myoneural junctions. *Ann. N.Y. Acad. Sci.* **135**: 8–19.

BIRKS, R. I. and COHEN, M. W. (1965) Effects of sodium pump inhibitors on myoneural transmission in the frog. In: *Muscle, its Structure and Function*, pp. 403–20. Daniel, E. E. (ed.). Pergamon Press, New York.

BIRKS, R., HUXLEY, H. E. and KATZ, B. (1960a) The fine structure of the neuromuscular junction of the frog. *J. Physiol.* **150**: 134–44.

BIRKS, R., KATZ, B. and MILEDI, R. (1960b) Physiological and structural changes at the amphibian myoneural junction in the course of nerve degeneration. *J. Physiol.* **150**: 145–68.

BIRKS, R. and MACINTOSH, F. C. (1961) Acetylcholine metabolism of a sympathetic ganglion. *Canad. J. Biochem. Physiol.* **39**: 787–827.

BLACKMAN, J. G., GINSBORG, B. L. and RAY, C. (1963) On the quantal release of the transmitter at a sympathetic synapse. *J. Physiol.* **167**: 402–15.

BOYD, I. A. and MARTIN, A. R. (1956a) Spontaneous subthreshold activity at mammalian neuromuscular junctions. *J. Physiol.* **132**: 61–73.

BOYD, I. A. and MARTIN, A. R. (1956b) The end-plate potential in mammalian muscle. *J. Physiol.* **132**: 74–91.

BOYD, I. A. and MARTIN, A. R. (1959) Membrane constants of mammalian muscle fibres. *J. Physiol.* **147**: 450–7.

BOYLE, P. J. and CONWAY, E. J. (1941) Potassium accumulation in muscle and associated changes. *J. Physiol.* **100**: 1–63.

BRAUN, M. and SCHMIDT, R. F. (1966) Potential changes recorded from the frog motor nerve terminal during its activation. *Pflüg. Arch. Ges. Physiol.* **287**: 56–80.

BRAUN, M., SCHMIDT, R. F. and ZIMMERMANN, M. (1966) Facilitation at the frog neuromuscular junction during and after repetitive stimulation. *Pflüg. Arch. Ges. Physiol.* **287**: 41–55.

BREEMEN, V. L., ANDERSON, E. and REGER, J. F. (1958) An attempt to determine the origin of synaptic vesicles. *Exp. Cell Res.*, Suppl. **5**, 153–67.

BRINKMAN, R. and RUITER, M. (1924) Die humorale Ubertragung der neurogenen Skelettmuskelerregung auf den Darm. *Pflüg. Arch. Ges. Physiol.* **204**: 766–8.

BRINKMAN, R. and RUITER, M. (1925) Die humorale Ubertragung der Skelettmuskelreizung eines ersten den Darm eines zueiten Frosches. *Pflüg. Arch. Ges. Physiol.* **208**: 58–62.

BROOKS, V. B. (1954) The action of botulinum toxin on motor-nerve filaments. *J. Physiol.* **123**: 501–15.

BROOKS, V. B. (1956) An intracellular study of the action of repetitive nerve volleys and of botulinum toxin on miniature end-plate potentials. *J. Physiol.* **134**: 264–77.

BROOKS, V. B. and THIES, R. E. (1962) Reduction of quantal content during neuromuscular transmission. *J. Physiol.* **162**: 298–310.

BROWN, G. L., DALE, H. H. and FELDBERG, W. (1936) Reactions of the normal mammalian muscle to acetylcholine and to eserine. *J. Physiol.* **87**: 394–424.

BUCHTHAL, F. and LINDHARD, J. (1937) Direct application of acetylcholine to motor endplates of voluntary muscle fibres. *J. Physiol.* **90**: 82–3P.

BURKE, W. (1957) Spontaneous potentials in slow muscle fibres of the frog. *J. Physiol.* **135**: 511–21.

BURKE, W. and GINSBORG, B. L. (1956a) The electrical properties of the slow muscle fibre membrane. *J. Physiol.* **132**: 586–98.

BURKE, W. and GINSBORG, B. L. (1956b) The action of the neuromuscular transmitter on the slow fibre membrane. *J. Physiol.* **132**: 599–610.

BURN, J. H. and RAND, M. J. (1959) The cause of the supersensitivity of smooth muscle to noradrenaline after sympathetic degeneration. *J. Physiol.* **147**: 135–43.

BURNSTOCK, G. and HOLMAN, M. E. (1962a) Spontaneous potentials at sympathetic nerve endings in smooth muscle. *J. Physiol.* **160**: 446–60.

BURNSTOCK, G. and HOLMAN, M. E. (1962b) Effect of denervation and of reserpine treatment on transmission at sympathetic nerve endings. *J. Physiol.* **160**: 461–9.

CANEPA, F. G. (1964) Acetylcholine quanta. *Nature (Lond.)* **201**: 184–5.

CANNON, W. B. and BACQ, Z. M. (1931) Studies on the conditions of activity in endocrine organs. XXVI. A hormone produced by sympathetic action on smooth muscle. *Amer. J. Physiol.* **96**: 392–412.

CANNON, W. B. and ROSENBLUETH, A. (1933) Studies on conditions of activity in endocrine organs XXIX. Sympathin E and Sympathin I. *Amer. J. Physiol.* **104**: 557–74.

COSTANTIN, L. L. and PODOLSKY, R. J. (1966) Evidence for depolarization of the internal membrane system in activation of frog semitendinosus muscle. *Nature* **210**: 483–6.

COUTEAUX, R. (1958) Morphological and cytochemical observations on the post-synaptic membrane at motor end-plates and ganglionic synapses. *Exp. Cell Res.*, Suppl. **5**, 294–322.

CSILLIK, B. (1965) *Functional Stucture of the Postsynaptic Membrane in the Myoneural Junction*, pp. 62–74. Academy Press, Budapest.

CURTIS, H. J. and COLE, K. S. (1938) Transverse electric impedance of the squid giant axon. *J. Gen. Physiol.* **21**: 757–65.

DALE, H. H. and DUDLEY, H. W. (1929) The presence of histamine and acetylcholine in the spleen of the ox and the horse. *J. Physiol.* **68**: 97–123.

DALE, H. H., FELDBERG, W. and VOGT, M. (1936) Release of acetylcholine at voluntary motor nerve endings. *J. Physiol.* **86**: 353–80.

DEL CASTILLO, J. and ENGBAEK, L. (1954) The nature of the neuromuscular block produced by magnesium. *J. Physiol.* **124**: 370–84.

DEL CASTILLO, J. and KATZ, B. (1954a) The effect of magnesium on the activity of motor nerve endings. *J. Physiol.* **124**: 553–9.

DEL CASTILLO, J. and KATZ, B. (1954b) Quantal components of the endplate potential. *J. Physiol.* **124**: 560–73.

DEL CASTILLO, J. and KATZ, B. (1954c) Statistical factors involved in neuromuscular facilitation and depression. *J. Physiol.* **124**: 574–85.

DEL CASTILLO, J. and KATZ, B. (1954d) Changes in endplate activity produced by presynaptic polarization. *J. Physiol.* **124**: 586–604.

DEL CASTILLO, J. and KATZ, B. (1954e) The membrane change produced by the neuromuscular transmitter. *J. Physiol.* **125**: 546–65.

DEL CASTILLO, J. and KATZ, B. (1955a) On the localization of acetylcholine receptors. *J. Physiol.* **128**: 157–81.

DEL CASTILLO, J. and KATZ, B. (1955b) Local activity at a depolarised nerve-muscle junction. *J. Physiol.* **128**: 396–411.

DEL CASTILLO, J. and KATZ, B. (1957a) A study of curare action with an electrical micro-method. *Proc. Roy. Soc.* B **146**: 339–56.

DEL CASTILLO, J. and KATZ, B. (1957b) The identity of "intrinsic" and "extrinsic" acetylcholine receptors in the motor end-plate. *Proc. Roy. Soc.* B **146**: 357–61.

DEL CASTILLO, J. and KATZ, B. (1957c) Interaction at end-plate receptors between different choline derivatives. *Proc. Roy. Soc.* B **146**: 369–81.

DEL CASTILLO, J. and KATZ, B. (1957d) La base "quantale" de la transmission neuromusculaire. In: *Microphysiologie comparée des elements excitables*, No. 67, pp. 245–58. Coll. Internat. C.N.R.S., Paris.

DEL CASTILLO, J. and STARK, L. (1952) The effect of calcium ions on the motor endplate potentials. *J. Physiol.* **116**: 507–15.

DENZ, F. A. (1953) On the histochemistry of the myoneural junction. *Brit. J. Exp. Path.* **34**: 329–39.

DE ROBERTIS, E. (1958) Submicroscopic morphology and function of the synapse. *Exp. Cell Res.*, Suppl. **5**: 347–69.

DE ROBERTIS, E. (1964) *Histophysiology of Synapses and Neurosecretion*, 1st ed., pp. 76–77. Pergamon Press, Oxford.

DE ROBERTIS, E. and FERREIRA, A. V. (1957) Submicroscopic changes of the nerve endings in the adrenal medulla after stimulation of the splanchnic nerve. *J. Biophys. Biochem. Cytol.* **3**: 611–14.

DE ROBERTIS, E. and FRANCHI, C. M. (1956) Electron microscope observations on synaptic vesicles in synapses of the retinal rods and cones. *J. Biophys. Biochem. Cytol.* **2**: 307–18.

DIAMOND, J. and MILEDI, R. (1962) A study of foetal and new-born rat muscle fibres. *J. Physiol.* **162**: 393–408.

DUDEL, J. and KUFFLER, S. W. (1961) The quantal nature of transmission and spontaneous miniature potentials at the crayfish neuromuscular junction. *J. Physiol.* **155**: 514–29.

ECCLES, J. C., KATZ, B. and KUFFLER, S. W. (1941) Nature of the "end-plate potential" in curarized muscle. *J. Neurophysiol.* **4**: 363–87.

ECCLES, J. C., KATZ, B. and KUFFLER, S. W. (1942) Effect of eserine on neuromuscular transmission. *J. Neurophysiol.* **5**: 211–30.

ECCLES, J. C. and JAEGER, J. C. (1958) The relationship between the mode of operation and the dimensions of the junctional regions at synapses and motor end-organs. *Proc. Roy. Soc.* B **148**: 38–56.

ECCLES, J. C. and MACFARLANE, W. V. (1949) Action of anti-cholinesterases on endplate potential of frog muscle. *J. Neurophysiol.* **12**: 59–80.

EDMUNDS, C. W. and ROTH, G. B. (1908) Concerning the action of curare and physostigmine upon nerve endings or muscle. *Amer. J. Physiol.* **23**: 28–45.

EHRENPREIS, S. (1960) Isolation and identification of the acetylcholine receptor protein of electric tissue. *Biochim. Biophys. Acta* **44**: 561–77.

EHRENPREIS, S. (1961) Isolation and properties of a drug binding protein from electric tissue of electric cell. *Proc. 1st Int. Pharmacol. Meeting*, Vol. 7. *Modern Concepts in the Relationship between Structure and Pharmacological Activity*, pp. 119–33.

EHRENPREIS, S. (1966) Possible nature of the cholinergic receptor. *Proc. N.Y. Acad. Sci.* **144**: 720–34.

ELLIOTT, T. R. (1904) On the action of adrenalin. *J. Physiol.* **31**: 20–1P.

ELLIOTT, T. R. (1905) The action of adrenalin. *J. Physiol.* **32**: 401–67.

ELMQVIST, D., HOFMANN, W. W., KUGELBERG, T. and QUASTEL, D. M. J. (1964) An electrophysiological investigation of neuromuscular transmission in myasthenia gravis. *J. Physiol.* **174**: 417–34.

ELMQVIST, D. and FELDMAN, D. S. (1965a) Calcium dependence of spontaneous acetylcholine release at mammalian motor nerve terminals. *J. Physiol.* **181**: 487–97.

ELMQVIST, D. and FELDMAN, D. S. (1965b) Spontaneous activity at a mammalian neuromuscular junction in tetrodotoxin. *Acta Physiol. Scand.* **64**: 475–6.

ELMQVIST, D., JOHNS, T. R. and THESLEFF, S. (1960) A study of some electrophysiological properties of human intercostal muscle. *J. Physiol.* **154**: 602–7.

ELMQVIST, D. and QUASTEL, D. M. J. (1965a) Presynaptic action of hemicholinium at the neuromuscular junction. *J. Physiol.* **177**: 463–82.

ELMQVIST, D. and QUASTEL, D. M. J. (1965b) A quantitative study of endplate potentials in isolated human muscle. *J. Physiol.* **178**: 505–29.

EMMELIN, N. and MACINTOSH, F. C. (1956) The release of acetylcholine from perfused sympathetic ganglia and skeletal muscle. *J. Physiol.* **131**: 477–96.

ENDO, M. (1966) Entry of fluorescent dyes into the sarcotubular system of the frog muscle. *J. Physiol.* **185**: 224–38.

FALK, G. and FATT, P. (1964) Linear electrical properties of striated muscle fibres observed with intracellular electrodes. *Proc. Roy. Soc.* B **160**: 69–123.

FALK, G. and FATT, P. (1965) Electrical impedance of striated muscle and its relation to contraction. In: *Studies in Physiology*, pp. 64–70. Curtis, D. R. and McIntyre, A. A. (eds.). Springer-Verlag, Berlin.

FATT, P. (1950) The electromotive action of acetylcholine at the motor end-plate. *J. Physiol.* **111**: 408–22.

FATT, P. and KATZ, B. (1950) Some observations on biological noise. *Nature (Lond.)* **166**: 597–8.

FATT, P. and KATZ, B. (1951) An analysis of the end-plate potential recorded with an intracellular electrode. *J. Physiol.* **115**: 320–70.

FATT, P. and KATZ, B. (1952) Spontaneous subthreshold activity at motor nerve endings. *J. Physiol.* **117**: 109–28.

FELDBERG, W. and VOGT, M. (1948) Acetylcholine synthesis in different regions of the central nervous system. *J. Physiol.* **107**: 372–81.

FELLER, W. (1950) *An Introduction to Probability Theory and its Applications*, 2nd ed., pp. 214. John Wiley & Sons Ltd., New York and London.

FENG, T. P. (1941) Studies on the neuromuscular junction. XXVI. The changes of the end-plate potential during and after prolonged stimulation. *Chin. J. Physiol.* **16**: 341–72.

FENG, T. P. and TING, Y. C. (1938) Studies on the neuromuscular junction. XI. A note on the local concentration of cholinesterase at motor nerve endings. *Chin. J. Physiol.* **13**: 141–3.

FRANZINI-ARMSTRONG, C. and PORTER, K. R. (1964) Sarcolemmal invaginations constituting the T system in fish muscle fibres. *J. Cell Biol.* **22**: 675–96.

FURSHPAN, E. J. (1956) The effects of osmotic pressure changes on the spontaneous activity at motor nerve endings. *J. Physiol.* **134**: 689–97.

GAGE, P. W. and HUBBARD, J. I. (1965) Evidence for a Poisson distribution of miniature end-plate potentials and some implications. *Nature (Lond.)* **208**: 395–6.

GAGE, P. W. and HUBBARD, J. I. (1966a) The origin of post-tetanic hyperpolarization in mammalian motor nerve terminals. *J. Physiol.* **184**: 335–52.

GAGE, P. W. and HUBBARD, J. I. (1966b) An investigation of the post-tetanic potentiation of end-plate potentials at a mammalian neuromuscular junction. *J. Physiol.* **184**: 353–75.

GAGE, P. W. and QUASTEL, D. M. J. (1965) Dual effect of potassium on transmitter release. *Nature (Lond.)* **206**: 625–6.

GAGE, P. W. and QUASTEL, D. M. J. (1966) Competition between sodium and calcium ions in transmitter release at a mammalian neuromuscular junction. *J. Physiol.* **185**: 95–123.

GINETZINSKY, A. G. and SHAMARINA, N. M. (1942) The tonomotor phenomenon in denervated muscle. *Uspekhi Sourenenoj Biologii.* **15**: 283–94.

GINSBORG B. L. (1960a) Spontaneous activity in muscle fibres of the chick. *J. Physiol.* **150**: 707–17.

GINSBORG, G. L. (1960b) Some properties of avian skeletal muscle fibres with multiple neuromuscular junctions. *J. Physiol.* **154**: 581–98.

GOLDSMITH, T. H. (1963) Rates of action of bath applied drugs at the neuromuscular junction of the frog. *J. Physiol.* **165**: 368–86.

GOPFERT, H. and SCHAEFER, H. (1938) Uber den direkt und indirekt erregten Aktionsstrom und die Function der motorischen Endplatte. *Pflüg. Arch. Ges. Physiol.* **239**: 597–619.

GUTH, L., ALBERS, R. W. and BROWN, W. C. (1964) Quantitative changes in cholinesterase activity of denervated muscle fibres and sole plates. *Exp. Neurol.* **10**: 236–50.

GUTH, L. and BROWN, W. C. (1965) The sequence of changes in cholinesterase activity during reinnervation of muscle. *Exp. Neurol.* **12**: 329–36.

GUTH, L. and ZALEWSKI, A. A. (1963) Disposition of cholinesterase following implantation of nerve into innervated and denervated muscle. *Exp. Neurol.* **7**: 316–26.

GWYNN, D. G. and VRBOVA, G. (1966) Changes in the histochemical appearance of cholinesterase at the neuromuscular junction in atrophic muscles. *J. Physiol.* **185**: 7–8P.

HASSELBACH, W. (1964) Relaxing factor and the relaxation of muscle. *Progr. Biophys.* **14**: 167–222.

HAYES, A. H. and RIKER, W. F. (1963) Acetylcholine release by denervated muscle. *Fed. Proc.* **22**: 215.

HEBB, C. (1963) Formation, storage and liberation of acetylcholine. In: *Cholinesterases and Anticholinesterase Agents*, pp. 55–88. Koelle, G. B. (ed.) (*Handbuch der Experimentellen Pharmakologie*, vol. 15). Springer-Verlag, Berlin.

HEBB, C. O., KRNJEVIĆ, K. and SILVER, A. (1964) Acetylcholine and choline acetyltransferase in the diaphragm of the rat. *J. Physiol.* **171**: 504–13.

HEBB, C. O. and SILVER, A. (1963) The effect of transection on the level of choline acetylase in the goat's sciatic nerve. *J. Physiol.* **169**: 10–11P.

HEBB, C. O. and WAITES, G. M. H. (1956) Choline acetylase in antero- and retro-grade degeneration of a cholinergic nerve. *J. Physiol.* **132**: 667–71.

HEIDENHAIN, R. (1883) Ueber pseudomotorische Nervenwirkungen. *Arch. Anat. Physiol., Lpz.*, Suppl. **7**: 133–77.

HESS, A. and PILAR, G. (1964) Slow fibres in the extraocular muscles of the cat. *J. Physiol.* **169**: 780–98.

HODGKIN, A. L. and HOROWICZ, P. (1959) The influence of potassium and chloride ions on the membrane potential of single muscle fibres. *J. Physiol.* **148**: 127–60.

HODGKIN, A. L. and HUXLEY, A. F. (1952a) The dual effect of membrane potential on sodium conductance in the giant axon of Loligo. *J. Physiol.* **116**: 497–506.

HODGKIN, A. L. and HUXLEY, A. F. (1952b) A quantitative description of membrane current and its application to conduction and excitation in nerve. *J. Physiol.* **117**: 500–44.

HODGKIN, A. L. and RUSHTON, W. A. H. (1946) The electrical constants of a crustacean nerve fibre. *Proc. Roy. Soc.* B **133**: 444–79.

HUBBARD, J. I. (1961) The effect of calcium and magnesium on the spontaneous release of transmitter from mammalian motor nerve endings. *J. Physiol.* **159**: 507–17.

HUBBARD, J. I. (1963) Repetitive stimulation at the mammalian neuromuscular junction and the mobilisation of transmitter. *J. Physiol. (Lond.)* **169**: 641–62.

HUBBARD, J. I., JONES, S. and LANDAU, E. (1967) The relationship between nerve terminal polarization and the liberation of acetylcholine. *Proc. N.Y. Acad. Sci.* **144**: 459–69.

HUBBARD, J. I., JONES, S. F. and LANDAU, E. M. (1968) An examination of the effects of osmotic pressure changes upon transmitter release from mammalian motor nerve terminals. *J. Physiol. (Lond.)* **197**: 636–59.

HUBBARD, J. I. and LØYNING, Y. (1966) The effects of hypoxia on neuromuscular transmission in a mammalian preparation. *J. Physiol.* **185**: 205–23.

HUBBARD, J. I. and SCHMIDT, R. F. (1963) An electrophysiological investigation of mammalian motor nerve terminals. *J. Physiol.* **166**: 145–67.

HUBBARD, J. I., SCHMIDT, R. F. and YOKOTA, T. (1965) The effect of acetylcholine upon mammalian motor nerve terminals. *J. Physiol.* **181**: 810–29.

HUBBARD, J. I. and WILLIS, W. D. (1962) Hyperpolarization of mammalian motor nerve terminals. *J. Physiol.* **163**: 115–37.

HUGHES, J. R. (1958) Post-tetanic potentiation. *Physiol. Rev.* **38**: 91–113.

HUTTER, O. F. (1952) Post-tetanic restoration of neuromuscular transmission blocked by d-tubocurarine. *J. Physiol.* **118**: 216–27.

HUTTER, O. F. and NOBLE, D. (1960) The chloride conductance of frog skeletal muscle. *J. Physiol.* **151**: 89–102.

HUTTER, O. F. and TRAUTWEIN, W. (1956) Neuromuscular facilitation by stretch of motor nerve endings. *J. Physiol.* **133**: 610–25.

HUXLEY, H. E. (1964) Evidence for continuity between the central elements of the triads and extracellular space in frog sartorius muscle. *Nature (Lond.)* **202**: 1067–71.

HUXLEY, A. F. and TAYLOR, R. E. (1958) Local activation of striated muscle fibres. *J. Physiol.* **144**: 426–41.

JENERICK, H. P. and GERARD, R. W. (1953) Membrane potential and threshold of single muscle fibres. *J. Cell. Comp. Physiol.* **42**: 79–95.

JENKINSON, D. H. (1957) The nature of the antagonism between calcium and magnesium ions at the neuromuscular junction. *J. Physiol.* **138**: 438–44.

KARCZMAR, A. (1963) Ontogenesis of cholinesterase. In: *Cholinesterases and Anticholinesterase Agents*, pp. 129–86. Koelle, G. B. (ed.) (*Handbuch der Experimentellen Pharmakologie*, vol. 15). Springer-Verlag, Berlin.

KATZ, B. (1948) The electrical properties of the muscle fibre membrane. *Proc. Roy. Soc.* B **135**: 506–34.

KATZ, B. (1962) The transmission of impulses from nerve to muscle, and the subcellular unit of synaptic action. *Proc. Roy. Soc.* B **155**: 455–77.

KATZ, B. and MILEDI, R. (1964) Further observations on the distribution of acetylcholine-reactive sites on skeletal muscle. *J. Physiol.* **170**: 379–88.

KATZ, B. and MILEDI, R. (1965a) Propagation of electric activity in motor nerve terminals. *Proc. Roy. Soc.* B **161**: 453–82.

KATZ, B. and MILEDI, R. (1965b) The measurement of synaptic delay, and the time course of acetylcholine release at the neuromuscular junction. *Proc. Roy. Soc.* B **161**: 483–95.

KATZ, B. and MILEDI, R. (1965c) The effect of calcium on acetylcholine release from motor nerve endings. *Proc. Roy. Soc.* B **161**: 496–503.

KATZ, B. and MILEDI, R. (1965d) Release of acetylcholine from a nerve terminal by electric pulses of variable strength and duration. *Nature (Lond.)* **207**: 1097–8.

KATZ, B. and MILEDI, R. (1965e) The quantal release of transmitter substances. In: *Studies in Physiology*, pp. 118–25. Curtis, D. R. and McIntyre, A. A. (eds.). Springer-Verlag, Berlin.

KATZ, B. and THESLEFF, S. (1957a) On the factors which determine the amplitude of the "miniature end-plate potential". *J. Physiol.* **137**: 267–78.

KATZ, B. and THESLEFF, S. (1957b) A study of the "desensitization" produced by acetylcholine at the motor end-plate. *J. Physiol.* **138**: 63–80.

KELLY, J. S. (1965) Antagonism between Na^+ and Ca^{++} at the neuromuscular junction. *Nature (Lond.)* **205**: 296–7.

KOELLE, G. B. (1963) Cytological distributions and physiological functions of cholinesterases. In: *Cholinesterases and Anticholinesterase Agents*, pp. 186–298. Koelle, G. B. (ed.) (*Handbuch der Experimentellen Pharmakologie*, vol. 15.) Springer-Verlag, Berlin.

KOREY, S., DE BRAGANZA, B. and NACHMANSOHN, D. (1951) Choline acetylase V. Esterifications and transacetylations. *J. Biol. Chem.* **189**: 705–15.

KRNJEVIĆ, K. and MILEDI, R. (1958a) Acetylcholine in mammalian neuromuscular transmission. *Nature (Lond.)* **182**: 805–6.

KRNJEVIĆ, K. and MILEDI, R. (1958b). Motor units in the rat diaphragm. *J. Physiol.* **140**: 427–39.

KRNJEVIĆ, K. and MITCHELL, J. F. (1961) The release of acetylcholine in the isolated rat diaphragm. *J. Physiol.* **155**: 246–62.

KRNJEVIĆ, K. and STRAUGHAN, D. W. (1964) The release of acetylcholine from the denervated rat diaphragm. *J. Physiol.* **170**: 371–8.

KUFFLER, S. W. (1942) Further study of transmission in an isolated nerve-muscle fibre preparation. *J. Neurophysiol.* **5**: 309–22.

KUFFLER, S. W. (1943) Specific excitability of the end-plate region in normal and denervated muscle. *J. Neurophysiol.* **6**: 99–110.

KUFFLER, S. W. and VAUGHAN WILLIAMS, E. M. (1953a) Small nerve junctional potentials. The distribution of small motor nerves to frog skeletal muscle, and the membrane characteristics of the fibres they innervate. *J. Physiol.* **121**: 289–317.

KUFFLER, S. W. and VAUGHAN WILLIAMS, E. M. (1953b) Properties of the "slow" skeletal muscle fibres of the frog. *J. Physiol.* **121**: 318–40.

KUPFER, C. and KOELLE, G. B. (1951) A histochemical study of cholinesterase during the formation of the motor endplate of the albino rat. *J. Exp. Zool.* **116**: 399–413.

LANGLEY, J. N. (1905) On the reaction of cells and of nerve-endings to certain poisons, chiefly as regards the reaction of striated muscle to nicotine and to curari. *J. Physiol.* **33**: 374–413.

LANGLEY, J. N. (1907) On the contraction of muscle, chiefly in relation to the presence of "receptive" substances. Part I. *J. Physiol.* **36**: 347–84.

LANGLEY, J. N. (1908) On the contraction of muscle, chiefly in relation to the presence of "receptive" substances. Part III. The reaction of frog's muscle to nicotine after denervation. *J. Physiol.* **37**: 285–300.

LANGLEY, J. N. (1909) On the contraction of muscle, chiefly in relation to the presence of "receptive" substances. Part IV. The effect of curari and of some other substances on the nicotine response of the sartorius and gastrocnemius muscles of the frog. *J. Physiol.* **39**: 235–95.

LANGLEY, J. N. (1914) The antagonism of curari and nicotine in skeletal muscle. *J. Physiol.* **48**: 73–108.

LEE, K. S., LADINSKY, H., CHOI, S. J. and KASUYA, Y. (1966) Studies on the *in vitro* interaction of electrical stimulation and Ca^{++} movement in sarcoplasmic reticulum. *J. Gen. Physiol.* **49**: 689–715.

LEVINE, L. (1966) An electrophysiological study of chelonian skeletal muscle. *J. Physiol.* **183**: 683–713.

LILEY, A. W. (1956a) An investigation of spontaneous activity at the neuromuscular junction of the rat. *J. Physiol.* **132**: 659–66.

LILEY, A. W. (1956b) The quantal components of the mammalian end-plate potential. *J. Physiol.* **133**: 571–87.

LILEY, A. W. (1956c) The effects of presynaptic polarization on the spontaneous activity at the mammalian neuromuscular junction. *J. Physiol.* **134**: 427–43.

LILEY, A. W. (1957) Spontaneous release of transmitter substance in multiquantal units. *J.Physiol.* **136**: 595–605.

LILEY, A. W. and NORTH, K. A. K. (1953) An electrical investigation of effects of repetitive stimulation on mammalian neuromuscular junction. *J. Neurophysiol.* **16**: 509–27.

LOEWI, O. (1921) Uber humorale Uberträgbarkeit der Herznervenwirkung. *Pflüg. Arch. Ges. Physiol.* **189**: 239–42.

LUNDBERG, A. and QUILISCH, H. (1953) Presynaptic potentiation and depression of neuromuscular transmission in frog and rat. *Acta Physiol. Scand.*, Suppl. 111, **30**: 111–20.

LUTTGAU, H. C. and NIEDERGERKE, R. (1958) The antagonism between Ca and Na ions on the frog's heart. *J. Physiol.* **143**: 486–505.

MACINTOSH, F. C. (1961) Effect of HC-3 on acetylcholine turnover. *Fed. Proc.* **20**: 562–8.

MACINTOSH, F. C., BIRKS, R. I. and SASTRY, P. B. (1956) Pharmacological inhibition of acetylcholine synthesis. *Nature (Lond.)* **178**: 1181.

MCINTYRE, A. R. (1959) Neuromuscular transmission and normal and denervated muscle sensitivity to curare and acetylcholine. In: *Curare and Curare-like Agents*, pp. 211–18. Bovet, D., Bovet-Nitti, F. and Marini-Bettolo, G. B. (eds.). Elsevier, Amsterdam.

MAENO, T. (1966) Analysis of sodium and potassium conductances in the procaine end-plate potential. *J. Physiol.* **183**: 592–606.

MAMBRINI, J. and BENOIT, P. R. (1964) Action du calcium sur la jonction neuromusculaire chez la Grenouille. *C.R. Soc. Biol. (Paris)* **158**: 1454–8.

MANTHEY, A. A. (1966) The effect of calcium on the desensitization of membrane receptors at the neuromuscular junction. *J. Gen. Physiol.* **49**: 963–76.

MARNAY, A. and NACHMANSOHN, D. (1938) Choline esterase in voluntary muscle. *J. Physiol.* **92**: 37–47.

MARTIN, A. R. (1955) A further study of the statistical composition of the end-plate potential. *J. Physiol.* **130**: 114–22.

MARTIN, A. R. (1966) Quantal nature of synaptic transmission. *Physiol. Rev.* **46**: 51–66.

MARTIN, A. R. and PILAR, G. (1964) Quantal components of the synaptic potential in the ciliary ganglion of the chick. *J. Physiol.* **175**: 1–16.

MILEDI, R. (1960a) The acetylcholine sensitivity of frog muscle fibres after complete or partial denervation. *J. Physiol.* **151**: 1–23.

MILEDI, R. (1960b) Junctional and extra-junctional acetylcholine receptors in skeletal muscle fibres. *J. Physiol.* **151**: 24–30.

MILEDI, R. (1960c) Properties of regenerating neuromuscular synapses in the frog. *J. Physiol.* **154**: 190–205.

MILEDI, R. (1962a) Induced innervation of end-plate free muscle segments. *Nature (Lond.)* **193**: 281–2.

MILEDI, R. (1962b) Induction of receptors. In: *Ciba Foundation Symposium on Enzymes and Drug Action*, pp. 220–35. Mongar, J. L. and de Reuch, A. V. S. (eds.). J. and A. Churchill, London.

MITCHELL, J. F. and SILVER, A. (1963) The spontaneous release of acetylcholine from the denervated hemidiaphragm of the rat. *J. Physiol.* **165**: 117–29.

MOUNTFORD, S. (1963) Effects of light and dark adaptation on the vesicle population of receptor bipolar synapses. *J. Ultrastruct. Res.* **9**: 403–16.

MUSCHOLL, E. (1957) Elektrophysiologische Untersuchung der einzelnen Faseranteile des isolierten Rattenzwerchfelles. *Pflüg. Arch. Ges. Physiol.* **264**: 467–83.

NACHMANSOHN, D. (1939) Choline esterase in voluntary muscle. *J. Physiol.* **95**: 29–35.

NACHMANSOHN, D. (1959) *Chemical and Molecular Basis of Nerve Activity*, 1st ed., pp. 143–4. Academic Press, New York.

NACHMANSOHN, D. (1963) Choline acetylase. In: *Cholinesterases and Anticholinesterase Agents*, pp. 40–54. Koelle, G. B. (ed.). (*Handbuch der Experimentellen Pharmakologie*, Vol. 15.) Springer-Verlag, Berlin.

NACHMANSOHN, D. and MACHADO, A. L. (1943) The formation of acetylcholine. A new enzyme "choline acetylase". *J. Neurophysiol.* **6**: 397–403.

NAKAMURA, Y., NAKAJIMA, S. and GRUNDFEST, H. (1965) The action of tetrodotoxin on electrogenic components in squid giant axons. *J. Gen. Physiol.* **48**: 985–96.

NARAHASHI, T., DEGUCHI, T., URAKAWA, N. and OHKUBO, Y. (1960) Stabilization and rectification of muscle fiber membrane by tetrodotoxin. *Amer. J. Physiol.* **198**: 934–8.

NARAHASHI, T., MOORE, J. W. and SCOTT, W. R. (1964) Tetrodotoxin blockage of sodium conductance increase in lobster giant axons. *J. Gen. Physiol.* **47**: 965–74.

NASTUK, W. L. (1951) Membrane potential changes at a single muscle end-plate produced by acetylcholine. *Fed. Proc.* **10**: 96.

NASTUK, W. L. (1953) The electrical activity of the muscle cell membrane at the neuromuscular junction. *J. Cell. Comp. Physiol.* **42**: 249–72.

NASTUK, W. L. (1966) Fundamental aspects of neuromuscular transmission. *Ann. N. Y. Acad. Sci.* **135**: 110–35.

NASTUK, W. L. and HODGKIN, A. L. (1950) The electrical activity of single muscle fibres. *J. Cell. Comp. Physiol.* **35**: 39–74.

NOBLE, D. (1966) Applications of the Hodgkin–Huxley equations to excitable tissues. *Physiol. Rev.* **46**: 1–50.

OGSTON, A. G. (1955) Removal of acetylcholine from a limited volume by diffusion. *J. Physiol.* **128**: 222–3.

OTSUKA, M., ENDO, M. and NONOMURA, Y. (1962) Presynaptic nature of neuromuscular depression. *Jap. J. Physiol.* **12**: 573–84.

PAGE, S. (1964) The organisation of the sarcoplasmic reticulum in frog muscle. *J. Physiol.* **175**: 10–11.

PEACHEY, L. D. (1965) The sarcoplasmic reticulum and transverse tubules of the frog's sartorius. *J. Cell Biol.* **25**: 209–31.

PELLEGRINO DE IRALDI, A. and DE ROBERTIS, E. (1961) Action of reserpine on the submicroscopic morphology of the pineal gland. *Experientia* **17**: 122–4.

ROBERTSON, J. D. (1956) The ultrastructure of a reptilian myoneural junction. *J. Biophys. Biochem. Cytol.* **2**: 381–94.

ROGERS, A. W., DARZYNKIEWICZ, Z., BARNARD, E. A. and SALPETER, M. M. (1966) Number and location of acetylcholinesterase molecules at motor end-plates of the mouse. *Nature (Lond.)* **210**: 1003–6.

SCHMITT, F. O. and DAVISON, P. F. (1965) Role of protein in neural function. *Neurosciences Research Programme*, Bulletin 3, No. 6, pp. 55–77.

SCHUELER, F. W. (1960) The mechanism of action of the hemicholiniums. *Int. Rev. Neurobiol.* **2**: 77–97.

114

SHERRINGTON, C. S. (1897) The central nervous system. In: *A Textbook of Physiology*, vol. 3, 7th ed. Foster, M. (ed.). Macmillan, London.

STRAUGHAN, D. W. (1960) The release of acetylcholine from mammalian motor nerve endings. *Brit. J. Pharmacol.* **15**: 417–24.

TAKEUCHI, A. (1958) The long-lasting depression in neuromuscular transmission of frog. *Jap. J. Physiol.* **8**: 102–13.

TAKEUCHI, A. (1959) Neuromuscular transmission of fish skeletal muscles investigated with intracellular microelectrodes. *J. Cell. Comp. Physiol.* **54**: 211–70.

TAKEUCHI, A. and TAKEUCHI, N. (1959) Active phase of frog's end-plate potential. *J. Neurophysiol.* **22**: 395–411.

TAKEUCHI, A. and TAKEUCHI, N. (1960) On the permeability of end-plate membrane during the action of the transmitter. *J. Physiol.* **154**: 52–67.

TAKEUCHI, N. (1963a) Some properties of conductance changes at the end-plate membrane during the action of acetylcholine. *J. Physiol.* **167**: 128–40.

TAKEUCHI, N. (1963b) Effects of calcium on the conductance change of the end-plate membrane during the action of transmitter. *J. Physiol.* **167**: 141–55.

THESLEFF, S. (1955a) The mode of neuromuscular block caused by acetylcholine, nicotine, decamethonium and succinylcholine. *Acta Physiol. Scand.* **34**: 218–31.

THESLEFF, S. (1955b) The effect of acetylcholine, decamethonium and succinylcholine on neuromuscular transmission in the rat. *Acta Physiol. Scand.* **34**: 386–92.

THESLEFF, S. (1959) Motor end-plate "desensitization" by repetitive nerve stimuli. *J. Physiol.* **148**: 659–64.

THESLEFF, S. (1960) Supersensitivity of skeletal muscle produced by botulinum toxin. *J. Physiol.* **151**: 598–607.

THESLEFF, S. and QUASTEL, D. M. J. (1965) Neuromuscular pharmacology. *Ann. Rev. Pharmacol.* **5**: 263–84.

THIES, R. E. (1965) Neuromuscular depression and apparent depletion of transmitter in mammalian muscle. *J. Neurophysiol.* **28**: 427–42.

USHERWOOD, P. N. R. (1963) Spontaneous miniature potentials from insect muscle fibres. *J. Physiol.* **169**: 149–60.

VERE-JONES, D. (1966) Simple stochastic models for the release of quanta of transmitter from a nerve terminal. *Aust. J. Statistics* **8**: 53–63.

WASER, P. G. (1960) The cholinergic receptor. *J. Pharm. (Lond.)* **12**: 577–94.

WASER, P. G. (1967) Receptor localization by autoradiographic techniques. *Proc. N.Y. Acad. Sci.* **144**: 737–53.

WILSON, I. B. (1952) Acetylcholinesterase XII. Further studies of binding forces. *J. Biol. Chem.* **197**: 215–25.

WILSON, I. B. and BERGMANN, F. (1950a) Studies on cholinesterase VII. The active surface of acetylcholine esterase derived from the effects of pH on inhibitors. *J. Biol. Chem.* **185**: 479–89.

WILSON, I. B. and BERGMANN, F. (1950b) Acetylcholinesterase VIII. Dissociation constants of the active groups. *J. Biol. Chem.* **186**, 683–92.

WILSON, I. B., BERGMANN, F. and NACHMANSOHN, D. (1950) Acetylcholinesterase X. Mechanism of the catalysis of acylation reactions. *J. Biol. Chem.* **186**: 781–90.

WILSON, I. B. and CABIB, E. (1956) Acetylcholinesterase: enthalpies and entropies of activation. *J. Amer. Chem. Soc.* **78**: 202–7.

WINEGRAD, S. (1965a) Autoradiographic studies of intracellular calcium in frog skeletal muscle. *J. Gen. Physiol.* **48**: 455–79.

WINEGRAD, S. (1965b) The location of muscle calcium with respect to the myofibrils. *J. Gen. Physiol.* **48**: 997–1002.

WOOLF, A. L. (1966) Morphology of the myasthenic neuromuscular junction. *Ann. N.Y. Acad. Sci.* **135**: 35–56.

SUPPLEMENTARY REFERENCE LIST

ASHLEY, C. C. and RIDGWAY, E. B. (1970) On the relationships between membrane potential, calcium transient and tension in single barnacle muscle fibers. *J. Physiol.* (*Lond.*) **209**: 105–30.

BIRKS, R. I., BURSTYN, P. G. R. and FIRTH, D. R. (1968) The form of sodium–calcium competition at the frog myoneural junction. *J. Gen. Physiol.* **52**: 887–908.

BLIOCH, Z. L., GLAGOLEVA, I. M., LIBERMAN, E. A. and NENASHEV, V. A. (1968) A study of the mechanism of quantal transmitter release at a chemical synapse. *J. Physiol.* (*Lond.*) **199**: 11–37.

DODGE, F. A. JR. and RAHAMIMOFF, R. (1967) Co-operative action of calcium ions in transmitter release at the neuromuscular junction. *J. Physiol.* (*Lond.*) **193**, 419–33.

EBASHI, S. and ENDO, M. (1968) Calcium ion and muscle contraction. *Prog. Biophys. Mol. Biol.* **18**: 123–83.

FELTZ, A. and MALLART, A. (1970) Differences in the action of acetylcholine on the denervated muscle fiber and on the normal end-plate. *Brain Res.* **22**: 264–7.

GAGE, P. W. (1967) Depolarization and excitation-secretion coupling in presynaptic terminals. *Fedn. Proc.* **26**, 1627–33.

GAGE, P. W. and EISENBERG, R. S. (1969a) Capacitance of the surface and transverse tubular membranes of frog sartorius muscle fibers. *J. Gen. Physiol.* **53**: 265–78.

GAGE, P. W. and EISENBERG, R. S. (1969b) Action potential, after potentials, and excitation contraction coupling in frog sartorius fibers without transverse tubules. *J. Gen. Physiol.* **53**: 298–310.

GINSBORG, B. L. (1967) Ion movements in junctional transmission. *Pharmacol. Rev.* **19**: 289–316.

GUTH, LLOYD (1968) "Trophic" influences of nerve on muscle. *Physiol. Rev.* **48**: 645–87.

HESS, A. (1970) Vertebrate slow muscle fibres. *Physiol. Rev.* **50**: 40–62.

HOWELL, J. N. (1969) A lesion of the transverse tubules of skeletal muscle. *J. Physiol.* (*Lond.*) **201**: 515–33.

HUBBARD, J. I. (1970) Mechanism of transmitter release. *Prog. Biophys. Mol. Biol.* **21**: 33–124.

HUBBARD, J. I., JONES, S. F. and LANDAU, E. M. (1968a) On the mechanism by which calcium and magnesium affect the spontaneous release of transmitter from mammalian motor nerve terminals. *J. Physiol.* (*Lond.*) **194**: 381–407.

HUBBARD, J. I., JONES, S. F. and LANDAU, E. M. (1968b) On the mechanism by which calcium and magnesium affect the release of transmitter by nerve impulses. *J. Physiol.* (*Lond.*) **196**: 75–87.

HUBBARD, J. I. and KWANBUNBUMPEN, S. (1968) Evidence for the vesicle hypothesis. *J. Physiol.* (*Lond.*) **194**: 407–21.

HUBBARD, J. I., LLINAS, R. and QUASTEL, D. M. J. (1969) *Electrophysiological Analysis of Synaptic Transmission* (Physiological Society monograph). Edward Arnold Ltd., London.

HUBBARD, J. I. and WILLIS, W. D. (1968) The effects of depolarization of motor nerve terminals upon the release of transmitter by nerve impulses. *J. Physiol.* (*Lond.*) **194**: 381–407.

HUXLEY, H. E. (1969) The mechanism of muscular contraction. *Science* **164**: 1356–66.

JONES, S. F. and KWANBUNBUMPEN, S. (1970a) Some effects of nerve stimulation and hemicholinium on quantal transmitter release at the mammalian neuromuscular junction. *J. Physiol.* (*Lond.*) **207**: 31–50.

JONES, S. F. and KWANBUNBUMPEN, S. (1970b) The effects of nerve stimulation and hemicholinium on synaptic vesicles at the mammialian neuromuscular junction. *J. Physiol.* (*Lond.*) **207**: 51–62.

KAO, C. T. (1966) Tetrodotoxin, saxitoxin and their significance in the study of excitation phenomena. *Pharmac. Rev.* **18**: 997–1049.

KATZ, B. (1969) *The Release of Neural Transmitter Substances*. Charles C. Thomas: Springfield, Ill.

KATZ, B. and MILEDI, R. (1967a) Modification of transmitter release by electrical interference with motor nerve endings. *Proc. Roy. Soc. (London)* B **167**: 1–7.

KATZ, B. and MILEDI, R. (1967b) Tetrodotoxin and neuromuscular transmission. *Proc. Roy. Soc. (London)* B **167**: 8–22.

KATZ, B. and MILEDI, R. (1967c) The release of acetylcholine from nerve endings by graded electric pulses. *Proc. Roy. Soc. (London)* B **167**: 23–28.

KATZ, B. and MILEDI, R. (1967d) The timing of calcium action during neuromuscular transmission. *J. Physiol. (Lond.)* **189**: 535–44.

KATZ, B. and MILEDI, R. (1967e) A study of synaptic transmission in the absence of nerve impulses. *J. Physiol. (Lond.)* **192**: 407–36.

KATZ, B. and MILEDI, R. (1968) The effect of local blockage of motor nerve terminals. *J. Physiol. (Lond.)* **199**: 729–43.

KATZ, B. and MILEDI, R. (1969a) Tetrodotoxin-resistant electric activity in presynaptic terminals. *J. Physiol. (Lond.)* **203**: 459–87.

KATZ, B. and MILEDI, R. (1969b) Spontaneous and evoked activity of motor nerve endings in calcium Ringer. *J. Physiol. (Lond.)* **203**: 689–706.

KHROMOV-BORISOV, N. V. and MICHELSON, M. J. (1966) The mutual disposition of cholinoreceptors of locomotor muscles, and the changes in their disposition in the course of evolution. *Pharmacol. Rev.* **18**, 1051–90.

LAMBERT, D. H. and PARSONS, R. L. (1970) Influence of polyvalent cations on the activation of muscle end-plate receptors. *J. Gen. Physiol.* **56**: 309–21.

LEUZINGER, W. and BAKER, A. L. (1967) Acetylcholinesterase. I. Large scale purification, homogeneity and amino acid analysis. *Proc. Nat. Acad. Sci. U.S.* **57**: 446–51.

LEUZINGER, W., BAKER, A. L. and CAUVIN, E. (1968) Acetylcholinesterase. II. Crystallization, absorption spectra, isoionic point. *Proc. Nat. Acad. Sci. U.S.* **59**: 620–3.

LEUZINGER, W., GOLDBERG, M. and CAUVIN, E. (1969) Molecular properties of acetylcholinesterase. *J. Mol. Biol.* **40**: 217–25.

LIÈVREMONT, M., CZAJKA, M. and TAZIEFF-DEPIERRE, F. (1968) Étude in situ d'une fixation de calcium et de sa liberation à la jonction neuromusculaire. *C.R Acad. Sci. (Paris)* **267D**: 1988–90.

LIÈVREMONT, M., CZAJKA, M. and TAZIEFF-DEPIERRE, F. (1969) Cycle du calcium à la jonction neuromusculaire. *C.R. Acad. Sci. (Paris)* **268D**: 379–82.

MALLART, A. and MARTIN, A. R. (1967) An analysis of facilitation of transmitter release at the neuromuscular junction of the frog. *J. Physiol. (Lond.)* **193**: 679–95.

MALLART, A. and MARTIN, A. R. (1968) The relation between quantum content and facilitation at the neuromuscular junction of the frog. *J. Physiol. (Lond.)* **196**: 593–604.

MANTHEY, A. A. (1970) Further studies of the effect of calcium on the time course of action of carbamylcholine at the neuromuscular junction. *J. Gen. Physiol.* **56**: 407–19.

NASTUK, W. L. and PARSONS, R. L. (1970) Factors in the inactivation of postjunctional membrane receptors of frog skeletal muscle. *J. Gen. Physiol.* **56**: 218–49.

PADYKULA, H. A. and GAUTHIER, G. F. (1967) The ultrastructure of neuromuscular junctions of mammalian red, white, and intermediate skeletal muscle fibres. *J. Cell. Biol.* **46**: 27–41.

PATON, W. D. M. and WAUD, D. R. (1967) The margin of safety of neuromuscular transmission. *J. Physiol. (Lond.)* **191**: 59–90.

PODOLSKY, R. J. and TEICHHOLZ, L. E. (1970) The relation between calcium and contraction kinetics in skinned muscle fibres. *J. Physiol. (Lond.)* **211**: 19–35.

117

POTTER, L. T. (1970) Synthesis, storage and release of [^{14}C] acetylcholine in isolated rat diaphragm muscles. *J. Physiol. (Lond.)* **206**: 145–66.

RAHAMIMOFF, R. (1968) A dual effect of calcium ions on neuromuscular facilitation. *J. Physiol. (Lond.)* **195**: 471–81.

ROGERS, A. W., DARZYNKIEWICZ, Z., SALPETER, M. M., OSTROWSKI, K. and BARNARD, E. A. (1969) Quantitative studies on enzymes in structures in striated muscles by labeled inhibitor methods. I. The number of acetylcholinesterase molecules and of other DFP- reactive sites at motor endplates, measured by radioautography. *J. Cell. Biol.* **41**: 665–85.

SAITO, A. and ZACKS, S. (1970) Ultrastructure of Schwann and perineural sheaths at the mouse neuromuscular junction. *Anat. Rec.* **164**: 379–90.

SCHMIDT, D. E., SZILAGYI, P. I. A., ALKON, D. L. and GREEN, J. P. (1970) A method for measuring nanogram quantities of acetylcholine by pyrolysis-gas chromatography: The demonstration of acetylcholine in effluents from the rat phrenic-nerve–diaphragm preparation. *J. Pharmacol.* **174**: 337–45.

TERAVAINEN, J. (1969) Localization of acetylcholinesterase in the rat myoneural junction. *Histochemie* **17**: 162–9.

CHAPTER 4

PHYSIOPATHOLOGY OF NEUROMUSCULAR TRANSMISSION

J. E. Desmedt

Brussels

IN SEVERAL clinical conditions in man, the neuromuscular transmission can be impaired without there being any significant anomaly either in the muscle fibers or in the motor nerve. Myasthenia gravis, the most widely known of these diseases, results from a presynaptic defect probably involving the synthesis of acetylcholine (Desmedt, 1958a, 1966; Elmqvist *et al.*, 1965). In the Lambert–Eaton syndrome which is generally associated with a bronchogenic carcinoma, the defect involves the electrosecretory process whereby the presynaptic action potential triggers the release of acetylcholine quanta from the motor endings (Eaton and Lambert, 1957; Lambert and Rooke, 1965; Lambert, 1966; Elmqvist and Lambert, 1968). The acetylcholine ejection is also involved in botulinum intoxication (Brooks, 1956; Thesleff, 1960; Zacks *et al.*, 1962), and in the recently identified syndrome resulting from intoxication with certain antibiotics (Pittinger and Long, 1958; Corrado *et al.*, 1959; Timmerman *et al.*, 1959; Bush, 1962; Elmqvist and Josefsson, 1962; McQuillen *et al.*, 1968).

Proper identification of these disorders which involve different processes of neuromuscular transmission relies essentially on electrophysiological studies applied to human patients. The progress in that area received considerable help from recent progress in biophysical concepts of synaptic mechanisms (Fatt and Katz, 1951; Fatt, 1954; Castillo and Katz, 1956; Takeuchi and Takeuchi, 1960, 1962; Katz, 1962, 1966; Hubbard and Schmidt, 1963; Katz and Miledi, 1965, 1967; Martin, 1966; Nastuk, 1966, 1967). The approach is twofold:

1. *Nerve stimulation studies on intact patients.* Supramaximal electric pulses are delivered to a motor nerve according to various programs and the electrical (and mechanical) responses of the corresponding muscles

are recorded and measured (Desmedt, 1958b, 1966; Lambert, 1960, 1966). Characteristic anomalies of the muscle responses to single or repetitive motor nerve volleys are recorded and allow the identification of the various disorders (cf. Figs. 2,5).

2. *Studies of muscle biopsies* in vitro. Small bundles of intercostal muscles are removed with their tendon ends intact under regional or general anesthesia (Creese *et al.*, 1957; Elmqvist *et al.*, 1960; Herrmann *et al.*, 1966). These bundles are set up in Locke or Krebs solution and can be stimulated directly or indirectly; microtechniques such as introduced by Fatt and Katz (1951) and Nastuk (1953) as well as mechanical recording are then readily applied.

4.1. POST-SYNAPTIC BLOCKS

Muscle weakness in myasthenia gravis has been interpreted in several ways along the years. At one time superficial similarities between myasthenic block and a partial curare block led to the suggestion of a postsynaptic causative disorder. According to these views the acetylcholine transmitter is released in normal amounts from the motor terminals but the chemoreceptors of the muscle end-plate are disordered and react abnormally with the acetylcholine (Churchill-Davidson and Richardson, 1953, 1961; Johns *et al.*, 1956; Grob *et al.*, 1956). Animal experiments showing that prolonged exposure to depolarizing cholinergic compounds, including acetylcholine itself, may desensitize the end-plate chemoreceptors (Zaimis, 1953; Thesleff, 1955; Katz and Thesleff, 1957; Taylor, 1959; Gissen and Nastuk, 1966; Nastuk, 1967) led to an increased concern with the potential role of altered cholinoceptivity in a variety of conditions. This trend proved useful for stimulating experimentation along new lines. However, it must now be recognized that no neurological disease has yet been consistently related to intrinsic chemoreceptor anomalies (Desmedt, 1965). In any case studies on myasthenic muscle *in vitro* indicate that the end-plates react normally to depolarizing drugs (carbachol, acetylcholine) and that the chemoreceptive area tested by microiontophoresis of acetylcholine is restricted to an end plate of 0.1–0.2 mm as in normal muscle (Dahlback *et al.*, 1961; Elmqvist *et al.*, 1964).

It must be appreciated that the above-quoted experiments on chemo-receptor desensitization indicate consistently that such a postsynaptic block requires exposure of the end-plate to depolarizing compounds for times much longer than the normal duration of transmitter action. In the absence of anticholinesterase drugs, the effect of acetylcholine released by the nerve is quickly terminated in 1–2 msec by hydrolysis and diffusion and the end-plate chemosensitivity does not change sufficiently for the neuro-muscular transmission to be blocked. Post-synaptic desensitization only becomes appreciable when the end plates are exposed for 1 second or more to depolarizing compounds, e.g. as a result of direct bath or iontophoretic applications *in vitro* (Katz and Thesleff, 1957; Katz, 1962) or in man after the i.v. injection of depolarizing inhibitors such as decamethonium in anesthesiology. Intoxications with large doses of anticholinesterase compounds also result in a postsynaptic block of that type (Grob and Johns, 1958). Such "cholinergic crisis" with severe respiratory insufficiency and generalized muscle weakness can occur in myasthenia gravis patients if overtreated with anticholinesterase drugs (Osserman, 1958; Osserman and Genkins, 1966; Glaser, 1966), and in normal man after accidental exposure to organophosphorus anticholinesterase insecticides (parathion or E 605, hexaethyl tetraphosphate) or chemical warfare agents (tabun, sarin . . .) (Grob, 1956; Holmstedt, 1959; Namba and Hiraki, 1958). All such intoxications or therapeutic hazards belong to a class of neuro-muscular blocks induced by extrinsic pharmacological effects and they should be differentiated from the specific neurological diseases involving the neuromuscular junction; in the latter no chemoreceptor disorder has yet been identified as of causative significance.

On the other hand, the possibility that a local increase in cholinesterase might interfere with the transmitter action in myasthenia has not been substantiated. In myasthenic muscle the cholinesterase content appears to be normal (Goodman *et al.*, 1939; Jones and Stadie, 1939; Wilson *et al.*, 1951; Fardeau, 1961; Zacks, 1964). The time course of the myasthenic end-plate potential is not different from normal in untreated myasthenic muscle which suggests that the released acetylcholine is normally hydro-lyzed by end-plate cholinesterase (Elmqvist *et al.*, 1964).

4.2. PRESYNAPTIC BLOCKS

It is now clear that changes in synaptic efficacy, i.e. facilitation or depression of neuromuscular transmission, are to be related to variations in the amounts of acetylcholine released from the motor nerve endings (Castillo and Katz, 1954, 1956; Katz, 1962, 1966; Brooks and Thies, 1962; Otsuka *et al.*, 1962; Hubbard, 1963; Thies, 1965; Martin, 1966). The underlying biophysical processes are only partially understood. For the purpose of the present pathophysiological discussion it is convenient to group these processes under two main headings:

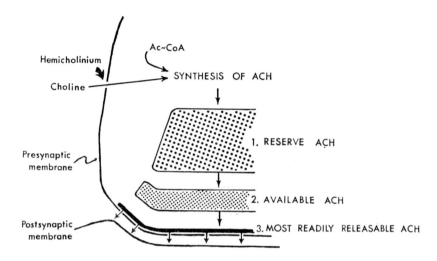

FIG. 1. Flow diagram of the acetylcholine metabolism in cholinergic nerve terminals, essentially based on the data of Birks and MacIntosh (1961). In the presynaptic terminals the acetylcholine is synthetized from acetyl-coenzyme A and choline. Choline is taken up from the extracellular fluid and its utilization is interfered with by hemicholinium HC-3 (MacIntosh, 1963). The acetylcholine is stored in several compartments arranged in series. (From Desmedt, 1966, fig. 2.)

1. *Electro-secretory processes* whereby the nerve action potential triggers the ejection of a certain number of acetylcholine quanta (Katz and Miledi, 1965, 1967, 1968); these processes are located within and/or close to the presynaptic membrane and require the participation of calcium ions from the extracellular fluid (Castillo and Katz, 1956; Katz and Miledi, 1967, 1968; Dodge and Rahamimoff, 1967; Jones and Landau, 1968). During repetitive activation at rates from about 5/sec the capacity of the motor axon spike to eject quanta increases with the frequency (postactivation facilitation).

2. *Metabolic and packaging processes* which manufacture acetylcholine quanta in the axoplasm and make them available for the surface electro-secretory mechanism. The stock of quanta appears to be organized in several subsystems, arranged in series, and only a fraction of the transmitter stocked in the endings is immediately available for release (Fig. 1) (Perry, 1953; Birks and MacIntosh, 1961; MacIntosh, 1963). The most readily releasable compartment no. 3 is partially depleted by activity, even indeed

after a single volley and it is then reloaded through mobilization (Eccles, 1964) of quanta from the compartment no. 2. This in turn stimulates the synthesis of new acetylcholine. Thus in neuromuscular activity a high rate of discharge of acetylcholine quanta is matched by a powerful metabolic response which is triggered by the partial depletion of the subsystems arranged in series (MacIntosh, 1963). As a consequence the number of quanta immediately available to the electrosecretory mechanism will thus be maximum in the junctions at rest and it can only decrease during activity. The number of quanta released by any motor axon volley (or the quantum content of the end-plate potential elicited thereby) is a function of the state of facilitation of the surface electrosecretory process and the state of depletion of the compartment of immediately available quanta. In normal muscles the safety factor of neuromuscular transmission is 3 or 4 (Paton and Waud, 1967) and the end-plate potentials remain suprathreshold in spite of such changes in quantum content during repetitive activation.

4.2.1. MYASTHENIA GRAVIS

In the clinically weak muscles of a myasthenic patient who is deprived of anticholinesterase drug therapy, the belly-tendon electrical response and the mechanical response to a supramaximal motor nerve volley are within normal limits or only slightly reduced (Harvey and Masland, 1941; Botelho *et al.*, 1952; Johns *et al.*, 1956; Desmedt, 1957, 1959, 1961, 1966; Lambert *et al.*, 1961). When the motor nerve is stimulated at low rates the muscle responses disclose a characteristic short-term decrement which levels off with the fifth response (Fig. 2, C). At 20/sec the decrement also appears but it is followed by a relative increase in the muscle responses (Fig. 2, D). After the intramuscular injection of 3 mg Prostigmine (Neostigmine), adequate to relieve the clinical weakness, the decrement is considerably attenuated (Fig. 2, E, F) so that the pattern of responses now approximates to those in normal man (Fig. 2, A, B). These variations of the muscle responses with repetitive activation correspond to variations in the number of neuromuscular junctions blocked in the recorded muscle since the supramaximal electric stimuli elicit an action potential in all the motor axons throughout the series. Similar features including the short-term decrement are recorded in normal human muscles partially curarized with d-tubocurarine (Desmedt, 1967). They can be ascribed in both cases to a reduced safety margin of transmission whereby normal changes in the quantum content of the end-plate potentials determine failure or recruitment in the population of neuromuscular junctions tested (Desmedt, 1966).

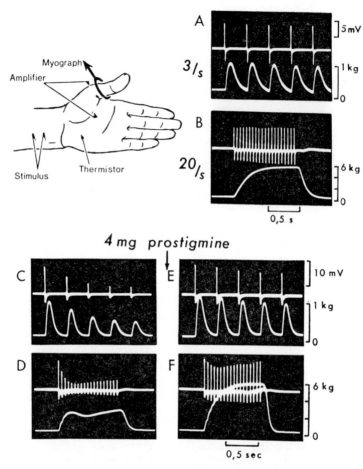

FIG. 2. Responses to nerve stimulation in normal adductor pollicis muscle (A, B) and in myasthenic muscle before (C, D) and after (E, F) the administration of a therapeutic dose of prostigmine. The arrangement of the electrodes appears in the diagram. The stimulation rate is 3/second in A, C, and E, and 20/second in B, D and F. (From Desmedt, 1962b, figs. 3 and 6.)

The decrement of successive responses both in myasthenic and in normal partially curarized muscles results from a progressive decrease in quantum content of the end-plate potentials as the compartment of immediately releasable quanta is depleted (Otsuka *et al.*, 1962; Wakabayashi and Iwasaki, 1964; Thies, 1965; Desmedt, 1966). The secondary facilitation at higher rates of stimulation is related to a potentiation of the surface electrosecretory process (Castillo and Katz, 1956; Eccles, 1964; Mallart and Martin, 1967, 1968; Katz and Miledi, 1968).

In the partially curarized normal muscle, the volley output of acetylcholine is not modified by the competitive inhibitor but a fraction of the end-plate chemoreceptors no longer react with the transmitter. In the myasthenic muscle the postsynaptic chemosensitivity and the pattern of quantal ejection are both normal but the quantum size is reduced (Elmqvist *et al.*, 1964). Each quantum contains presumably a smaller number of acetylcholine molecules and produces a smaller end-plate depolarization, as indicated by the small voltage of the spontaneous miniature end-plate potentials, which are about 0.2 mV instead of about 0.9 mV (Elmqvist and Lambert, 1968). Roughly speaking, the synaptic kinetics in terms of number of quanta released would be fairly normal in myasthenia gravis but the safety margin is reduced by devaluation of the quantal currency.

The next question is related to the differences between myasthenic block and the block induced in normal muscles by competitive inhibitors such as d-tubocurarine (Desmedt, 1957). Myasthenic block indeed presents characteristic features which determine the specific manifestations of the disease. In myasthenic patients the amount of muscle weakness is not constant throughout the day: it increases as the muscles are used in voluntary or reflex contractions and it recovers as the muscles are rested (Goldflam, 1893; Osserman, 1958). This is related to a peculiar lability of the neuromuscular mechanism whereby periods of activity increase the synaptic failure. To demonstrate the long-term changes in amount of block one must use infrequent stimulations in order to secure a reasonable base line. Five supramaximal stimuli delivered to the motor nerve at 3/second every minute or so provide an adequate program (Fig. 3, A). The short-term decrement seen in the successive responses at 3/second permits an estimate of the amount of block. When a faradic exercise is produced by stimulating the same motor nerve at, say, 50/second for 2–10 seconds (Fig. 3, B) the neuromuscular transmission improves for about 20 seconds and the short-term decrement is reduced (Fig. 3, C). Thereafter the block increases more and more beyond the initial level and it is most marked 2 to 4 minutes after the exercise (Fig. 3, D). From then on recovery is observed over the next 10 to 20 minutes (Fig. 3, E). The delayed and reversible increase in block after a brief exercise has been called "postactivation exhaustion" (Desmedt, 1957). This phenomenon is also recorded after a voluntary exercise, i.e. when the patient is instructed to contract maximally the muscle under study for 10–40 seconds and then relax while the amount of block is tested by 3/second test stimulations of

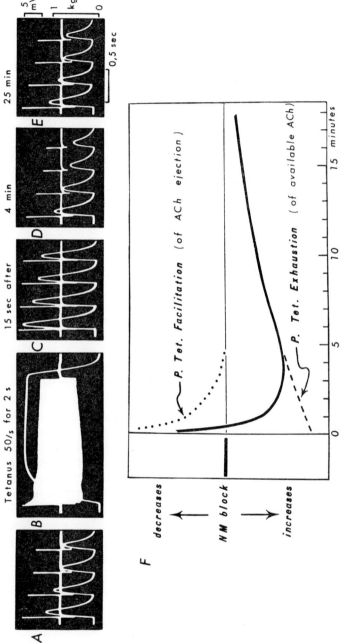

FIG. 3. The postactivation cycle of neuromuscular transmission in myasthenic muscle. Same electrode arrangement as in Fig. 2. Test stimulations of the ulnar nerve at 3/second are presented first in the rested muscle (A), and then at various times after a brief faradization of the nerve (B). Postactivation facilitation is seen in C, 15 seconds after the faradization. Postactivation exhaustion appears maximally in D, 4 minutes after the faradization. F, variations in neuromuscular block (estimated from the percentage decrement in 3/second test trains) after a brief exercise which occurs at time zero. The solid curve is analysed into two components as explained in the text. (From Desmedt, 1966, fig. 13.)

the motor nerve (Desmedt, 1961a, 1961b, 1966). Since the exhaustion phenomenon also follows a voluntary exercise, it can be made responsible for the long-lasting component of the activity-dependent clinical paresis (Desmedt, 1957, 1962, 1966).

The myasthenic post-activation cycle can obviously be analysed into a facilitation component and an exhaustion component, as suggested in (Fig. 3, F) and it has indeed proved possible to dissociate the two components by appropriate stimulation programs (Desmedt, 1966). In partially curarized normal muscles, only the postactivation facilitation component is present (Fig. 4, C) (Desmedt, 1967). On the other hand, the myasthenic type of postactivation cycle can be produced in cat muscle by administration of hemicholinium HC-3 (Schueler, 1960), an inhibitor of acetylcholine synthesis (MacIntosh *et al.*, 1956; Birks and MacIntosh, 1961; MacIntosh, 1963) provided the stocks of transmitter have been depleted by prolonged repetitive activity (Fig. 4, B) (Desmedt, 1958, 1966). This substantiates the view that myasthenic block results from a defect in acetylcholine synthesis. In hemicholinium block the end-plate potential and the miniature end-plate potentials are reduced in voltage and the quantum size decreases as a result of previous activity (Elmqvist and Quastel, 1965). That the quantum size varies after hemicholinium is clearly established because the voltage of the spontaneous miniature end-plate potentials is normal initially and decreases much below 0.9 mV as the stocks are depleted. Elmqvist thinks that in myasthenic muscle the quantum size is "reduced but fixed". However, this proposition is more difficult to substantiate because in myasthenic muscle the voltage of miniature end-plate potentials is very small throughout (Elmqvist and Lambert, 1968) and technical limitations make it difficult to assess any variations. On the other hand, the exhaustion phenomenon recorded in whole muscles demonstrates a reversible deterioration of synaptic efficacy after exercise. Since this is absent in normal curarized muscle it does not reflect the normal kinetics of quantal release and therefore it cannot be explained by a "reduced but fixed" quantum size. The proposed working hypothesis is that an inadequate rate of replenishment of transmitter after depletion determines a subnormal loading of quanta in acetylcholine, and thus a further devaluation of the quanta currency for several minutes after an exercise (Desmedt, 1966). Anticholinesterase drugs only represent a symptomatic therapy for myasthenic patients and they do not improve the underlying disorder. They provide an indirect means of augmenting the neuromuscular safety margin by prolonging the duration of action of the released acetylcholine.

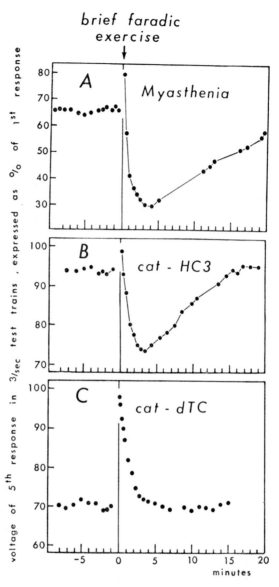

FIG. 4. Comparison of the postactivation cycles in human myasthenic muscle (A), in normal cat muscle treated with hemicholinium HC-3 and after depletion of transmitter stores through prolonged activation (B), and in normal cat muscle in a steady state of partial curarization with d-tubocurarine (C). Abscissa, time in minutes with the zero corresponding to the faradization of the motor nerve at 50/second for 2 to 10 seconds. Ordinate, percentage decrement of the fifth electrical muscle response in the 3/second test trains. (From Desmedt, 1958a.)

4.2.2. THE LAMBERT–EATON SYNDROME

This rare neuromuscular disease sometimes associated with a broncho-genic carcinoma has been differentiated from classical myasthenia gravis by electrophysiological studies on the patients (Lambert *et al.*, 1961; Lambert and Rooke, 1965). The proximal muscles of the limbs present some degree of weakness but the ocular and bulbar muscles are spared. There is no evidence of abnormal function either in the peripheral nerves or in the muscles. When a motor nerve is stimulated by supramaximal electric pulses the muscle electric response is found much smaller than in normals (Fig. 5). Administration of tensilon or of other anticholinesterase drug does not improve the responses. However, voluntary exercise of the muscle will induce a marked facilitation which is seen both in the increased voltage of the motor unit potentials during the latter part of the exercise

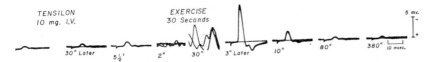

Fig. 5. Patient with the Lambert–Eaton syndrome. Electric responses of the muscle to supramaximal electric pulses delivered to the motor nerve, before and after 10 mg tensilon i.v., and then after a voluntary contraction of the same muscle for 30 seconds. (Courtesy of E. H. Lambert.)

and in the increased muscle responses to the nerve volley (Fig. 5). The facilitation then dissipates. When the nerve is stimulated at rates higher than about 5/second the muscle responses increase progressively and eventually reach about a normal voltage (Lambert and Rooke, 1965; Lambert, 1966). Microphysiological studies on intercostal muscle biopsies *in vitro* show that quantal size is fairly normal but that the quantum content of the end-plate potential is markedly reduced (Elmqvist and Lambert, 1968). The frequency of spontaneous release of quanta is not increased when the potassium concentration in the medium is raised to 20 mM; this indicates a defect in the electrosecretory process (Elmqvist and Lambert, 1968). In normal or myasthenic muscles the frequency of quantal release increases about 100-fold under such conditions, thus confirming that the release process itself is not involved in true myasthenia gravis. By contrast the Lambert–Eaton syndrome involves the electro-secretory process rather than the formation or synthesis of acetylcholine quanta. Therapeutic effects are indeed observed in the latter for calcium and guanidine (Lambert, 1966) which are both known to potentiate the release mechanism (Castillo and Katz, 1956; Otsuka and Endo, 1960). Anticholinesterase drugs are not effective because the amounts of acetylcholine released in the rested muscle are much too small.

4.2.3. OTHER NEUROMUSCULAR DISORDERS

In botulinium intoxication the number of acetylcholine quanta released by the motor nerve action potential is also reduced, as well as the spontaneous release (Brooks, 1956; Thesleff, 1960). This accounts for the clinical weakness which has not yet been analysed in detail in the human patients. The muscle electric response to motor nerve stimulation is reduced and can be augmented by the administration of guanidine (Cherington and Ryan, 1968).

Several antibiotics such as kanamycin, streptomycin, dihydrostreptomycin, neomycin, can also produce neuromuscular block (Pittinger and Long, 1958; Corrado *et al.*, 1959). Most of the human cases have been observed after intraperitoneal administration of large doses of such antibiotics and when renal function was inadequate. Mild paralysis can be improved by anticholinesterase drugs but these are no longer effective in the more severe cases; calcium administration will then relieve the block. *In vitro* studies indicate that the neuromuscular block by antibiotics is related to a reduction in the quantum content of the end-plate potential. Furthermore, an increase of potassium concentration in the medium does not augment the spontaneous quantal release (Elmqvist and Josefsson, 1962). This indicates that the antibiotics concerned interfere with the electrosecretory process.

REFERENCES

BIRKS, R. and MACINTOSH, F. C. (1961) Acetylcholine metabolism of a sympathetic ganglion. *Canad. J. Biochem. Physiol.* **39**: 787–827.

BOTELHO, S. Y., DEATERLY, C. F. and COMROE, J. H. (1952) Electromyogram from orbicularis oculi in normal persons and in patients with myasthenia gravis. *Arch. Neurol. Psychiat.* **67**: 348–53.

BROOKS, V. B. (1956) An intracellular study of the action of repetitive nerve volleys and of botulinum toxin on miniature end plate potentials. *J. Physiol.* **134**: 264–77.

BROOKS, V. B. and THIES, R. E. (1962) Reduction of quantum content during neuromuscular transmission. *J. Physiol.* **162**: 298–310.

BUSH, G. H. (1962). Antibiotic paralysis. *Brit. Med. J.* **2**: 1062–3.

CASTILLO, J. DEL and KATZ, B. (1954) Statistical factors involved in neuromuscular facilitation and depression. *J. Physiol.* **124**: 574–85.

CASTILLO, J. DEL and KATZ, B. (1956) Biophysical aspects of neuro-muscular transmission. *Progr. Biophys. Biophys. Chem.* **6**: 121–70.

CHERINGTON, M. and RYAN, D. W. (1968) Botulism and guanidine. *New Engl. J. Med.* **278**: 931–3.

CHURCHILL-DAVIDSON, H. C. and RICHARDSON, A. T. (1953) Neuromuscular transmission in myasthenia gravis. *J. Physiol.* 122: 252–63.

CHURCHILL-DAVIDSON, H. C. and RICHARDSON, A. T. (1961) A study of neuromuscular transmission in 100 cases of myasthenia gravis. In: *Myasthenia Gravis*, pp. 199–207. Viets, H. R. (ed.). Ch. Thomas, Springfield.

CORRADO, A. P., RAMOS, A. O. and DEESCOBAR, C. T. (1959) Neuromuscular blockade by neomycine potentiation by ether anesthesia and d-tubocurarine and antagonism by calcium and prostigmine. *Arch. Int. Pharmacodyn.* 121: 380–94.

CREESE, R., DILLON, J. B., MARSHALL, J., SABAWALA, P. B., SCHNEIDER, D. J., TAYLOR, D. B. and ZINN, D. E. (1957) The effect of neuromuscular blocking agents on isolated human intercostal muscles. *J. Pharmacol. Exp. Ther.* 119: 485–94.

DAHLBÄCK, O., ELMQVIST, D., JOHNS, T. R., RADNER, S. and THESLEFF, S. (1961) An electrophysiologic study of the neuromuscular junction in myasthenia gravis. *J. Physiol.* 156: 336–43.

DESMEDT, J. E. (1957) Nature of the defect of neuromuscular transmission in myasthenic patients: "post-tetanic exhaustion". *Nature* 179: 156–67.

DESMEDT, J. E. (1958a) Myasthenic-like features of neuromuscular transmission after administration of an inhibitor of acetylcholine synthesis. *Nature* 182: 1673–4.

DESMEDT, J. E. (1958b) Méthodes d'étude de la fonction neuromusculaire chez l'homme. Myogramme isométrique, électromyogramme d'excitation et topographie de l'innervation terminale. *Acta Neurol. Psychiat. Belg.* 58: 977–1017.

DESMEDT, J. E. (1959) The physiopathology of neuromuscular transmission and the trophic influence of motor innervation. *Amer. J. Physical Med.* 38: 248–61.

DESMEDT, J. E. (1961a) Neuromuscular defect in myasthenia gravis: electrophysiological and histopathological evidence. In: *Myasthenia Gravis*, pp.150–176. Viets, H. R. (ed.). Ch. Thomas, Springfield.

DESMEDT, J. E. (1961b) Les phénomènes de facilitation et d'épuisement de postactivation dans la myasthénie grave et leur signification physio-pathologique. *Pathologie-Biologie* 9: 1149–56.

DESMEDT, J. E. (1962a) Identification and titration of myasthenic defect by nerve stimulation. *Electroenceph. Clin. Neurophysiol.*, suppl 22: 63–64. Premier Congrès International d'Electromyographie, Pavie. Elsevier, Amsterdam.

DESMEDT, J. E. (1962b) Données récentes sur la pathogénie de la myasthénie. *Bull. Acad. Roy. Med. Belg.*, VIIe série, 2: 213–67.

DESMEDT, J. E. (1965) Le diagnostic électromyographique des maladies neuromusculaires. *VIIIe Congrès International de Neurologie*, Vienne, Tome S, pp. 13–27.

DESMEDT, J. E. (1966) Presynaptic mechanisms in myasthenia gravis. Third Symposium on Myasthenia Gravis. *Ann. N.Y. Acad. Sci.* 135: 209–46.

DESMEDT, J. E. (1967) Problèmes physiopathologiques posés par la myasthénie grave. *Actualités Pharmacologiques*, 20e série, pp. 201–16. Hazard, P. and Cheymol, J. (eds.).

DODGE, F. A. and RAHAMIMOFF, R. (1967) Co-operative action of calcium ions in transmitter release at the neuromuscular junction. *J. Physiol.* 193: 419–32.

EATON, L. M. and LAMBERT, E. H. (1957) Electromyography and electric stimulation of nerves in diseases of motor unit: observations on myasthenic syndrome associated with malignant tumors. *J.A.M.A.* 163: 1117–24.

ECCLES, J. C. (1964) *The Physiology of Synapses*. Springer Verlag.

ELMQVIST, D., JOHNS, T. R. and THESLEFF, S. (1960) A study of some electrophysiological properties of human muscle. *J. Physiol.* 154: 602–7.

ELMQVIST, D. and JOSEFSSON, J. O. (1962) The nature of the neuromuscular block produced by neomycine. *Acta Physiol. Scand.* 54: 105–10.

ELMQVIST, D., HOFMANN, W. W., KUGELBERG, J. and QUASTEL, D. M. J. (1964) An electrophysiological investigation of neuromuscular transmission in myasthenia gravis. *J. Physiol.* **174**: 417–34.

ELMQVIST, D. and LAMBERT, E. H. (1968) Detailed analysis of neuromuscular transmission in a patient with the myasthenic syndrome sometimes associated with bronchogenic carcinoma. *Mayo Clinic Proc.* **43**: 689–713.

ELMQVIST, D. and QUASTEL, D. M. J. (1965) Presynaptic action of hemicholinium at the neuromuscular junction. *J. Physiol.* **177**: 463–82.

FARDEAU, M. (1961) Anatomo-pathologie du muscle squelettique dans la myasthénie. *Pathologie-Biologie* **9**: 1141–7.

FATT, P. (1954) Biophysics of junctional transmission. *Physiol. Rev.* **34**: 674–710.

FATT, P. and KATZ, B. (1951) An analysis of the end plate potential recorded with an intra-cellular electrode. *J. Physiol.* **115**: 320–70.

GISSEN, A. J. and NASTUK, W. L. (1966) The mechanisms underlying neuromuscular block following prolonged exposure to the depolarizing agents. *Ann. N.Y. Acad. Sci.* **135**: 184–94.

GLASER, G. H. (1966) Crisis, precrisis and drug resistance in myasthenia gravis. *Ann. N.Y. Acad. Sci.* **135**: 335–49.

GOLDFLAM, S. (1893) Ueber einen Schemibar heilbaren bulbärparalytischen Symptonen-complex mit Betheiligung der Extremitäten. *Dtsch. Z. Nervenheilk.* **4**: 312–52.

GOODMAN, L., CARLSON, R. I. and GILMAN, A. (1939) Muscle and blood cholinesterase in myasthenia gravis: case study. *J. Pharmacol.* **66**: 15–16.

GROB, D. and JOHNS, R. J. (1958) Use of oximes in the treatment of intoxication by anticholinesterase compounds in normal subjects. *Amer. J. Med.* **24**: 497–511.

GROB, D., JOHNS, R. J. and HARVEY, A. M. (1956) Stimulating and depressant effects of acetylcholine and choline in patients with myasthenia gravis and their relationship to the defect in neuromuscular transmission. *Bull. Johns Hopkins Hosp.* **99**: 153–81.

HARVEY, A. M. and MASLAND, R. L. (1941) The electromyogram in myasthenia gravis. *Bull. Johns Hopkins Hosp.* **69**: 1–13.

HERRMAN, C., SABAWALA, P. B., BARKER, W. F. and DILLON, J. B. (1966) Reappraisal of "in vitro" muscle biopsy in myasthenia gravis. *Ann. N.Y. Acad. Sci.* **135**: 302–11.

HUBBARD, J. I. (1963) Repetitive stimulation at the mammalian neuromuscular junction and the mobilisation of transmitter. *J. Physiol.* **169**: 641–62.

HUBBARD, J. I., JONES, S. F. and LANDAU, E. M. (1968) On the mechanism by which calcium and magnesium affect the release of transmitter by nerve impulses. *J. Physiol.* **196**: 75–86.

HUBBARD, J. I. and SCHMIDT, R. F. (1963) An electrophysiological investigation of mammalian motor nerve terminals. *J. Physiol.* **166**: 145–67.

JOHNS, R. J., GROB, D. and HARVEY, A. M. (1956) Studies in neuromuscular function. *Bull. Johns Hopkins Hosp.* **99**: 125–35.

JONES, M. S. and STADIE, W. C. (1939) The choline-esterase content of the muscle of myasthenia gravis and the serum of four other groups of clinical conditions. *Quart. J. Exp. Physiol.* **29**: 63–67.

KATZ, B. (1962) The transmission of impulses from nerve to muscle and the subcellular unit of synaptic action. *Proc. Roy. Soc. Biol.* **155**: 455–77.

KATZ, B. (1966) *Nerve, Muscle and Synapse.* McGraw-Hill, New York.

KATZ, B. and MILEDI, R. (1965) The effect of temperature on the synaptic delay at the neuromuscular junction. *J. Physiol.* **181**: 656–70.

KATZ, B. and MILEDI, R. (1967) The timing of calcium action during neuromuscular transmission. *J. Physiol.* **189**: 535–44.

KATZ, B. and MILEDI, R. (1968) The role of calcium in neuromuscular facilitation. *J. Physiol.* **195**: 481–92.

KATZ, B. and THESLEFF, S. (1957) A study of the "desensitization" produced by acetylcholine at the motor end plate. *J. Physiol.* **138**: 63–80.

LAMBERT, E. H. (1960) Neurophysiological techniques useful in the study of neuromuscular disorders. *Res. Publ. Ass. Nerv. Ment. Dis.* **38**: 247–73.

LAMBERT, E. H. (1966) Defects of neuromuscular transmission in syndromes other than myasthenia gravis. *Ann. N.Y. Acad. Sci.* **135**: 367–84.

LAMBERT, E. H. and ROOKE, E. D. (1965) Myasthenic state and lung cancer. In: *The Remote Effects of Cancer on the Nervous System*, pp. 67–80. Brain, W. R. and Norris, F. H. (eds.). Grune & Stratton, New York.

LAMBERT, E. H., ROOKE, E. D., EATON, L. M. and HODGSON, C. H. (1961) Myasthenic syndrome occasionally associated with bronchial neoplasm: neurophysiologic studies. In: *Myasthenia Gravis*, pp. 362–410. Viets, H. R. (ed.). Ch. Thomas, Springfield.

MACINTOSH, F. C. (1963) Synthesis and storage of acetylcholine in nervous tissue. *Canad. J. Biochem. Physiol.* **41**: 2555–71.

MACINTOSH, F. C., BIRKS, R. I. and SASTRY, P. B. (1956) Pharmacological inhibition of acetylcholine synthesis. *Nature* **178**: 1181.

McQUILLEN, M. P., CANTOR, H. E. and O'ROURKE, J. R. (1968) Myasthenic syndrome associated with antibiotics. *Arch. Neurol.* **18**: 402–15.

MALLART, A. and MARTIN, A. R. (1967) An analysis of facilitation of transmitter release at the neuromuscular junction of the frog. *J. Physiol.* **193**: 679–94.

MALLART, A. and MARTIN, A. R. (1968) The relation between quantum content and facilitation at the neuromuscular junction of the frog. *J. Physiol.* **196**: 593–604.

MARTIN, A. R. (1966) Quantal nature of synaptic transmission. *Physiol. Rev.* **46**: 51–66.

NAIMAN, J. G., SAKURAI, K. and MARTIN, J. D. (1965) The antagonism of calcium and neostigmine to kanamycin-induced neuromuscular paralysis. *J. Surg. Res.* **5**: 323–8.

NASTUK, W. L. (1953) Membrane potential changes at a single muscle end plate produced by transitory application of acetylcholine with an electrically controlled microjet. *Fed. Proc.* **12**: 102.

NASTUK, W. L. (1966) Fundamental aspects of neuromuscular transmission. *Ann. N.Y. Acad. Sci.* **135**: 110–35.

NASTUK, W. L. (1967) Activation and inactivation of muscle post-junctional receptors. *Fed. Proc.* **26**: 1639–46.

OSSERMAN, K. E. (1958) *Myasthenia Gravis*. Grune & Stratton, New York.

OSSERMAN, K. E. (1966) Myasthenia gravis. In: *Ann. N.Y. Acad. Sci.* **135**: 680 pp.

OSSERMAN, K. E. and GENKINS, G. (1966) Critical reappraisal of the use of edrophonium (Tensilon) chloride tests in myasthenia gravis and significance of clinical classification. *Ann. N.Y. Acad. Sci.* **135**: 312–34.

OTSUKA, M. and ENDO, M. (1960) The effect of guanidine on neuromuscular transmission. *J. Pharmacol.* **128**: 273–82.

OTSUKA, M., ENDO, M. and NONOMURA, Y. (1962) Presynaptic nature of neuromuscular depression. *Jap. J. Physiol.* **12**: 573–84.

PATON, W. D. M. and WAUD, D. R. (1967) The margin of safety of neuromuscular transmission. *J. Physiol.* **191**: 59–90.

PERRY, W. L. M. (1953) Acetylcholine release in the cat's superior cervical ganglion. *J. Physiol.* **119**: 439–54.

PITTINGER, C. B. and LONG, J. P. (1958) The neuromuscular blocking action of neomycine sulfate. *Antibiot. Chemother.* **8**: 198–203.

SCHUELER, F. W. (1960) The mechanism of action of the hemicholiniums. *Int. Rev. Neurobiol.* **2**: 77–97.

TAKEUCHI, A. and TAKEUCHI, N. (1960) On the permeability of end plate membrane during the action of transmitter. *J. Physiol.* **154**: 52–67.

TAKEUCHI, A. and TAKEUCHI, N. (1962) Electrical changes in pre- and post-synaptic axons of the giant synapse of Loligo. *J. Gen. Physiol.* **45**: 1181–93.

TAYLOR, D. B. (1959) The mechanism of action of muscle relaxants and their antagonists. *Anesthesiology* **20**: 439–52.

THESLEFF, S. (1955) The mode of neuromuscular block caused by acetylcholine, nicotine, decamethonium and succinylcholine. *Acta Physiol. Scand.* **34**: 218–31.

THESLEFF, S. (1960) Supersensitivity of skeletal muscle produced by botulinum toxin. *J. Physiol.* **151**: 598–607.

THIES, R. E. (1965) Neuromuscular depression and the apparent depletion of transmitter in mammalian muscle. *J. Neurophysiol.* **28**: 427–42.

TIMMERMAN, J. C., LONG, J. P. and PITTINGER, C. B. (1959) Neuromuscular blocking properties of various antibiotic agents. *Toxic. Appl. Pharmacol.* **1**: 299–303.

WAKABAYASHI, T. and IWASAKI, S. (1964) Successive epp pattern and presynaptic factors in neuromuscular transmission. *Tohoku J. Exp. Med.* **83**: 225–36.

WILSON, A., MAW, G. A. and GEORGHEGAN, H. (1951) Cholinesterase activity of blood and muscle in myasthenia gravis. *Quart. J. Med.* **20**: 13–19.

ZACKS, S. I. (1964) *The Motor End Plate.* Saunders, W. B. (ed.). Philadelphia.

ZACKS, S. I., METZGER, J. F., SMITH, C. W. and BLUMBERG, J. M. (1962) Localization of ferritin-labelled botulinus toxin in the neuromuscular junction of the mouse. *J. Neuropath.* **21**: 610–33.

ZAIMIS, E. J. (1953) Motor end plate differences as a determining factor in the mode of action of neuromuscular blocking substances. *J. Physiol.* **122**: 238–51.

CHAPTER 5

POINTS OF IMPACT OF MODIFIERS
OF NEUROMUSCULAR TRANSMISSION

J. Cheymol and F. Bourillet

Paris

THE neuromuscular synapse has been the subject of a great number of pharmacodynamic studies, mainly owing to the strong and growing interest in the peripheral motor activity of living beings, but also when it is considered as a model of a relatively simple synapse, by reason of the experimental advantages that it has over the central nervous system synapses. The ever-growing number of new reactive chemical molecules, and the introduction of microscopic, electrophysiological, radioisotopic and iontophoretic techniques, have brought about new insights into the mechanism of action of these molecules, and into the physiology of this synapse.

One can summarize* the transmission at the neuromuscular junction in the following schematic manner:

1. *Presynaptic phase.* Acetylcholine is synthesized and stored at the level of the terminal axon in ways which allow its more or less easy liberation. It is accepted that the synaptic vesicles observed by means of electron microscopy correspond to the units of reserve, or "quanta".†

The arrival of nerve impulses at the motor nerve ending triggers a synchronized liberation of a certain number of "quanta"‡ of acetylcholine, which diffuse across the synaptic cleft.

2. *Postsynaptic phase.* These molecules of ACh reach the specific receptors of the postsynaptic membrane or motor end-plate, and there cause a depolarization, the end-plate potential, which is limited in space to the motor end-plate, and in time by the effect of cholinesterase concentrated at this level.§

---

* For details, see the preceding chapters.
† Several thousand molecules of acetylcholine.
‡ Several hundred quanta.
§ The presence of cholinesterase at the level of the nerve endings has been demonstrated, but in a smaller quantity than at the motor end-plate.

When the amplitude of the end-plate potential reaches the excitation threshold of the adjacent resting membrane, a muscle action potential is generated; this spreads by conduction over the length of the muscle fibers and causes the activation of the contractile mechanism.

The different steps that assure transmission can be either blocked or, conversely, facilitated by many molecules, most of which have the principal characteristic of being strongly ionized cations. Their activity is in fact explained by the interference which they can produce with regard to ions playing an essential role in transmission at the level of the receptors or of the membranes: acetylcholine, and also Na and K ions. Three factors determine the intensity of their activity: the degree of ionization, the size of the ion, and also the ease of access to membranes and receptors. At the level of the muscle and its neural zone, the motor end-plate, there is no special protection; on the contrary, the nerve on the greater portion of the axon is shrouded in myelin, which is particularly impermeable to strongly ionized molecules. Only the Ranvier's nodes and the terminal part of the nerve fiber which is deprived of myelin constitute unprotected zones, and are therefore the most sensitive areas of the motor neurone.

In Table 1, and the comments that follow, is given a clear review of the different points at the level of which various molecules can modify events at the neuromuscular junction.

5.1. POSSIBILITIES OF PRESYNAPTIC ACTION

5.1.1. ACTION ON THE TRANSMITTER

(a) *BIOSYNTHESIS*

While it is possible to imagine direct inhibitors of cholinacetylase or of acetylcoenzyme A, it is by competition with choline, or by interference with its transport, that the currently known inhibitors of the biosynthesis of acetylcholine, such as hemicholinium and triethylcholine, act. These substances produce a slow progressive paralysis, due to the exhaustion of the reserves of ACh and the lessening of the ACh content of each quantum. This process is reversed by choline.

(b) *STORES—MOBILIZATION*

The storage of acetylcholine in forms more and more directly available and the changing of one form into the other (mobilization–demobilization)

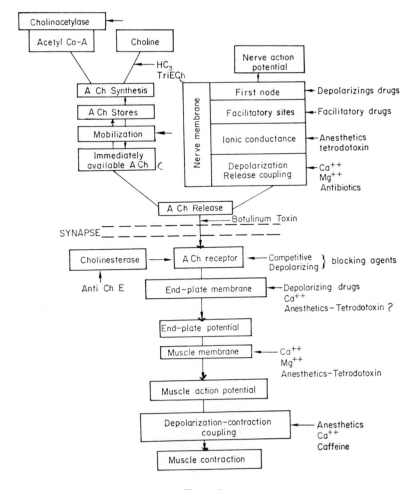

TABLE 1.

have hitherto been altered only by varying the degree of nervous stimulation. It is quite possible, however, that chemical agents could intervene at this level of transmission.

Presynaptic cholinesterases, and hence anti-ChE drugs, would also act at this level.

5.1.2. NERVE MEMBRANE

Different compounds can affect the nerve membrane at the level either of the Ranvier's nodes, or of the nerve endings (areas deprived of myelin) and can alter either their permeability to ions, or the polarization itself.

(a) *PERMEABILITY TO IONS*

Depolarization of the nerve membrane is the manifestation of a variation (limited in time) in the permeability of this membrane to certain ions, especially Na, which tends to re-enter the cell, and K, which tends to leave it. Certain compounds can block this "conductance" to ions in a more or less specific manner, and in consequence can also block depolarization. This is the case with local anesthetics which affect both Na and K ions, and with tetrodotoxin and saxitoxin,* which affect Na ions only.

(b) *DEPOLARIZATION*

The existence of cholinoceptive receptors at the level of the nerve endings, and of the Ranvier's node, is very probable. Certain depolarizing and facilitating quaternary ammonium compounds stimulate these receptors, and also produce antidromic discharges, either spontaneously or in response to an orthodromic stimulus. These discharges show themselves by facilitating transmission.

Depolarizing compounds (acetylcholine, decamethonium) work on the first Ranvier's node. Facilitating drugs, working on a facilitatory site, include the derivatives of hydroxyanilinium, oxamides, etc.

5.1.3. DEPOLARIZATION—LIBERATION COUPLING

The liberation of the directly available transmitter when depolarization reaches the nerve ending is affected by means of a "coupling" mechanism, in which the Ca ions play an essential role. Mg ions and certain antibiotics are able to inhibit this mechanism, and can cause a blocking of transmission by lessening the number of quanta liberated by the influx. Ca ions, on the other hand, oppose this type of blocking.

5.1.4. LIBERATION

Analysis of the paralysis produced by the botulinus toxin leads to the conclusion that the toxin works by inhibiting the liberation of acetylcholine.

* See Chapter 8.

5.2. POSSIBILITY OF POSTSYNAPTIC ACTION

5.2.1. CHOLINOCEPTIVE RECEPTORS OF THE MOTOR END-PLATE

These are specific receptors on to which molecules of acetylcholine, liberated and diffused across the synaptic cleft, attach themselves. Most of the stimulants and blocking drugs act on these receptors as agonists or antagonists, either competitive or not.

5.2.2. CHOLINESTERASIC SITES

These enzymes, localized in the folds of the postsynaptic membrane, limit the action of acetylcholine by hydrolyzing it. This activity is inhibited by most anticholinesterase drugs.

5.2.3. MEMBRANE OF THE MOTOR END-PLATE

The variations in the conductance of ions which are normally shown by this depolarizable, chemically excitable membrane, can be inhibited by certain toxic substances (such as tetrodotoxin in the cat or anesthetics), which thus oppose the onset of the end-plate potential.

A prolonged depolarization brings about insensitivity in this membrane (the mechanism of action of depolarizants).

5.2.4. MUSCLE MEMBRANE

As in the case of nerve membrane, the conductance of ions permitting depolarization can be blocked by different compounds (anesthetics or tetrodotoxin), which hinder the production of the muscle action potential.

5.2.5. EXCITATION–CONTRACTION–RELAXATION COUPLING

The activation of the contractile mechanisms on the arrival of the muscle action potential is brought about by a complex mechanism of coupling due to specialized structures (T tubules and sacs of the sarcoplasmic reticulum forming triads), in which the liberation and exhaustion of Ca ions successively intervene.

Different compounds are able to act directly or indirectly on this coupling mechanism: Ca ions, caffeine, certain ions such as NO_3^-, Zn^{2+}, etc.

139

5.2.6. CONTRACTILE ELEMENTS

Some highly toxic substances can produce paralysis by disturbing the muscle contraction (mono-iodoacetic acid), or by necrotic damage of the fibrillary system of the skeletal muscles (antimalarial derivatives of methoxyquinoline).

CONCLUSION

This listing of different "points of impact" of neuromuscular transmission is not exhaustive. Progress in our knowledge of the detailed mechanisms of transmission, and the discovery of new molecules that present new actions at the neuromuscular junction, will add to the list.

In addition, it is important to note that a compound can generally act on several different points, either in the same doses or in different ones; and that the effects thus produced can act together or in opposition.

Finally, one must not forget the variations that can be exhibited by the functioning of a neuromuscular junction, and therefore the mechanisms of action of the compounds that modify it, as a function of the animal species, the different muscles of the same animal, and the pathological or experimental conditions under which this function is studied.

Subsection II

INHIBITORS OF THE NEUROMUSCULAR JUNCTION

A. NATURAL INHIBITORS

CHAPTER 6

VENOMS: THEIR INHIBITORY ACTION ON NEUROMUSCULAR TRANSMISSION

O. Vital-Brazil

Sao Paulo

MOTOR disturbances are commonly observed in poisonings by venoms. In most cases, their origin is peripheral, neuromuscular or muscular. This is certainly due to the fact that the membrane of the motor nerve terminals and of the post-junctional structures are easily accessible to both fat-soluble and fat-insoluble substances, while normally the interstitial fluid in the central nervous system is protected against penetration of the latter. This review analyses the incidence, nature and importance of snake venom inhibitory action on neuromuscular transmission. Some references are made as well, to the neuromuscular action of venoms from amphibia, molluscs, scorpions, spiders and hymenoptera. The muscular actions of those venoms which exert neuromuscular blocking actions are also discussed.

6.1. SNAKE VENOMS

Muscular and neuromuscular actions are of particular importance in the genesis of the effects produced by the venoms from the proteroglyph, Elapidae and Hydrophiidae. Venoms from the solenoglyph, Viperidae and Crotalidae, usually do not cause, in mammals, paralysis or other motor disturbances due to an action on myoneural junction or skeletal muscle. Nevertheless, venoms from several Crotalidae (Houssay and Pave, 1922; Peng, 1960) and from at least one Viperidae, *Echis carinata* (Kellaway and Holden, 1932), exhibit a weak neuromuscular activity demonstrable only, in most instances, in experiments on amphibia. The South American rattlesnake (*Crotalus durissus terrificus*) venom constitutes an exception being, as the venom from proteroglyph, intensely neurotoxic (Brazil and

145

Pestana, 1909; Brazil, 1914; Wajchenberg *et al.*, 1954). It causes neuro-muscular block in mammals (Barrio and Vital Brazil, 1951; Cheymol *et al.*, 1966) and also in frogs, in which it exhibits an activity similar to that of the venom of *Naja naja* (Houssay and Pave, 1922).

6.1.1. ELAPIDAE VENOMS

INCIDENCE

All studied venoms from members of this family, with the exception only of *Pseudechis australis* (Kellaway and Holden, 1932; Kellaway *et al.*, 1932) from Australia, have shown a potent neuromuscular blocking activity. They are: (i) Venoms from the cobras of Asia like the Indian cobra, *Naja naja* (Brunton and Fayrer, 1874; Ragotzi, 1890; Arthus, 1910; Cushny and Yagi, 1918; Houssay and Pave, 1922; Kellaway *et al.*, 1932; Gautrellet *et al.*, 1934; Vital Brazil and Barrio, 1950a, 1950b; Schmidt *et al.*, 1964; Vick *et al.*, 1965; Cheymol *et al.*, 1966), Formosan cobra, *N. naja atra* (Su, 1960; Lee and Peng, 1961), King cobra or hamadryad, *Ophiophagus hannah* (Rogers, 1905; Arthus, 1912a; Houssay and Pave, 1922), and of Africa, like the Cape cobra, *Naja nivea* (Epstein, 1930), Egyptian cobra, *N. haja* (Cheymol *et al.*, 1966) and spitting cobra, *N. nigricollis* (Cheymol *et al.*, 1966). (ii) Venoms from the Asiatic kraits like the common Indian krait, *Bungarus coeruleus* (Rogers, 1905; Arthus, 1912a) and the banded kraits, *B. fasciatus* (Rogers, 1905), from India, and *B. multicinctus* (Chang, 1960a; Chang, 1960b) from Formosa. (iii) Venom from the African ringhals, *Hemachatus haemachatus* (Fraser and Gunn, 1909). (iv) Venom from the Egyptian black snake, *Walterinnesia aegyptia* (Mohamed and Zaki, 1957) from Egypt, Arabia and Asia Minor. (v) Venoms from Australian Elapidae, like the tiger snake, *Notechis scutatus* (Arthus, 1912b; Houssay and Pave 1922; Kellaway *et al.*, 1932), red-bellied black snake, *Pseudechis porphyriacus* (Arthus, 1912b; Houssay and Pave, 1922; Kellaway *et al.*, 1932), death adder, *Acantophis antarcticus* (Kellaway *et al.*, 1932), brown snake, *Demansia textilis* (Kellaway *et al.*, 1932), copperhead, *Denisonia superba* (Kellaway *et al.*, 1932), and taipan, *Oxyuranus scutellactus* (Kellaway *et al.*, 1932). (vi) Venoms from the American coral snakes, like *Micrurus frontalis* (Vital Brazil and Barrio, 1950a, 1950b) and *M. lemniscatus* (Vital Brazil, 1963).

MUSCULAR ACTION

Besides the neuromuscular blocking action proper, some elapidic venoms, like the Indian cobra venom, also act directly on the skeletal muscle causing loss of excitability and, in some preparations, contracture and/or fibrillations which are not abolished by curare (Cushny and Yagi, 1918; Houssay *et al.*, 1922; Kellaway and Holden, 1932). However, this muscular action is seen predominantly in amphibian muscles, specially in isolated preparations. In neuromuscular preparations *in situ*, direct excitability is usually preserved after neuromuscular block and no fibrillation or contracture occurs. In the rat isolated phrenic nerve-diaphragm preparation cobra venom, in relatively high doses, causes contracture (Su, 1960; Cheymol *et al.*, 1966) and depresses direct muscle excitability (Su, 1960). These effects are not observed with venoms from the banded krait from Formosa (Chang, 1960a) and the South American coral snake (Vital Brazil, 1963). The muscular action of *Naja naja atra* venom is due to a different component (cardiotoxin) than that (cobra neurotoxin) which produces block of neuromuscular transmission (Lee and Chang, 1966).

CHARACTERISTICS AND MECHANISM OF THE NEUROMUSCULAR ACTION

The neuromuscular blocking action caused by the several Elapidae venoms is very similar. The following characteristics are common to the action of all these venoms on the myoneural junctions: (i) Onset after a more or less prolonged latent period, depending on the dose employed, and slow progress of the block (Fig. 1). (ii) Absence of potentiation of the maximal twitch and, in the *in vivo* experiments, of fasciculations or contracture. (iii) Partial and transitory antagonism by neostigmine and other anticholinesterasic drugs (Vital Brazil and Barrio, 1950b; Chang, 1960a; Su, 1960; Vital Brazil, 1963; Cheymol *et al.*, 1966). (iv) No influence of Ca^{++} (Vital Brazil and Barrio, 1950b; Chang, 1960a) or of choline (Chang, 1960a; Cheymol *et al.*, 1966) on the block. (v) Synergism with the competitive neuromuscular blocking drugs either in causing neuromuscular block (Schmidt *et al.*, 1964; Cheymol *et al.*, 1966) or in the inhibition of end-plate depolarization by acetylcholine (Peng, 1960). (vi) Inhibition of the effect caused by acetylcholine and by other cholinomimetic substances (Fig. 2) in striated muscles, such as contracture of the frog rectus abdominis (Chang, 1960b; Su, 1960; Cheymol *et al.*, 1966) or the rat isolated and denervated hemidiaphragm (Vital Brazil, 1963; Cheymol *et al.*, 1966), depolarization of the end-plates in the frog sartorius muscle (Peng, 1960) and responses of the cat anterior tibial muscle to intra-arterial injection (Cheymol *et al.*, 1966). However, contracture caused by K^+ either in the frog rectus abdominis (Chang, 1960b; Su, 1960) or in the rat isolated

147

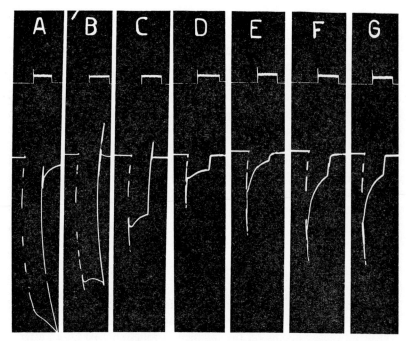

FIG. 1. Isolated rat phrenic nerve-diaphragm. Phrenic nerve stimulation with supramaximal square wave pulses of 0.5 msec and 50 c/sec for periods of 3 seconds timed from 30 to 30 minutes. A, response prior to the addition of *Micrurus lemniscatus* venom to the bath. B, C and D, responses 30, 60 and 90 minutes after addition of 10 mcg/ml of *M. lemniscatus* venom to the bath. Immediately after D, the preparation was repeatedly washed. E, F and G, responses 30, 60 and 90 minutes after D. Tyrode solution, 80 ml bath at 36–37°C, oxygenation with 95% and 5% CO_2. (From Vital Brazil, 1963.)

denervated hemidiaphragm (Vital Brazil, 1963) is not depressed. (vii) Irreversibility or extremely slow and difficult reversibility of the neuro-muscular action. Block due to *B. multicinctus* venom in the phrenic nerve-diaphragm preparation is irreversible (Chang, 1960a) as well its inhibitory effect on acetylcholine contracture in the frog rectus abdominis (Chang, 1960b). On the other hand, the action of coral snake and Formo-san cobra venoms (Vital Brazil, 1963; Su, 1960) is reversible, although only partially, in the rat phrenic nerve-diaphragm (Fig. 1). Their inhibitory effects on acetylcholine contracture of the rat denervated hemidiaphragm and the frog rectus abdominis are also partially reversible. *In vivo*, respir-atory and motor paralysis caused by Indian cobra venom and, therefore, its neuromuscular blocking action, is reversible. Arthus (1910) demon-

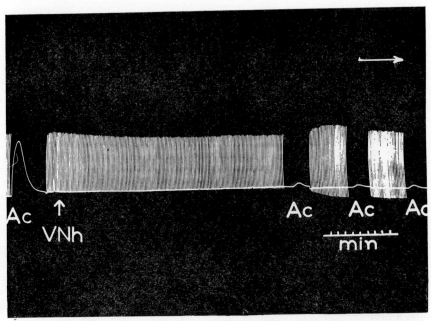

FIG. 2. Isolated and denervated rat hemidiaphragm. Muscle stimulation with square wave pulses of 0.1 c/sec, 0.1–0.2 msec and 60–80 V. The electric stimulation was interrupted for 30 seconds every time acetylcholine was added to the bath. After acetylcholine, the preparation was continuously washed for 9.5 minutes. Acetylcholine (0.75 mcg/ml) was added before and 30, 45 and 60 minutes after the addition (at VNh) of 1 mcg/ml of *Naja haja* venom to the bath. Between each addition of acetylcholine (at Ac) direct stimulation was carried out for the 5 minutes that preceded the chemical stimulation. Tyrode solution, 50 ml bath at 36–37°C oxygenation with 95% O_2 and 5% CO_2. (From Cheymol, Bourillet and Roch-Arveiller, 1966.)

strated such reversibility by injecting cobra antivenom in rabbits already paralysed and by using artificial respiration until recovery of motor function and spontaneous respiration occurred. According to Kellaway (1932) the *in vivo* reversibility of the neuromuscular action of venoms from the Australian snakes *Denisonia superba* and *Notechis scutatus* is more difficult to demonstrate than that of *Naja naja* venom. According to Campbell (1964) respiratory and motor paralysis in humans caused by New Guinea snake (*Oxyuranus scutellatus canni, Acantophis antarcticus rugosus, Pseudechis papuanus*) bites are reversible.

Venoms from *B. multicinctus* (Chang, 1960a) and from *N. naja atra* (Lee and Chang, 1964) depress the release of acetylcholine by nervous

149

impulses. Depression caused by *B. multicinctus* is seen in the rat phrenic nerve-diaphragm preparation only after complete neuromuscular block. This effect is caused by components (β- and γ-bungarotoxins, cardiotoxin) different from those (α-bungarotoxin, cobra neurotoxin) causing inhibition of acetylcholine action on striated muscle (Chang and Lee, 1963, 1966).

Characteristics referred to in (ii), (iii), (v) and (vi) show that Elapidae venom block is of the non-depolarizing type, mostly postjunctional and, in all probability, due to occupation of acetylcholine receptors at the end-plate. Arguments in favor of this last hypothesis are: (a) The protection offered by dimethyltubocurarine against the inhibition, caused by the venoms from *B. multicinctus* (Chang, 1960b) and *N. n. atra* (Su, 1960) on acetylcholine contracture of the frog rectus abdominis. (b) Selective localization of radioiodinated venom from *B. multicinctus* at the end-plate zone of mice diaphragms (Lee and Tseng, 1966). (c) The results of researches with α-bungarotoxin and cobra neurotoxin (Lee and Chang, 1966; Chang and Lee, 1966).

Characteristics referred to in (i) and (vii) differentiate the behavior of venoms from that of curarizing drugs. They seem to indicate a slow diffusion of molecules of the venom active components to the biophase and a firm fixation at the receptor sites.

ENZYMATIC ACTIVITIES

Elapidic, as ophidic venoms in general, are mixtures of proteins, most of which exhibit pharmacologic and/or enzymatic activities. Neuro-muscular effects, in contradistinction to other disturbances, are not caused by the activity of any enzyme present in the venoms. The following are in favor of such a view: (i) Neuromuscular (Vital Brazil, 1963) and toxic (Bragança and Quastel, 1953) activities are not abolished by heating elapidic venoms to 100°C for 15 minutes, whereas all enzymatic, except phospholipasic (Bragança and Quastel, 1953) and endonucleasic (Meldrum, 1965) activities, are destroyed by this treatment. (ii) The phospholipases A are very little toxic (Neumann and Habermann, 1956; Habermann, 1957b). (iii) Toxicity and enzymatic activity determination in components separated by electrophoresis, resin chromatography and other procedures, reveal that the toxicity of elapidic venoms is found in components without enzymatic activities (Radomski and Deichmann, 1958; Doery, 1958; Yang *et al.*, 1960; Master and Srinivasa Rao, 1961). (iv) Cobra neurotoxin, the component responsible for the neuromuscular blocking action of *N. n. atra* venom, is devoid of such enzymatic activities as protease, cholinesterase, phospholipase-A and hyaluronidase (Chang and Lee,

150

1966). (v) Of the four biologically active components separated from the Formosan banded krait venom, one is atoxic and exhibits the cholinesterasic activity of the venom (Chang and Lee, 1963).

POLYPEPTIDIC TOXINS

Elapidic neurotoxins are proteic substances of small molecular weight. They can be grouped (Meldrum, 1965) under the denomination of "polypeptidic toxins" with others, also obtained from venoms, which show similar characteristics such as small molecular weight, generally high isoelectric point and high pharmacologic activity not associated with enzymatic activities of their own.

Neuromuscular and muscular actions of polypeptidic toxins from *B. multicinctus* (a-, β- and γ-bungarotoxins) and from *Naja naja atra* (cobra neurotoxin and cardiotoxin) were studied by Lee and his group (Chang and Lee, 1963; Lee and Tseng, 1966; Lee and Chang, 1966; Chang and Lee, 1966). Their studies confirm and enlarge the above-mentioned findings on the mode of action of elapidic venoms.

a-Bungarotoxin and cobra neurotoxin do not modify the release of acetylcholine by the nervous impulses. Its neuromuscular blocking action is entirely of postjunctional origin. Both these toxins do not change the resting potential of the fiber membrane, or the amplitude and timecourse of the action potential elicited after complete blockade, by direct stimulation of muscle fibers. They progressively diminish the amplitudes of the miniature end-plate potentials, which disappear before completion of neuromuscular block. Neostigmine increases the height and duration of the end-plate potential in preparations submitted to the action of a-bungarotoxin or cobra neurotoxin. The height of some of these e.p.p. reaches again the excitation threshold of the fiber membrane, eliciting propagated responses. Terminal nerve spikes are not affected. Antidromic activities in the phrenic nerve elicited by isolated shocks in preparations maintained in Tyrode solution with neostigmine are abolished by both toxins. All these effects are elicited by d-tubocurarine from which the toxins differ by the slow reversibility of their action (cobra neurotoxin) or by their irreversibility (a-bungarotoxin). Lee and Tseng (1966) observed also that radioiodinated a-bungarotoxin localizes at the end-plate zone of the diaphragm in mice, like drugs that act through combination with the cholinergic receptors in the motor end-plate (Waser, 1959).

β-Bungarotoxin acts solely at a prejunctional site blocking the liberation of acetylcholine whether spontaneous, or caused by a nervous impulse. It does not abolish, however, the terminal nerve spikes. This toxin causes initially an increase in the frequency of the miniature end-plate potentials followed by a decrease without reduction in their amplitude. The miniature end-plate potentials disappear after the end-plate potential. Choline does not antagonize β-bungarotoxin block. The signs and symptoms it elicits in mice are different from those caused by α-bungarotoxin. Initially it produces hyperirritability. Limb paralysis appears at a later stage. Respiration becomes rapid and superficial assuming a gasping character and the animal usually dies suddenly after convulsive movements. γ-Bungarotoxin, and very probably the toxin obtained from *Walterinnesia aegyptia* venom by Mohamed and Zaki (1957), act like β-bungarotoxin.

Cardiotoxin depolarizes the muscle fiber membrane, an effect which is potentiated, but not elicited by phospholipase A from *N. n. atra* venom. It causes contracture of muscle fibers, abolishes the terminal nerve spikes and, consequently, the liberation of acetylcholine. It finally renders the muscle inexcitable.

RESPIRATORY PARALYSIS AND ITS CAUSE

Respiratory paralysis usually is the primary cause of death in envenomation caused by small or moderate doses of elapidic venoms. Large doses can produce severe cardiovascular disturbances, and even death by circulatory failure. The same can occur with small doses of venom from certain species such as *N. nigricollis* (Cheymol *et al.*, 1966) and, in some animal species, such as the cat, with venom from *N. nivea* (Epstein, 1930) and *N. n. atra* (Lee and Peng, 1961). Apart from these cases, artificial respiration allows maintenance of life for many hours after cessation of spontaneous respiration, a fact already described by Brunton and Fayrer (1874). Nevertheless, death usually occurs by circulatory failure before spontaneous respiration returns.

Paralysis is exclusively of peripheral origin. This is proven by the following experimental findings: (i) Rhythmic discharges of action potentials along the phrenic nerve persist after respiratory paralysis in animals—rabbits (Kellaway *et al.*, 1932), dogs (Lee and Peng, 1961; Vick *et al.*, 1965) or cats (Lee and Peng, 1961)—injected with venom from cobra and other Elapidae and kept alive with artificial respiration. (ii) Cessation of artificial respiration for several minutes or administration of 5% CO_2, 95% O_2 increases and prolongs phrenic nerve discharges. (iii) Discharges are synchronous with artificial respiration when the vagi are intact, and become slow and prolonged after vagal section (Lee and Peng, 1961). This last finding shows that the Hering–Breuer reflex is not abolished after cessation of spontaneous respiration.

Elapidic venoms can cause apnea when deposited directly on the floor of the 4th ventricle (Elliot, 1905; Kellaway *et al.*, 1932) or injected in the cisterna magna (Ouyang, 1950). However, studies using I^{131} tagged venom (Lee and Tseng, 1966) reveal an extremely small penetration of its components into the cerebral spinal and brain interstitial fluids, thus explaining the absence of action of these venoms on the respiratory centers when introduced by the usual routes of parenteral administration.

Before the use of electrophysiological methods, opinions varied as to the cause of respiratory paralysis. For instance, Ragotzi (1890); Arthus (1910); Cushny and Yagi (1918); Gautrelet *et al.* (1934) believed it to be due exclusively to "curarization" of the diaphragm. Others, like Rogers (1905) and Elliot (1905) believed that the primary cause was central and due to an hypothetical action of the venom on the respiratory centers. Still others, like Brunton and Fayrer (1874) and Epstein (1930), believed that respiratory paralysis could have both origins.

SIGNS AND SYMPTOMS OF ENVENOMATION

Certain signs and symptoms are common to elapidic envenomation in general whether caused by the bite of American coral snakes (Brazil and Brazil Filho, 1933), Australian (Tisdall and Sewell, 1913) and New Guinea (Campbell 1964), snakes, cobras (Reid, 1964; Ahuja and Singh, 1956) and kraits (Beli Ram, 1923; Ahuja and Singh, 1956) from Asia or African Elapidae (Christensen, 1955). These symptoms and signs are identical to those caused by competitive neuromuscular blocking drugs in man and monkey (Fig. 5) and can be confidently attributed to the curare-like action of elapidae venoms. They consist in (i) Visual disturbances, characterized by blurring of vision and diplopia. (ii) Bilateral lidptosis. (iii) Paralysis of other facial and cervical muscles ("broken-neck syndrome" of Reid) as well as paralysis of pharyngeal and laryngeal muscles. (iv) Loss of muscle power causing incoordinated gait and sometimes inability to stand up. (v) Complete paralysis of the locomotor apparatus and diaphragmatic respiration in severe cases.

6.1.2. HYDROPHIIDAE VENOMS

INCIDENCE

All Hydrophiidae venoms investigated so far show, like those from Elapidae, a potent neuromuscular blocking activity. The venom from the following species were studied: (i) *Enhydrina schistosa* (Fraser and Elliot, 1904; Kellaway *et al.*, 1932; Carey and Wright, 1961; Cheymol *et al.*,

153

1966). (ii) *Lapemis hardwickii* (Cheymol *et al.*, 1966). (iii) *Hydrophis cianocinctus* (Cheymol *et al.*, 1966). (iv) *Laticauda semifasciata* (Tamiya and Arai, 1966).

MUSCULAR ACTION

Direct muscle excitability usually is preserved after complete neuromuscular block caused by Hydrophiidae venom. No fibrillations or contractures are observed in several preparations submitted to their action. The only experimental indication of muscular action was obtained by Carey and Wright (1961) using a special method of administering the venom in the femoral artery of rabbits. Some animals developed irreversible limb paralysis associated with degenerative changes in the muscles. Reid (1961), however, considers the Hydrophiidae venoms primarily myotoxic in man. He observed the following symptoms and signs in cases of bites by these sea snakes: generalized muscular pains, causing resistance to passive movements of limbs and head, trismus, myoglobinuria, hyperpotassemia, and scattered generalized necrosis of muscle fibers (Marsden and Reid, 1961).

CHARACTERISTICS AND MECHANISM OF NEUROMUSCULAR ACTION

The characteristics of neuromuscular action of Hydrophiidae venom (Cheymol *et al.*, 1966, Carey and Wright, 1961) are similar to those described for the Elapidae venom. The block is also of the nondepolarizing type, partially or totally postjunctional. As in Elapidae venom, it is probable that the polypeptidic toxins of Hydrophiidae venoms occupy the cholinergic receptors at the end-plate causing the block. However, a prejunctional mechanism has not been investigated and cannot, therefore, be dismissed.

POLYPEPTIDIC TOXINS

Toxicity of *Enhydrina schistosa* venom and, therefore, its neuromuscular blocking action is associated with a basic, dialyzable toxin, with no phospholipase activity (Carey and Wright, 1961, 1962). On the other hand, Tamiya and Arai (1966) separated from *Laticauda semifasciata* venom two basic crystallized toxins (erabutoxins a and b), with a molecular weight around 7000. These toxins are responsible for 95% of the venom toxicity. They produce an irreversible neuromuscular block in the frog sciatic-sartorius preparations and inhibit irreversibly the acetylcholine contracture

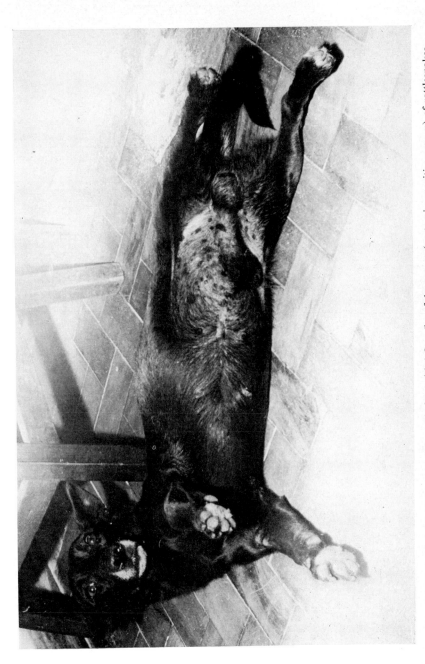

Fig.3. This dog was injected i.m. 1½–2 hours before with 1.5 mg/kg of the venom (crotamine-positive venom) of rattlesnakes from Santiago del Estero, Argentina. It shows the symptoms elicited by crotamine, that is, stiffness of the skeletal muscles, especially of those of the limbs.

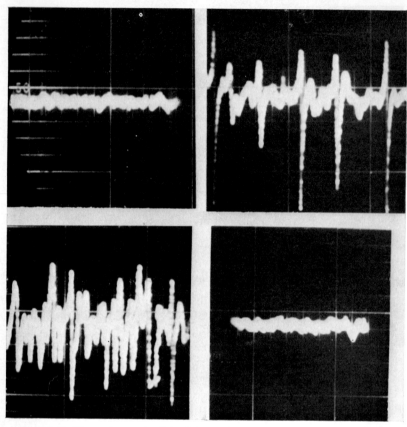

Fig. 4. Oscillograph records of the tibialis anterior muscle action potentials of a dog anesthetized with sodium pentobarbital (30 mg/kg, i.v.). The peroneal nerve was sectioned. Upper left, trace shows absence of muscle action potentials before crotamine administration. Upper right and lower left, trace shows repetitive firing of muscle action potentials following the injection (i.v.) of 2 mg/kg of crotamine. Lower right, trace shows the disappearance of the muscle action potentials following the intra-arterial (arteria tibialis) injection of 3 mg/kg of quinine hydrochloride. (From Vital Brazil, J. Lacaz de Morais and R. Ferri, unpublished.)

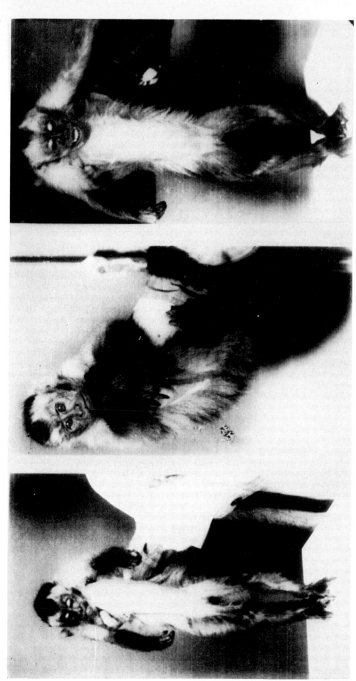

FIG. 5. From left to right: (1) a monkey 15 hours after receiving 100 mcg/kg of crotoxin i.v., (2) the same monkey 30 hours later after nearly complete recovery and (3) another *Cebus* sp. 3 to 5 minutes after being intravenously injected with 300 mcg/kg of gallamina (Flaxedil). Ptosis of the eyelids and of the jaw, paralysis of the muscles of the neck as well as generalized loss of muscle strength occurred in both monkeys. They also became aphonic, could not swallow and presented diaphragm respiration. Consciousness in both animals seemed to be preserved. (From Vital Brazil, Franceschi and Waisbich, 1966.)

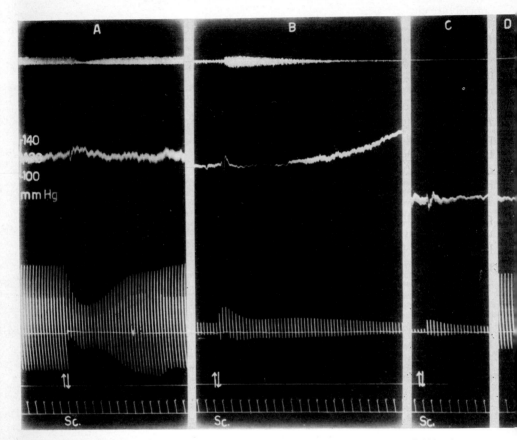

FIG. 6. Cat, 2.4 kg, sodium pentobarbital. Records of respiration, arterial blood pressure and contraction of tibialis anterior muscle. The peroneal nerve was continuously stimulated with supramaximal square wave pulses of 0.2 msec duration delivered at a rate of 6 per minute. Direct stimulation of the muscle (at D) was done after complete neuromuscular block had occurred, with pulses of 100 V, 2 msec, timed 10 seconds apart. Immediately after A, 1 mg/kg of crotoxin was intravenously injected. B and C are records taken 105 and 122 minutes after the administration of crotoxin. At Sc, 0.05 mg/kg of succinylcholine chloride were intravenously injected. Artificial respiration (at C and D) was given after spontaneous respiration had ceased. Time: 30/30 sec.
(From Vital Brazil, 1966.)

of the rectus abdominis of frog although they do not antagonize the contracture elicited by K^+.

RESPIRATORY PARALYSIS

The primary cause of death in Hydrophiidae envenomation is, at least in animals, respiratory paralysis. Differently from cobra venom it causes no hypotension (Cheymol *et al.*, 1966).

Kellaway *et al.* (1932) observed in rabbits injected with venom from *E. schistosa*, and kept alive by artificial respiration, discharge of action potentials along the phrenic nerve after cessation of spontaneous respiration, just as they found in experiments with Elapidae venom. On the other hand, Carey and Wright (1961) showed that in rabbits the injection of very small doses of *E. schistosa* venom in the medulla produces apnoea. This effect, however, is caused by the phospholipase fraction, which is practically atoxic (5% of the venom toxicity) when administered by the usual parenteral routes. The toxic component was inactive by intramedullary injection. These results show the peripheral nature of respiratory paralysis caused by Hydrophiidae venom.

6.1.3. *Crotalus Durissus Terrificus* VENOM

Two regional varieties (Barrio and Vital Brazil, 1951) can be identified in *C. d. terrificus* venom: (i) Type I venom (Brazil, Argentina) induces in an earlier phase spasmodic attacks in mice and rats, and muscular rigidity in dogs (Fig. 3) and, in a later phase, muscular hypotonia and flaccid paralysis. (ii) Type II venom (Brazil) produces only muscular hypotonia and flaccid paralysis. These varieties can be called (Schenberg, 1959) "crotamino-positive" and "crotamino-negative", since their different pharmacological behavior is entirely due (Barrio, 1954) to the presence or absence of crotamine (Gonçalves and Polson, 1947; Gonçalves and Vieira, 1950; Gonçalves, 1956) in the venom.

Crotamine is a polypeptidic toxin, strongly basic, with a minimum molecular weight (Gonçalves *et al.*, 1966) of 6000.

MUSCULAR ACTION

Type I venom (Barrio and Vital Brazil, 1951) and crotamine (Cheymol *et al.*, 1966) act directly on skeletal muscle. Under its influence a single stimulus produces a normal twitch followed by sustained contraction. These, as well as other effects, are antagonized by Ca^{++}, Mg^{++}, quinidine and quinine. High doses of venom, or of crotamine, cause sustained contraction of skeletal muscle and discharge of muscle action potentials (Fig. 4) which are not abolished by curare. Muscular responses to single maximal impulses may be depressed at first, but they are potentiated later on. Both the venom (Moussatché and Vieira, 1953) and crotamine (Cheymol *et al.*, 1966) sensitize the frog rectus abdominis to K^+ and to a much lesser degree to acetylcholine. In the author's opinion the responses under the action of crotamine may be classified in the group of veratrinic responses. Others (Cheymol *et al.*, 1966) do not share this opinion. Only with the elucidation of the crotamine responses, i.e. whether contractures or tetanic, can this question be solved.

NEUROMUSCULAR ACTION

It is difficult to study the blocking action of the whole venom on neuromuscular transmission. When small doses of it are employed, paralysis and block developed after many hours. With larger doses there is severe cardiovascular disturbances as well as depressor effects on skeletal muscles (Cheymol *et al.*, 1966). These effects do not occur when cristalline crotoxin is used. This is the component which is responsible (Vital Brazil *et al.*, 1966) for the paralysis and the block of neuromuscular transmission elicited by the crude venom whether of type I or type II.

CROTOXIN

This toxin, isolated by Slotta and Fraenkel-Conrat (1938), has molecular weight (Gralén and Svedberg, 1938) of 30,000. It exhibits phospholipase and hyaluronidase activities. It is formed (Neumann and Habermann, 1955; Habermann, 1957 a, b) by an acid polypeptidic toxin and a basic and little toxic phospholipase A, possibly in ionic combination. It induces muscular hypotonia and flaccid paralysis. In most animal species the order of involvement of the various groups is identical to that caused by curarizing drugs (Fig. 5). The diaphragm is the last, or one of the last, muscles to become paralysed. In this event, artificial respiration keeps the animals alive for hours. Consciousness seems preserved during paralysis. When administered by intra (cerebro) ventricular route in cats, crotoxin evokes convulsions.

The characteristics of the neuromuscular action of crotoxin are as follows: (i) Onset after a prolonged latent period and slow progress of block. (ii) Partial and evanescent antagonism produced by edrophonium and by succinylcholine. The action of this last compound is reversed during the partial block produced by crotoxin in the cat (Fig. 6). (iii) Shift to the right of the dose-response curve for acetylcholine in the isolated and denervated rat hemidiaphragm. (iv) Extremely slow reversibility of the paralysis and, therefore of the neuromuscular action. The block is of the nondepolarization type, probably predominantly or exclusively post-junctional. The type of the shift produced in the dose response curve for acetylcholine suggests crotoxin blocks the action of that substance by reacting with specific receptors and also at some other point of the muscle fiber membrane. An action on the acetylcholine receptors is also hinted by the similarity of the order of involvement of the various muscular groups in the animals injected with crotoxin and curare.

SIGNS AND SYMPTOMS OF ENVENOMATION

Patients bitten by the South American rattlesnake have shown, in general, the signs and symptoms described for elapidic intoxication, particularly, visual disturbances, bilateral lidptosis, paralysis of other face and neck muscles, difficulty in swallowing and, in some cases, total paralysis. These effects can, confidently, be attributed to the inhibitory action of crotoxin on neuromuscular transmission. Rigidity of skeletal muscles a short time after the bite has been referred to by some patients (Wajchenberg *et al.*, 1954). It could be due to the action of crotamine.

6.2. OTHER VENOMS

Some Indian tribes in the Chocó region, situated in the north-west of Colombia, between the Pacific coast and the Cordillera Occidental, use as an arrow poison the cutaneous secretion of a very small frog *Dendrobates tinctorius* (*Phyllobates bicolor*). This venom, called "kokoi" by the Indians (the same name is given to the frog), possesses high toxicity (Marki and Witkop, 1963). It elicits cardiac and central nervous system actions and it also inhibits neuromuscular transmission and acts directly on skeletal muscles. Using a purified venom, Fries and Duranti (1963) observed in the rat phrenic nerve-diaphragm preparation, abolition of indirect excitability followed by gradual depression of responses to direct excitation and, finally, abolition of direct excitability and strong muscle contracture. On the other hand, Tasaki (1963) observed, in the frog sciatic-sartorius preparation, that the venom does not interfere with conduction of nervous impulses. Spontaneous repetitive discharges of muscle action potentials were registered before complete neuromuscular block. The action of the venom is irreversible.

In Australian coastal waters, from Darwin, in the north, until Melbourne, in the south, lives a small octopus, *Octopus* (*Hapalochlaena*) *maculosus*, whose bite can induce paralysis, and occasionally death, in man (Simon *et al.*, 1964; Trethewie, 1965). Saline extract from the large posterior salivary glands (venom glands) of this octopus causes death in animals by respiratory failure although it also induces severe hypotension. Respiratory paralysis, however, has a central origin since electrical discharges in the phrenic nerve and in the diaphragm disappear simultaneously. In isolated neuromuscular preparations the venom blocks conduction of nervous impulses. There are some hints that it also inhibits neuromuscular transmission. Submitting acetone extracts of *Octopus maculosus* venom glands to one-dimensional paper chromatography, Simon *et al.* (1964) revealed the existence of one substance which produces conduction block and one or two components blocking neuromuscular transmission.

Pharmacological actions elicited by scorpion venoms, either from the various species of Buthidae or Scorpionidae, are very similar. Scorpion venom induces intense local pain and severe autonomic disturbances (hypertension, bradycardia, tachycardia, respiratory and temperature disturbances, diaphoresis, tearing, salivation, diarrhea, etc.). It also elicits effects on the locomotor apparatus such as spasms, fibrillations, tremors and convulsions. In frogs, after the convulsive phase there is complete motor paralysis. It is of peripheral origin, as originally demonstrated by Bert (1865) who performed Claude Bernard's experiment (ligature of the frog limb with exclusion of the sciatic nerve) using scorpion venom. Motor stimulatory effects are also, at least in part, of peripheral origin. In isolated preparations or following the intra-arterial injection of the venom, fibrillations, twitches and, with *Leiurus quinquestriatus* venom, contractures are observed (Houssay, 1919; Del Pozo, 1956; Adam and Weiss, 1959). Potentiation of the maximal twitch is also produced by scorpion venom (Del Pozo, 1956). These effects are abolished by curare (Houssay, 1919; Del Pozo, 1956) and are not observed in denervated muscles (Del Pozo, 1956). Scorpion venom is a potent liberator of acetylcholine from cholinergic nerve endings (Vital Brazil and Neder, 1967). This property explains all effects, described above, observed in isolated neuromuscular preparations or in *in vivo* experiments following intra-arterial injection of the venom. It also explains the decurarizing effect (Del Pozo, 1956) produced by the venom. On the other hand, the mechanism of the neuromuscular block produced by scorpion venoms is unknown. Houssay (1919) believed that the respiratory paralysis in mammals was caused by the block of neuromuscular transmission. However, Del Pozo (1956) kept animals alive after respiratory paralysis by artificial respiration applied by means of rhythmical stimulation of the phrenic nerves. This result precludes participation of neuromuscular block in the genesis of respiratory paralysis.

Bites from the Theraphosidae crab spiders elicit flaccid paralysis in small mammals, reptiles and amphibia. Houssay (1917) verified, in experiments in mice and small frogs, that the theraphose venom produces neuromuscular block which is responsible for the locomotor and respiratory paralysis.

Bee's venom (Hofmann, 1952a) induces, in the rat phrenic nerve-diaphragm preparation, a weak contracture followed by abolition of indirect excitability. The block is irreversible and not antagonized by neostigmine. Direct excitability is present at the moment of the block and abolished later on. Hofmann (1952a) suggests that the respiratory paralysis in bee's venom intoxication is of peripheral origin. In frog muscle the venom produces contracture and loss of excitability (Hofmann, 1952b).

The female wasps of some families of Hymenoptera immobilize their prey—a spider or an insect—with one or more stings. The paralysed animal will be the nourishment for the wasp larvae. The small *Habrobracon juglandis*, a braconid wasp, paralyses larvae of such insects as *Ephestia*, *Plodia* and *Galleria*, by injecting through the sting minute quantities of its very potent venom. The blood that oozes from the stings will nourish the female wasp and their larvae. Beard (1952), using electrophysiological techniques, was able to show that "the paralysis results from impairment of the excitatory process of the body wall musculature" (Beard, 1952). The site of action was therefore considered by Beard to be the neuromuscular junction. Rathmayer (1966) also brought evidence to show that the venom of *Philanthus* (sphecidae) paralyses the honeybee, its prey, by acting peripherally.

ADDENDUM

Since this chapter was written, important advances have been made on the chemistry of the neuromuscular blocking polypeptidic toxins (neurotoxins) from the Elapidae venoms (see the reviews of Lee, 1970 and Jiménez-Porras, 1970 or the original papers of Botes and Strydom, 1969; Chang, 1970; Hamaguchi *et al.*, 1968; Karlsson *et al.*, 1966; Nakai *et al.*, 1970; Narita and Lee, 1970; Porath, 1966; Yang, 1965, 1967; Yang *et al.*, 1968, 1969a, 1969b). Some very interesting papers on the mechanism of action of these Elapidae toxins on neuromuscular junction have also appeared. Tazieff-Depierre and Pierre (1966) investigated the neuromuscular action of toxin α, a neurotoxin of known amino acid composition (see Karlsson *et al.*, 1966) from *Naja nigricollis* venom, on the sciatic-gastrocnemius preparation *in situ* of the cat. The toxin, contrary to the crude venom, produced a reversible blockade and caused only a small fall in the arterial blood pressure. Neostigmine antagonized completely the neuromuscular blocking effect of the toxin and also restored spontaneous respiration. Toxin α inhibited the release of Ca^{++} from the isolated diaphragm of mice caused by acetylcholine (Tazieff-Depierre *et al.*, 1969), an effect also produced by d-tubocurarine. Lester (1970) investigated the effects of toxin T_3 [a neurotoxin of known aminoacid composition isolated from the Thailand cobra (*Naja naja siamensis*) venom] on the frog (*Rana pipiens*) neuromuscular junction. Toxin T_3 caused a decrease in the amplitude of the end-plate potential (e.p.p.) and miniature end-plate potentials (m.e.p.p.s); the quantal composition of the e.p.p. remained unaffected. On the other hand, the toxin blocked the response to micro-iontophoretic applications of acetylcholine and carbachol. The time course of the e.p.p., m.e.p.p. frequency and muscle fiber resting potential were not altered by Toxin T_3. Lester concluded that the toxin acts specifically with low reversibility on the acetylcholine receptor at the skeletal neuromuscular junction. Changeux *et al.* (1970) have reported some experiments carried out with α-bungarotoxin and various preparations derived from the electric organ of *Electrophorus electricus*. The toxin irreversibly blocked the electrical response of the isolated electroplax caused by carbachol. It also irreversibly inhibited the permeability change to sodium ions elicited by carbachol on purified membrane fragments (microsacs) prepared from the electric organ. d-Tubocurarine protected against the irreversible action of α-bungarotoxin. This finding shows that the toxin combines with the same macromolecule as does d-tubocurarine and carbachol, i.e. with the acetylcholine receptor. Finally Changeux and co-workers were able to demonstrate that α-bungarotoxin blocked the binding of radioactive decamethonium to a protein isolated from the electric organ which presents several characteristic properties of the cholinergic receptor macromolecule. β-Bungarotoxin, as it has been already referred to in this chapter, produces complete disappearance of m.e.p.p.s after a period of initial increase in their frequency. Chen and Lee (1970) have found that this toxin induces increase profiles of open synaptic vesicles at the axolemma, accompanied with decreased numbers of synaptic vesicles and subsequently almost complete depletion of the vesicles in the axon terminal of the motor end-plates. An identical depletion of synaptic vesicles in the nerve terminal of the motor end-plates is caused by black widow spider venom (Clark *et al.*, 1970) which initially also produces a great increase in m.e.p.p. frequency (Longenecker *et al.*, 1970). Both results support the idea that the acetylcholine *quanta* are stored in the synaptic vesicles.

According to Rübsamen *et al.* (1971), crotoxin can be resolved by chromatography on carboxymethyl cellulose in the following components: (i) a strongly basic phospholipase A; (ii) an acidic substance, named crotapotin; (iii) a mixture (called fraction III) of phospholipase A, crotapotin and an inactive basic substance present in small amounts only. Phospholipase A (LD_{50} i.v. 0.54 mg/kg in mice) was about five times less toxic than crotoxin (LD_{50} i.v. 0.108 mg/kg). In contrast, the specific enzymatic activity of phospholipase A was about four times higher than that of crotoxin. Crotapotin was devoid of toxicity (LD_{50} i.v. 50 mg/kg in mice) and phospholipase A activity. However, its recombination with phospholipase A increased 12-fold the toxicity and inhibited the *in vitro* enzymatic activity of phospholipase A. The former crotactin, according to Rübsamen and co-workers, was perhaps a complex between high amounts of crotapotin and relatively low amounts of phospholipase A.

Vital Brazil and Excell (1970) investigated the effects of crotoxin and crotactin* on the frog neuromuscular junction using the sciatic-sartorius preparation and, in most experiments, conventional microelectrode techniques. Both toxins caused spontaneous contractions prior to the blockade of neuromuscular transmission. The resting membrane potential was unaffected by the toxins. After an initial reduction in the m.e.p.p. frequency, crotoxin and crotactin evoked "large" spontaneous potentials (mostly 1–5 mV) which were followed by explosive bursts of m.e.p.p.s. Both toxins caused a rapid decrease in the quantal composition of the e.p.p. On the other hand, crotoxin reduced only to a small extent the sensitivity of the end-plate region to carbachol. The action of crotoxin (and crotactin) on the frog neuromuscular junction is, therefore, predominantly prejunctional while, on mammal neuromuscular junction, it seems to act mainly on the postjunctional membrane (Vital Brazil, 1966).

The cause of respiratory paralysis produced by crotoxin was investigated by recording in cats the bioelectric discharges along the phrenic nerve (Vital Brazil *et al.*, in preparation). The paralysis was found to be of peripheral origin as the discharges of action potentials increased in amplitude as respiration became depressed and persisted in cats kept alive with artificial respiration after complete cessation of spontaneous respiration. In consistency with this finding are the results obtained by Lomba (1969)

---

* Crotactin used in this study was obtained from crotoxin by chromatography in amberlite CG-50. It was devoid of phospholipase A activity in *in vitro* and *in vivo* experiments.

who studied the distribution in dogs of ^{131}I-labeled crotoxin. The concentration of the toxin in the cerebrospinal fluid and brain was found to be extremely low while it was relatively high in skeletal muscle.

REFERENCES

ADAM, K. R. and WEISS, C. (1959) Actions of scorpion venom on skeletal muscle. *Brit. J. Pharmacol.* **14**: 334–9.

AHUJA, M. L. and SINGH, G. (1956) Snakebite in India. In: *Venoms*, pp. 341–51. Buckley, E. E. and Porges, N. (eds.). Publ. no. 44 of the American Association for the Advancement of Sciences, Washington, D.C.

ARTHUS, M. (1910) Le venin de cobra est un curare. *Arch. Internat. Physiol.* **10**: 161–91.

ARTHUS, M. (1912a) De la spécificité des sérums antivenimeux. Sérum anticobraique et venins d'hamadryas (*Naja bungarus*) et de krait (*Bungarus coeruleus*). *Arch. Internat. Physiol.* **11**: 265–84.

ARTHUS, M. (1912b) Physiologie comparée des intoxications par les venins de serpents. *Arch. Internat. Physiol.* **11**: 285–316.

BARRIO, A. (1954) Estudio electroforetico del veneno de serpiente de cascabel. *Ciencia e Investigatión.* **10**: 368–70.

BARRIO, A. and VITAL BRAZIL, O. (1951) Neuromuscular action of the *Crotalus terrificus terrificus* (Laur.) poisons. *Acta Physiol. Latinoamericana* **1**: 291–308.

BEARD, R. L. (1952) *The Toxicology of Habrobracon Venom: A Study on a Natural Insecticide.* Connecticut Agricultural Experimental Station, New Haven, Bull. no. 562.

BELI RAM, M. B. (1923) Two fatal cases of snake bite. *The Indian Medical Gazette* **58**: 585–6.

BERT, P. (1865) Contribution à l'étude des venins: venin de scorpion. *C.R. Soc. Biol.* (4) D, pp. 136–9.

BOTES, D. P. and STRYDOM, D. J. (1969) A neurotoxin, toxin alfa, from Egyptian cobra (*Naja haje haje*) venom. *J. Biol. Chem.* **244**: 4147–57.

BRAGANÇA, B. M. and QUASTEL, J. H. (1953) Enzyme inhibitions by snake venoms. *Biochem. J.* **53**: 88–102.

BRAZIL, V. (1914) *La Défense contre l'Ophidisme*, pp. 148–279. Pocai-Weiss & Co., São Paulo.

BRAZIL, V. and BRAZIL FILHO, V. (1933) *Do envenenamento Elapineo em Confronto com o Choque Anaphylàtico.* Bol. Inst. Vital Brazil, no. 15.

BRAZIL, V. and PESTANA, B. R. (1909) Nova contribuição ao estudo do envenenamento ophídico. V. Ação physiologica. *Rev. Med. de S. Paulo* **12**: 415–25.

BRUNTON, T. L. and FAYRER, J. (1874) On the nature and physiological action of the poison of *Naja tripudians* and other Indian venomous snakes. *Proc. Roy. Soc.* (*London*) **22**: 68–133.

CAMPBELL, C. H. (1964) Venomous snake bite in Papua and its treatment with tracheotomy, artificial respiration and antivenom, *Trans. Roy. Soc. Trop. Med. Hyg.* **58**: 263–73.

CAREY, J. E. and WRIGHT, E. A. (1961) The site of action of the venom of the sea snake *Enhydrina schistosa. Trans. Roy. Soc. Trop. Med. Hyg.* **55**: 153–60.

CAREY, J. E. and WRIGHT, E. A. (1962) Studies on the fractions of the venom of the sea snake *Enhydrina schistosa. Australian J. Exper. Biol. Med. Sci.* **40**: 427–36.

CHANG, C. C. (1960a) Studies on the mechanism of curare-like action of *Bungarus multicinctus* venom. 1. Effect on the phrenic nerve-diaphragm preparation of the rat. *J. Formosan Med. Ass.* **59**: 315–22.

CHANG, C. C. (1960b) Studies on the mechanism of curare-like action of *Bungarus multicinctus* venom. II. Effect on response of rectus abdominis muscle of the frog to acetylcholine. *J. Formosan Med. Ass.* **59**: 416–26.

CHANG, C. C. (1970) Immunochemical studies on fluoresceinthiocarbamyl and reduced s-carboxymethylated cobrotoxin. *J. Biochem. (Tokyo)* **67** (3): 343–52.

CHANG, C. C. and LEE, C. Y. (1963) Isolation of neurotoxins from the venom of *Bungarus multicinctus* and their modes of neuromuscular blocking action. *Arch. Int. Pharmacodyn.* **144**: 241–57.

CHANG, C. C. and LEE, C. Y. (1966) Electrophysiological study of the neuromuscular blocking action of cobra neurotoxin. *Brit. J. Pharmacol.* **28**: 172–81.

CHANGEUX, J. P., KASAI, M. and LEE, C. Y. (1970) Use of snake venom toxin to characterize the cholinergic receptor protein. *Proc. Nat. Acad. Sci., U.S.A.* **67** (3): 1241–7.

CHEN, L. and LEE, C. Y. (1970) Ultrastructural changes in the motor nerve terminals caused by beta-bungarotoxin. *Virchows Arch. Abt. B Zellpath.* **6**: 318–25.

CHEYMOL, J., BOURILLET, F. and ROCH, M. (1966) Action neuromusculaire des venins des quelques *Crotalidae, Elapidae* et *Hydrophiidae. Mem. Inst. Butantan, Simp. Internac.* **33**: 541–54.

CHRISTENSEN, P. A. (1955) *South African Snake Venoms and Antivenoms.* The South African Institute for Medical Research, Johannesburg, South Africa.

CLARK, A. W., MAURO, A., LONGENECKER, H. E. and HURLBUT, W. P. (1970) Effects of black widow spider venom on the frog neuromuscular junction. Effects on the fine structure of the frog neuromuscular junction. *Nature* **225** (5234): 703–5.

CUSHNY, A. R. and YAGI, S. (1918) On the action of cobra venom, Parts I and II. *Phil. Trans. R. Soc. (London),* Ser. B, **208**: 1–36.

DEL POZO, E. C. (1956) Mechanism of pharmacological actions of scorpion venoms, In: *Venoms,* pp. 123–9. Buckley, E. E. and Porges, N. (eds.). Publ. no. 44 of the American Association for the Advancement of Sciences, Washington, D.C.

DOERY, H. M. (1958) The separation and properties of the neurotoxins from the venom of the tiger snake *Notechis scutatus scutatus. Biochem. J.* **70**: 535–43.

ELLIOTT, R. H. (1905) A contribution to the study of the action of Indian cobra venom. *Phil. Trans. Roy. Soc. (London),* Ser. B, **197**: 361–4.

EPSTEIN, D. (1930) The pharmacology of the venom of the Cape cobra (*Naja flava*). *Quart. J. Exper. Physiol.* **20**: 7–19.

FRASER, T. R. and ELLIOT, R. H. (1904) Contributions to the study of the action of sea-snake venoms. *Proc. Roy. Soc. (London)* **74**: 104–9.

FRASER, T. R. and GUNN, J. A. (1909) Quoted by EPSTEIN, D. (1930). In: The pharmacology of the venom of the Cape cobra (*Naja flava*). *Quart. J. Exper. Physiol.* **20**: 7–19.

FRIES and DURANTI (1963) Quoted by MARKI, F. and WITKOP, B. (1963). In: The venom of the Colombian arrow poison frog *Phyllobates bicolor. Experientia* **19**: 329–38.

GAUTRELET, J., HALPERN, N. and CORTEGGIANI, E. (1934) Du mécanisme d'action des doses physiologiques de venin de cobra sur la circulation, la respiration et l'excitabilité neuro-musculaire. *Arch. Internat. Physiol.* **38**: 293–352.

GONÇALVES, J. M. (1956) Purification and properties of crotamine. In: *Venoms,* pp. 261–74. Buckley, E. E. and Porges, N. (eds.). Publ. no. 44 of the American Association for the Advancement of Sciences, Washington, D.C.

GONÇALVES, J. M., GIGLIO, J. R. and MANTOVANI, B. (1966) *Crotamine.* Abstracts of International Symposium on Animal Venoms, São Paulo, 17 a 23 de julho.

GONÇALVES, J. M. and POLSON, A. (1947) The electrophoretic analysis of snake venom. *Arch. Biochem.* **13**: 253–9.

GONÇALVES, J. M. and VIEIRA, L. G. (1950) Estudos sôbre venenos de serpentes brasileiras. I. Análise Electroforética. *An. Acad. Bras. Cienc.* **22**: 141–9.

163

GRALÉN, N. and SVEDBERG, T. (1938) The molecular weight of crotoxin. *Biochem. J.* **32**: 1375–7.

HABERMANN, E. (1957a) Gewinnung und Eigenschaften von Crotactin, Phospholipase A, Crotamin und "Toxin III" aus dem Gift der brasilianischen Klapperschlange. *Biochem. Zeitschr.* **329**: 405–15.

HABERMANN, E. (1957b) Zur Pharmakologie des Giftes der brasilianischen Klapperschlange. *Arch. Exper. Path. u. Pharmakol.* **232**: 244–5.

HAMAGUCHI, K., IKEDA, K. and LEE, C. Y. (1968) Optical rotatory dispersion and circular dichroism of neurotoxins isolated from the venom of *Bungarus multicinctus.* *J. Biochem. (Tokyo)* **64** (4): 503–6.

HOFMANN, H. T. (1952a) Über neuromuskuläre von Bienengift am isolierten Rattenzwechfell. *Arch. Exper. Path. u. Pharmakol.* **216**: 250–7.

HOFMANN, H. T. (1952b) Über neuromuskuläre Wirkungen von Bienengift am Skeletmuskel des Frosches. *Arch. Exper. Path. u. Pharmakol.* **214**: 523–33.

HOUSSAY, B. A. (1917) Datos complementarios sobre la acción fisiologica del veneno de las a rañas Theraphose. *La Prensa Medica Argentina* **4**: 18–19.

HOUSSAY, B. A. (1919) Action physiologique du venin des scorpions (*Buthus quinquestriatus* et *Tytius bahiensis*). *J. Physiol. Pathol. Générale* **18**: 305–17.

HOUSSAY, B. A., NEGRETE, J. and MAZZOCCO, P. (1922) Acción de los venenos de serpientes sobre el nervio y musculo aislados. *Rev. Asoc. Med. Arg.* **35**: 185–200.

HOUSSAY, B. A. and PAVE, S. (1922) Acción curarizante de los venenos de serpientes. I. Acción curarizante sôbre la rana. *Rev. Asoc. Med. Arg.* **35**: 166–84.

JIMÉNEZ-PORRAS, J. M. (1970) Biochemistry of snake venoms. *Clin. Toxicol.* **3** (3): 389–431.

KARLSSON, E., EAKER, D. L. and PORATH, J. (1966) Purification of a neurotoxin from the venom of *Naja nigricollis*. *Biochim. Biophys. Acta* **127**: 505–20.

KELLAWAY, C. H. (1932) The peripheral action of the Australian snake venoms. 3. The reversibility of the curare-like action. *Australian J. Exper. Biol. Med. Sci.* **10**: 195–202.

KELLAWAY, C. H. CHERRY, R. O. and WILLIAMS, F. E. (1932) The peripheral action of the Australian snake venoms. 2. The curare-like action in mammals. *Australian J. Exper. Biol. Med. Sci.* **10**: 181–94.

KELLAWAY, C. H. and HOLDEN, H. F. (1932) The peripheral action of the Australian snake venoms. 1. The curare-like action in frogs. *Australian J. Exper. Biol. Med. Sci.* **10**: 167–79.

LEE, C. Y. (1970) Elapid neurotoxins and their mode of action. *Clin. Toxicol.* **3** (3): 457–72.

LEE, C. Y. and CHANG, C. C. (1964) Quoted by MELDRUM, B. S. (1965b) In: The actions of snake venoms on nerve and muscle. The pharmacology of phospholipase A and of polypeptide toxins. *Pharmacol. Rev.* **17**: 393–445.

LEE, C. Y. and CHANG, C. C. (1966) Modes of actions of purified toxins from elapid venoms on neuromuscular transmission. *Mem. Inst. Butantan, Simp. Internac.* **33**: 555–72.

LEE, C. Y. and PENG, M. T. (1961) An analysis of the respiratory failure produced by the Formosan elapid venoms. *Arch. Int. Pharmacodyn.* **133**: 180–92.

LEE, C. Y. and TSENG, L. F. (1966) Distribution of *Bungarus multicinctus* venom following envenomation. *Toxicon* **3**: 281–90.

LESTER, H. A. (1970) Postsynaptic action of cobra toxin at the myoneural junction. *Nature* **227**(5259): 727–8.

LOMBA, M. G. (1969) Estudos sôbre a distribuição e excreção da crotoxina-^{131}I em cães. Doctoral thesis, State University of Campinas, Campinas, São Paulo, Brazil.

LONGENECKER, H. E., HURLBUT, W. P., MAURO, A. and CLARK, A. W. (1970) Effect of black widow spider venom on the frog neuromuscular junction. Effects on end-plate potential, miniature end-plate potential and nerve terminal spike. *Nature* **225** (5234): 701–3.

MARKI, F. and WITKOP, B. (1963) The venom of the Colombian arrow poison frog *Phyllobates bicolor. Experientia* **19**: 329–38.

MARSDEN, A. T. H. and REID, H. A. (1961) Pathology of sea-snake poisoning. *Brit. Med. J.* **1**: 1290–3.

MASTER, W. P. and SRINIVASA RAO, S. (1961) Identification of enzymes and toxins in venoms of Indian cobra and Russell's viper after starch gel electrophoresis. *J. Biol. Chem.* **236**: 1986–90.

MELDRUM, B. S. (1965) The actions of snake venoms on nerve and muscle. The pharmacology of phospholipase A and of polypeptide toxins. *Pharmacol. Rev.* **17**: 393–445.

MOHAMED, A. H. and ZAKI, O. (1957) Effect of the black snake toxin on the gastrocnemius-sciatic preparation. *J. Exper. Biol.* **35**: 20–26.

MOUSSATCHÉ, H. and VIEIRA, G. D. (1953) Sôbre o mecanismo da contratura produzida pelo veneno de cascavel (*Crotalus terrificus terrificus*). *An. Acad. Brasil. Cienc.* **25**: 249–58.

NAKAI, K., NAKAI, C., SASAKI, T., KAKIUCHI, K. and HAYASHI, K. (1970) Purification and some properties of Toxin A from the venom of the Indian cobra. *Naturwissenschaften* **57** (8): 387–8.

NARITA, K. and LEE, C. Y. (1970) The amino acid sequence of cardiotoxin from Formosan cobra (*Naja naja atra*) venom. *Biochem. Biophys. Research Commun.* **41** (2): 339–43.

NEUMANN, W. P. and HABERMANN, E. (1955) Über Crotactin, das Haupttoxin des Giftes der brasilianischen Klapperschlange (*Crotalus terrificus terrificus*). *Biochem. Zeitschr.* **327**: 170–85.

NEUMANN, W. P. and HABERMANN, E. (1956) Paper electrophoresis separation of pharmacologically and biochemically active components of bee and snake venoms. In: *Venoms*, pp. 171–4. Buckley, E. E. and Porges, N. (eds.). Publ. no. 44 of the American Association for the Advancement of Sciences, Washington, D.C.

OUYANG, C. (1950) Quoted by LEE, C. Y. and PENG, M. T. (1961). In: An analysis of the respiratory failure produced by the Formosan elapid venoms. *Arch. Int. Pharmacodyn.* **133**: 180–92.

PENG, M. T. (1960) Effect of Formosan snake venoms on the depolarizing action of acetylcholine at motor endplate. *J. Formosan Med. Ass.* **59**: 1073–82.

PORATH, J. (1966) Some preparation methods based on molecular size and charge and their application to purification of polypeptides and proteins in snake venoms. *Mem. Inst. Butantan, Symp. Internac.* **33** (2): 379–87.

OMSKI, J. L. and DEICHMANN, W. B. (1958) The relationship of certain enzymes in cobra and rattlesnake venom to the mechanism of action of these venoms. *Biochem. J.* **70**: 293–7.

OTZI, V. (1890) Ueber die Wirkung des Giftes der *Naja tripudans. Arch. für Path. Anat. u. Physiol. u. für Klin. Med.* **122**: 201–5.

RATHMAYER, W. (1966) The effect of the poison of spider and diggerwasps on their prey (Hymenoptera: *Pompilidae, Sphecidae*) *Mem. Inst. Butantan* **33**: 651–8.

REID, H. A. (1961) Myoglobinuria and sea-snake bite poisoning. *Brit. Med. J.* **1**: 1284–9.

REID, H. A. (1964) Cobra-bites. *Brit. Med. J.* **2**: 540–5.

ROGERS, L. (1905) The physiological action and antidotes of Colubrine and Viperine snake venoms. *Phil. Trans. Roy. Soc. (Lond.)*, Ser. B, **197**: 123–91.

RÜBSAMEN, K., BREITHAUPT, H. and HABERMANN, E. (1971) Biochemistry and pharmacology of the crotoxin complex. I. Subfractional and recombination of the crotoxin complex. (In the press.)

SCHENBERG, S. (1959) Análise da crotamina no veneno individual de cascaveis recebidas pelo Instituto Butantan. *Mem. Inst. Butantan* **29**: 213–26.

SCHMIDT, J. L., GOODSELL, E. B., BRONDYK, H. D., KUETER, K. E. and RICHARDS, R. K. (1964) The prolonged effect of cobra venom on the sensitivity to *d*-tubocurarine. *Arch. Int. Pharmacodyn.* **147**: 569–75.

SIMON, S. E., CAIRNCROSS, K. D., SATCHELL, D. G., GAY, W. S. and EDWARDS, S. (1964) The toxicity of *Octopus maculosus Hoyle* venom. *Arch. Int. Pharmacodyn.* **149**: 318–29.

SLOTTA, C. H. and FRAENKEL-CONRAT, H. L. (1938) Estudos quimicos sôbre os venenos ofídicos. 4. Purificação e cristaliza ção de veneno da cobra cascavel. *Mem. Inst. Butantan* **12**: 505–12.

SU, C. (1960) Mode of curare-like action of cobra venom. *J. Formosan Med. Ass.* **59**: 1083–91.

TAMIYA, N. and ARAI, H. (1966) Studies on sea-snake venoms. *Biochem. J.* **99**: 624–30.

TASAKI, I. Quoted by MARKI, F. and WITKOP, B. (1963). In: The venom of the Colombian arrow poison frog *Phyllobates bicolor. Experientia* **19**: 329–38.

TAZIEFF-DEPIERRE, F. and PIERRE, J. (1966) Action curarisante de la toxine alfa de *Naja nigricollis. C.R. Acad. Sci. Paris* **263**: Série D, pp. 1785–8.

TAZIEFF-DEPIERRE, F., CZAJKA, M. and LOWAGIE, C. (1969) Action pharmacologique de fractions pures de venin de *Naja nigricollis* et libération de calcium dans les muscles striés. *C.R. Acad. Sci. Paris* **268**: Série D, pp. 2511–14.

TISDALL, H. F. and SEWELL, J. E. (1913) Treatment anti-venin 24 hours after bite by tiger snake. *M.J. Australia* **1**: 604–5.

TRETHEWIE, E. R. (1965) Pharmacological effects of the venom of the common octopus *Hapalochlaena maculosa. Toxicon* **3**: 55–59.

VICK, J. A., CIUCHTA, H. P. and POLLEY, E. H. (1965) The effect of cobra venom on the respiratory mechanism of the dog. *Arch. Int. Pharmacodyn.* **153**: 424–9.

VITAL BRAZIL, O. (1963) *Ação Neuromuscular da Peçonha de Micrurus.* Tese de Doutoramento apresentada à Faculdade de Medicina da Universidade de São Paulo, São Paulo, Brasil, 77 pp.

VITAL BRAZIL, O. (1966) Pharmacology of crystalline crotoxin. II. Neuromuscular blocking action. *Mem. Inst. Butantan, Simp. Internac.* **33**: 981–92.

VITAL BRAZIL, O. and BARRIO, A. (1950a) Acción curarizante de las ponzoñas de Elapidae. I. Fenomenos de inhibicion y facilitacion en la union neuromuscular. *La Prensa Medica Argentina* **37**: 1249–56.

VITAL BRAZIL, O. and BARRIO, A. (1950b) Acción curarizante de las ponzoñas de Elapidae. II. Efectos de algunos antagonistas del curare. *La Prensa Medica Argentina* **37**: 1313–18.

VITAL BRAZIL, O. and EXCELL, B. J. (1970) Action of crotoxin and crotactin from the venom of *Crotalus durissus terrificus* (South American rattlesnake) on the frog neuromuscular junction. *J. Physiol.* **212**: 34–35P.

VITAL BRAZIL, O., FRANCESCHI, J. P. and WAISBICH, E. (1966) Pharmacology of crystalline crotoxin. I. Toxicity. *Mem. Inst. Butantan, Simp. Internac.* **33**: 973–92.

VITAL BRAZIL, O. and NEDER, A. C. (1967) Liberação farmacológica de acetilcolina. *Ciência e Cultura* **19**: 404.

WAJCHENBERG, L., SESSO, J. and INAGUE, T. (1954) Feições clínico-laboratoriais do envenenamento crotálico humano. *Rev. Ass. Med. Brasil.* **1**: 179–93.

WASER, P. G. (1959) Curare and cholinergic receptors in the motor endplate. In: *Curare and Curare-like Agents*, p. 219. Bovet, D., Bovet-Nitti, F. and Marini-Bettòlo, G. B. (eds.). Amsterdam.

YANG, C. C. (1965) Crystallization and properties of cobrotoxin from Formosan cobra venom. *J. Biol. Chem.* **240**: 1616–18.

YANG, C. C. (1967) The disulfide bonds of cobrotoxin and their relationship to lethality. *Biochim. Biophys. Acta* **133**: 346–55.

YANG, C. C., CHANG, C. C., HAYASHI, K., SUSUKI, T., IKEDA, K. and HAMAGUCHI, K.

(1968) Optical rotatory dispersion and circular dichroism of cobrotoxin. *Biochim. Biophys. Acta* **168**: 373–6.

YANG, C. C., CHANG, C. C., HAYASHI, K. and SUSUKI, T. (1969a) Amino acid composition and end group analysis of cobrotoxin. *Toxicon* **7**: 43–47.

YANG, C. C., KAO, L. C. and CHIU, W. C. (1960) Biochemical studies on the snake venoms. VIII. Electrophoretic studies on banded krait (*Bungarus multicinctus*) venom and the relation of toxicity with enzyme activities. *J. Biochem.* **48**: 714–22.

YANG, C. C., YANG, H. J. and HUANG, J. S. (1969b) The amino acid sequence of cobrotoxin. *Biochim. Biophys. Acta* **188**: 65–77.

CHAPTER 7

THE ACTION OF BOTULINUM TOXIN ON NEUROMUSCULAR TRANSMISSION

A. S. V. Burgen

London

THE toxin is an exotoxin produced by the saprophytic bacterium, *Clostridium botulinum*. Five major strains A, B, C, D, E are known which differ in the immunological characteristics of the toxins produced, although these do not differ qualitatively in their pharmacological effects. Culture on tryptic digest or casein media yields filtrates containing more than 10^6 mouse LD_{50} per ml. Toxins may be readily purified by acid precipitation; type A toxin has been obtained crystalline, and the others in apparently pure but amorphous form. All the toxins are proteins apparently composed solely of normal amino acids; their molecular weights are uncertain, initially a value of 1,000,000 was given for type A but subsequent evidence has suggested that this apparent value is due to aggregation of subunits of molecular weight $\sim 60,000$. These characteristics probably hold for the other toxin types as well.

The lethal dose of pure type A toxin for the mouse is 4.5×10^{-12} g ($\sim 2 \times 10^{-10}$ g/kg); the time taken for botulinum toxin to produce its effects depends on dose; at the LD_{50} level the mean time to death is about 24 hours and is approximately halved with tenfold increase in the dose. The minimum latency with large doses is 10–20 minutes.

There are considerable species differences in susceptibility to the toxins. The mouse, guinea pig and rabbit are about equally susceptible to all five types, but the rat is sensitive to types A and C but relatively resistant in types B and D. Dog, cat and the hen are highly resistant to type D. Human sensitivities are not known but reported cases have been due almost entirely to types A, B and E.

Type A and B toxins are rapidly inactivated by heating at over 80°C, but types C and D are more heat resistant. Botulinum toxin is very poorly

169

absorbed from the alimentary tract but due to its formidable toxicity a lethal dose is readily ingested (Lamanna, 1959; van Heyningen, 1950; Wright, 1955 and Stevenson, 1962).

Early workers with botulinum noted the extraordinary parallelism between the chemical mediator acting at synaptic junctions and the susceptibility of these junctions to the toxin—only cholinergic synapses being affected (Edmunds and Long, 1923; Dickson and Shevky, 1923 a and b). Ambache (1949, 1951) was unable to show block of sympathetic responses in the eye or nictitating membrane even with greatly elevated doses of toxin. Until recently the specificity for the cholinergic system was unquestioned but Rand and Whaler (1965) have claimed to find effects on the sympathetic fibers to the piloerector muscles, vas deferens and the small intestine. Even allowing this botulinum toxin is an unusually specific pharmacological agent.

The actions of the toxin may be studied *in vivo*, in which case the toxin is injected directly into the muscle to be studied in small distributed doses and the animal is protected from general effects by intravenous antitoxin (Ambache, 1949, 1951; Guyton and MacDonald, 1947). Alternatively the effect of the toxin may be studied *in vitro* on the phrenic-nerve diaphragm preparation (Burgen, 1949) or the guinea-pig serratus (Brooks, 1954, 1956), intercostal muscle (Elmqvist and Quastel, 1965a) or other mammalian nerve–muscle preparations. In the *in vitro* preparation following the addition of 1–5000 mouse LD_{50}/ml (~ 5–25×10^{-9} g/ml) type A toxin no changes are evident for 30–40 minutes following which there is a progressive decrease in the contractile response to nerve stimulation leading to complete block in 1–2 hours; the response to direct excitation of the muscle fibers remains unchanged. Similar results are obtained if the surface electrogram is studied (Brooks, 1954). When single fiber responses are observed no change is seen until late in the latent period when a progressive increase in the stimulus-response interval occurs passing abruptly into block. For a short period following the onset of block, conduction can be restored by a second shock delivered after 1–10 msec (Brooks, 1954), by doubling the Ca concentration or by the addition of tetraethylammonium (Thesleff, 1960). No effects of the toxin can be shown on the nerve trunk (Burgen *et al.*, 1949) but the output of acetylcholine from the nerve terminals on stimulation is reduced to less than 20% of that before poisoning. On the other hand, the sensitivity of the muscle to injected acetylcholine is not affected at all (Burgen *et al.*, 1949; Brooks, 1954).

Intracellular electrode studies have shown that when block has just developed the end-plate potential is still present but is subthreshold

(Brooks, 1956); it is e.p.p. summation that leads to temporary recovery with paired shocks. With further progress of poisoning the e.p.p. rapidly declines in size and finally is not detectable. In a normal muscle spontaneous miniature end-plate potentials (m.e.p.p.s) are continually being fired off and the frequency of these falls off in parallel with the decline in the e.p.p. but the mean size and distribution of sizes of the m.e.p.p.s are unaffected (Brooks, 1956; Thesleff, 1960). Following a brief tetanus the frequency of m.e.p.p. discharge is greatly increased; this effect is also depressed and finally extinguished by the toxin. That acetylcholine is still present in the terminals and can be released at a time when transmission is completely blocked is shown by two observations, firstly, slight damage to the nerve endings by pressure of a microelectrode leads to showers of m.e.p.p.s being set up (Thesleff, 1960) and secondly, stimulation of the muscle by massive shocks in the bath can lead to a release of acetylcholine comparable in amount to that released before poisoning (Brooks, 1954).

Following chronic poisoning *in vivo* the changes in the neuromuscular responses are identical to those in denervation. The muscle fibrillates and wastes (Guyton and MacDonald, 1947; Josefsson and Thesleff, 1961) and instead of a normal sensitivity to acetylcholine confined to applications made at the end-plate and its vicinity, the fiber becomes supersensitive and responds nearly equally to application of acetylcholine made anywhere along the length of the fiber (Thesleff, 1960). Perhaps the most striking phenomenon concerns reinnervation. If the cut end of a motor nerve is grafted into a normal muscle no innervation from the foreign motor fibers occurs, on the other hand, such a graft applied to a muscle whose intrinsic motor supply has degenerated leads to reinnervation. Motor nerve grafts take in botulinum-poisoned muscles as well as in denervated muscles and when recovery from poisoning occurs many fibers are doubly innervated with two spatial separated end-plates (Hofmann *et al.*, 1964).

In vivo the effects of botulinum toxin are very long-lasting and full recovery which eventually occurs may take 6–12 months (Guyton and MacDonald, 1947; Josefsson and Thesleff, 1961); this contrasts with the much more rapid recovery after nerve crushing. At no time in the poisoning are histological changes observable at the end-plate either with the light microscope or the electron microscope (Thesleff, 1960; Brooks, 1964); the muscle fibers show the characteristic atrophic changes of denervation.

The characteristics of botulinum poisoning of the neuromuscular junction leave no doubt that this is a pure presynaptic block with no direct effects on the end-plate. The block could be due to block of conduction in the terminal segment of the motor nerve or the end ramification or to an alteration in the release process, or to a reduction in synthesis or storage of acetylcholine. Attempts to demonstrate an inhibition of synthesis of acetylcholine have failed (Burgen *et al.*, 1949), but in any case either of these mechanisms is made improbable by the finding that the amplitude of the m.e.p.p.s is unaffected, whereas we should expect m.e.p.p. amplitude to decrease and m.e.p.p. frequency to be unaltered if synthesis was reduced [see, for instance, the effects of hemicholinium (Elmqvist and Quastel, 1965b)]; with impaired storage the effects should be similar, but m.e.p.p. frequency might even be increased. The fact that the m.e.p.p. frequency is so grossly affected is not consistent with a block of terminal conduction but is consistent with an interference with release. This matter could be finally settled by the techniques recently described by Katz and Miledi (1965a, b) in which it is possible to measure conduction of impulses in the terminal nerve fibers and to measure very localized release of acetylcholine. By the same technique it was possible to show that after nerve conduction was blocked with tetrodotoxin it was still possible to release acetylcholine by local depolarization. The continued release of acetylcholine by massive stimulation of the poisoned muscle is probably by this mechanism; it would be interesting to have confirmation of this by direct test. One of the unusual features of botulinum poisoning is the long latency before effects are produced and also the very high temperature coefficient of poisoning (Burgen *et al.*, 1949; Ambache and Martins-Ferreira, 1952). This can be judged by the effects on frogs which are very insensitive at a laboratory temperature of 17° but much more sensitive at 30°. This behavior might be construed as being in opposition to the postulate that the delay is due to slow diffusion of this macromolecule to the site of action, but diffusion does not necessarily have the $Q_{10} = 1.3$ found in free solution if it is occurring through a very restrictive medium such as the cell membrane. However, a major contribution of diffusion to the delay is made much less likely by the finding that removal of toxin from the muscle during the latent period of its action fails to prevent eventual paralysis (Burgen *et al.*, 1949). One can only speculate that the delay is due to the time taken after fixation of the toxin during which a metabolic process reaches threshold or during which the toxin undergoes a conformation change to an active state. The selectivity of the toxin for cholinergic endings is an interesting problem and one can visualize such a process occurring as a recognition of a somatotype surface comparable to the cell recognition that occurs in organogenesis and reassembly of disaggregated cell suspensions.

172

This brings us to the fascinating problem of receptor dispersal and hypersensitivity. The acetylcholine receptors on embryonic muscle before innervation have the dispersed pattern and localization of the receptors and induction of the end-plate follow innervation. It is possible that the inductive effect of innervation is due to release of transmitter but perhaps more plausible that it is a recognition induction; the effects of botulinum toxin would then be due to combination with the nerve endings and block of the recognition signal which is probably humoral (Grobstein, 1965). Since the toxin can evidently block the spontaneous release of acetylcholine from the ending, it may also block the release of such a humoral agent. A quite extraordinary feature of toxin action is its great persistence referred to above. It would be surprising to find the survival of a foreign protein for so long and it is therefore important to find out whether the toxin really does survive or whether it is the induced change that is so prolonged. Recently it has been found possible to label toxin by cross linkage to ferritin without loss of toxicity (Zacks *et al.*, 1962). This procedure offers some hope of settling this problem.

Finally we cannot conclude this review without pointing out the very high potency of the toxin. The toxic dose for a mouse is only about 4×10^7 molecules. If one estimates the number of muscle fibers in a mouse as $\sim 10^6$ this allows only 40 molecules per ending not taking into account the uptake of the toxin by other cholinergic fibers.

REFERENCES

AMBACHE, N. (1949) The peripheral action of *Cl. botulinum* toxin. *J. Physiol.* **108**: 127–41.

AMBACHE, N. (1951) A further survey of the action of *Clostridium botulinum* toxin upon different types of autonomic nerve fibre. *J. Physiol.* **113**: 1–16.

AMBACHE, N. and MARTINS-FERREIRA, H. (1952) Paralysis of the discharge in *Electrophorus electricus* produced by botulinum toxin. *Anais Acad. Brasil. Cienc.* **24**: 225–39.

BROOKS, V. B. (1954) The action of botulinum toxin on motor nerve filaments. *J. Physiol.* **123**: 501–15.

BROOKS, V. B. (1956) An intracellular study of the action of repetitive nerve volleys and of botulinum toxin on miniature end-plate potentials. *J. Physiol.* **134**: 264–77.

BROOKS, V. B. (1964) The pharmacological actions of botulinum toxin. In: *Botulism*. Lewis, K. H., and Cassell, K. (eds.) Public Health Service Publication. 999-FP-1. Washington.

BURGEN, A. S. V., DICKENS, F. and ZATMAN, L. J. (1949) The action of botulinum toxin on the neuromuscular junction. *J. Physiol.* **109**: 10–24.

DICKSON, E. C. and SHEVKY, R. (1923a) Botulism: studies on the manner in which the toxin of *Clostridium botulinum* acts on the body. I. The effect on the autonomic nervous system. *J. Exp. Med.* **37**: 711–31.

DICKSON, E. C. and SHEVKY, R. (1923b) Botulism: studies on the manner in which the

toxin of *Clostridium botulinum* acts on the body. II. The effect on the voluntary nervous system. *J. Exp. Med.* **38**: 327–46.

EDMUNDS, C. W. and LONG, P. W. (1923) Contributions to the pathologic physiology of botulinum. *J. Amer. Med. Ass.* **81**: 542–7.

ELMQVIST, D. and QUASTEL, D. M. (1965a) A quantitative study of endplate potentials in isolated human muscle. *J. Physiol.* **178**: 505–29.

ELMQVIST, D. and QUASTEL, D. M. (1965b) Presynaptic action of hemicholinium at the neuromuscular junction. *J. Physiol.* **177**: 463–82.

GROBSTEIN, C. (1965) Differentiation: environmental factors, chemical and cellular. In: *Cells and Tissues in Culture*. Willmer (ed.). Academic Press, London.

GUYTON, A. C. and MACDONALD, M. A. (1947) Physiology of botulinum toxin. *Arch. Neurol. Psych.* **57**: 578–92.

HEYNINGEN, W. E. VAN (1950) *Bacterial Toxins*. Blackwell, Oxford.

HOFMANN, W. W., THESLEFF, S. and ZELENA, J. (1964) Innervation of botulinum poisoned skeletal muscle by accessory nerves. *J. Physiol.* **171**: 27P.

JOSEFSSON, J. O. and THESLEFF, S. (1961) Electromyographic findings in experimental botulinum intoxication. *Acta Physiol Scand.* **51**: 163–8.

KATZ, B. and MILEDI, R. (1965a) Propagation of electric activity in motor nerve terminals. *Proc. Roy. Soc.* B **161**: 453–82.

KATZ, B. and MILEDI, R. (1965b) Release of acetylcholine from a nerve terminal by electric pulses of variable strength and duration. *Nature* **207**: 1097–8.

LAMANNA, C. (1959) The most poisonous poison. *Science* **130**: 763–72.

RAND, M. J. and WHALER, B. C. (1965) Impairment of sympathetic transmission by botulinum toxin. *Nature* **206**: 588–91.

STEVENSON, J. W. (1962) Bacterial neurotoxins. In: *Neurochemistry*, 2nd ed. Elliot, Page and Quastel (eds). Thomas, Springfield.

THESLEFF, S. (1960) Supersensitivity of skeletal muscle produced by botulinum toxin. *J. Physiol.* **151**: 598–607.

WRIGHT, G. P. (1955) The neurotoxins of *clostridium botulinum* and *clostridium tetanus*. *Pharmacol. Rev.* **7**: 413–65.

ZACKS, S. I., METZGER, J. F., SMITH, C. W. and BLUMBERG, J. M. (1962) Localisation of ferritin labelled botulinum toxin in the neuromuscular junction of the mouse. *J. Neuropath. Exp. Neurol.* **21**: 610–33.

CHAPTER 8

TETRODOTOXIN AND SAXITOXIN*

J. Cheymol and F. Bourillet

Paris

INTRODUCTION

Apart from those toxins of bacterial origin and protein nature which comprise the most toxic substances known, a new class of very active molecules of biological origin has been discovered and subjected to special study over the last 15 years. These substances are known at present as *Tetrodotoxin* and *Saxitoxin*; their characteristic property is an ability to block at the excitable membrane level the movement of sodium ions, essential for the initiation of electrical activity. Their structure is also characteristic: tetrodotoxin is the first known substance possessing a hemilactal function of an ortho acid; these are small nonprotein molecules, free from antigenicity. Is one therefore justified in calling them "toxins"?

The name "tetrodotoxin" given by Tawara in 1910 to an extract of the viscera of the fish *Fugu* (tetraodon) has been retained for the pure crystalline substance; it is now used in preference to terms such as spheroidin, fugutoxin, pufferfish poison, etc.

The term "saxitoxin", given by Schuett and Rapoport (1962), seems to be the one of choice for designating the poison of various shell-fish (particularly *Saxidomus giganteus*) and of poisonous phytoplanktons, in spite of the present incompleteness of our knowledge concerning its chemical structure.

These biotoxins have been the cause of a number of cases of food poisoning, the characteristic symptoms of which are usually anesthesia of the lips and extremities, together with vertigo and nausea; at the same time a progressive paralysis of the limbs and respiratory muscles develops which, in severe cases, leads to death by asphyxia. Because of these latter symptoms, this condition has been described for some time as a curarization.

* For a more thorough study of these toxins, see Section 71 of the *Encylopedia*.

175

8.1. ORIGIN—STRUCTURE—PROPERTIES

8.1.1. The tetrodotoxin obtained since 1950–2 in a crystallized form (Yokoo, 1950; Tsuda and Kawamura, 1952) is extracted from the viscera (ovaries, liver . . .) of various Japanese salt-water fish belonging principally to the genus *Fugu** of the tetraodontid family.

The toxin content of the various organs varies according to the season, rising particularly during spawning; it can reach 1000 mcg/g of fresh tissue.

The presence of toxin in the course of embryonic development of *Fugu* is proof of its endogenous origin (Suyama and Uno, 1957). Moreover another toxin with paralytic properties, tarichatoxin, has been discovered in the eggs and embryos of the Californian newt (*Taricha torosa*); it has been established that this toxin, obtained in crystalline form, is absolutely identical to tetrodotoxin (Mosher *et al.*, 1964).

The chemical structure of this molecule was firmly established in 1964 (Woodward).† Its basic molecular formula is $C_{11}H_{17}N_3O_8$, corresponding to a molecular weight of 319; it is a substituted aminoquinazoline, the side chain and hydroxyl groups of which form a hemilactal of the ortho-acid.

It is an amphoteric ion giving stable aqueous solutions in the form of an acid salt.

The preparation of derivatives of tetrodotoxin, and the study of their

* These poisonous fish are furnished with particularly hard ivory teeth (crab eaters) and can inflate themselves with air or water at the approach of danger (balloon fish, puffer fish).

† Four groups of workers have been engaged in determining the exact formula of tetrodotoxin: that of Tsuda and of Hirata in Japan, that of Woodward and of Mosher in the U.S.A.

toxicity and their activity on excitable membranes, has shown the importance of the hemilactal bond and of the hydroxyl group in position 4. Rupture of this bond and reduction or substitution of the hydroxyl in position 4 would alter the positive charge of the guanidinium group and result in loss of activity and toxicity (Tsuda *et al.*, 1964; Deguchi, 1967; Narahashi *et al.*, 1967c; Ranney *et al.*, 1968).

8.1.2. Saxitoxin can be extracted from various shell-fish (Schantz *et al.*, 1957; Mold *et al.*, 1957) (siphon of clams: *Saxidomus giganteus*; hepato-pancrease of mussels: *Mytilus californianus*, *M. edulis*; oysters: *Oestra edulis*, etc.) normally feeding on plankton which they collect by filtering large amounts of sea-water. In certain waters and at certain times, some species of toxic plankton develop in very large numbers and render poisonous, without killing them, the shell-fish which have absorbed them. The true producers of toxins, therefore, are these dinoflagellates, principally the genus *Gonyaulax* (*G. catenella* or *tamarensis*) (Sommer *et al.*, 1937), which are abundant along the Pacific and Atlantic coasts of North America.

From pure cultures of these planktons can be extracted a toxin identical to that obtained from poisonous shell-fish (Schantz *et al.*, 1966; Schantz, 1967).

Saxitoxin is a water soluble dibasic compound, dialyzable, giving salts with mineral acids and optically active. Unlike tetrodotoxin, however, saxitoxin has not been obtained in a crystalline form and its exact structure has yet to be determined. Its basic molecular formula is $C_{10}H_{17}N_7O_4$, 2HCl and molecular weight 372 (Schantz, 1960–1).

Two degradation products of saxitoxin are known:

by treatment in the warm with P + HI, one obtains 3-methyl,6,7-dihydro 5H-pyrrol (1-2c) pyrimidine-1, of molecular formula $C_8H_{10}N_{20}$ (Schuett and Rapoport, 1962);

by oxidation in alkaline medium, followed by reduction, a purine of the formula $C_9H_{10}O_2N_6$, HCl is obtained which is a 2-imino, 8-amino, 6-methyl, 3β-carboxyethylpurine (Rapoport *et al.*, 1964).

8.2. NEUROMUSCULAR EFFECTS

The symptoms of poisoning by the toxin of *Fugu* or of shell-fish, that is by tetrodotoxin or saxitoxin, are very similar and characterized by a progressive paralysis leading to asphyxia. The idea of a curarizing action has been accepted for a long time, but more advanced studies have shown that the paralysis produced by these toxins is much more complex than a simple curarization.

8.2.1. DESCRIPTION OF THE PARALYSIS

In man, the symptoms reported in the literature are very similar for tetrodotoxin and saxitoxin: rapid absorption, anesthesia of lips and tongue, tingling of the extremities, impaired taste, a curious sensation of lightness, restlessness particularly with tetrodotoxin, vertigo, nausea, vomiting, abdominal pain, finally general weakness, atonia of the muscles of neck and limbs, dyspnoea followed by death due to respiratory arrest within 8 to 24 hours. If one survives this period, the prognosis is favorable.

In intact unanesthetized animals, the intravenous injection of toxins (2–4 mcg/kg in the rabbit and chicken, 7–8 mcg/kg in the mouse) produces a muscular weakness with incoordinate movements coupled with respiratory difficulty and finally death in a state of flaccid paralysis, 1 to 2 minutes after injection.

It is important to note the early effect on the respiratory muscles (Cheymol *et al.*, 1961–8; Evans, 1965; Cheng *et al.*, 1968).

On an in situ nerve-muscle preparation in the cat or rabbit, following intravenous injection (6–7 µg/kg of tetrodotoxin and 5 mcg/kg of saxitoxin), a progressive paralysis develops without any latency and affects most powerfully the red muscles (soleus in the cat), being reversed only slowly and with difficulty. After intra-arterial injection, the effect is more intense and more easily reversible (Cheymol *et al.*, 1961–68; Kao and Nishiyama, 1965; Evans, 1965). The rat is less sensitive (Cheymol and Thach-Toan, 1969).

On an isolated nerve-muscle preparation (rat phrenic nerve-diaphragm preparation) the effects are comparable (0.02–0.1 mcg toxin per ml— Murtha, 1960; Cheymol *et al.*, 1961–8; Fleisher *et al.*, 1961).

The paralytic effect of these toxins is therefore peripheral, progressive without any latency and slowly reversible; it is not antagonized by neostigmine or edrophonium.

The sensitivity of different species of animals to these toxins varies considerably: the lower animals (unicellular, invertebrates, molluscs . . .) are insensitive; fish, amphibians, reptiles are somewhat more sensitive, and the higher species (birds, mammals) are very sensitive indeed to these toxins (Ishihara, 1918; Suyehiro, 1948; Woodward, 1961; Kao and Fuhrman, 1963). The fish *Fugu* and the newt are two exceptions; while being sensitive to saxitoxin, they are resistant to large doses of tetrodotoxin. This expected but very singular phenomenon has not yet been explained precisely (specific antibodies, special enzymic mechanism, or possibly some structural feature of the excitable membranes—Kao and Fuhrman, 1967).

8.2.2. MECHANISM OF THE PARALYTIC ACTION

This appears to be different from curarization, because it affects simultaneously the presynaptic nervous structures, the muscle fiber and possibly the motor end-plate.

(a) *PRESYNAPTIC STRUCTURES*

An initial piece of experimental evidence, namely the fall in the amount of acetylcholine liberated at the motor nerve terminals (Fleisher *et al.*, 1961; Cheymol *et al.*, 1962a), indicates that these toxins act at the presynaptic level. However, this does not show the exact site of action. The concept of an inhibition of the biosynthesis or release of transmitter has been discarded.* On the contrary, it has been shown experimentally and on a number of nerve fibers that these toxins blocked the conduction process along motor and sensory fibers, without the slightest depolarizing effect and by a noncompetitive mechanism (Higman and Bartels, 1961). They resemble, therefore, local anesthetics (Ogura and Mori, 1968) which reduce the permeability of excitable membranes to Na and K ions, but they are nearly 100,000 times more active than procaine and cocaine. Their action is also more selective since they inhibit the early and transient variations of permeability to Na ions† in most excitable membranes, a variation which initiates the first phase of the action potential by penetration of these Na ions; the permeability to K and Cl ions is not affected. This mechanism has been revealed by classical electrophysiological methods (Narahashi *et al.*, 1960; Dettbarn *et al.*, 1960, 1965; Kao and Fuhrman, 1963; Kao and Nishiyama, 1965b), etc., and shown directly by the use of voltage clamped axons (Narahashi *et al.*, 1964; Nakamura *et al.*, 1964, 1965; Takata *et al.*, 1966; Hille, 1968). Tetrodotoxin is inactive when injected inside the squid giant axon; its action is therefore mediated entirely at the outside surface of the cell membrane‡ (Moore, 1965; Moore *et al.*, 1966; Narahashi *et al.*, 1967a).

* In essence: increase in frequency of stimulation of a motor nerve does not increase the muscular paralysis; choline has no antagonistic action (Cheymol *et al.*, 1961–8). The frequency of spontaneous miniature potentials shows little or no modification (Ogura *et al.*, 1964; Kao and Nishiyama, 1965b; Elmquist and Feldman, 1965; Nishiyama, 1968). Local depolarization of nerve terminals again produces normal postsynaptic potentials, except in the absence of calcium (Katz and Miledi, 1966, 1967).

† Itokawa and Cooper (1969) suggest, in a recent paper, that tetrodotoxin blocks the inward current of Na ions by displacing thiamine phosphate and occupying its site in the membrane.

‡ In agreement with Kao and Nishiyama (1965b) the following basic mechanism can be accepted: the guanidinium group has a strong positive charge and a size very similar

In the intact organism it is likely that the motor nerve terminals will be affected before the larger nerve trunks. It has been shown experimentally that the end-plate potential disappears before the action potential of the nerve fiber several millimeters from the synapse (Cheymol *et al.*, 1962a, b and c); on the other hand it has been demonstrated that the diffusion of these toxins is particularly difficult and very often requires an aperture in the perineural sheaths (Fingerman *et al.*, 1953; Evans, 1964).

This poor diffusibility accounts for certain discrepancies according to experimental conditions: in nerve preparations *in situ*, blockade of the action potential is seen with doses of 0.5 to 3.0 mcg/kg i.v. (Watanabe, 1958); in isolated preparations (desheathed nerve fibers), the minimal active concentrations are 3 nM (Dettbarn *et al.*, 1960; Kao and Fuhrman, 1963) and much higher if they are intact (Fingerman *et al.*, 1953; Evans, 1964).

(b) *MUSCLE FIBERS*

As in the case of nerve fibers, these toxins block the propagation of the action potential without a depolarizing action (Furukawa *et al.*, 1959) by inhibiting the variations in permeability of the muscle membrane to sodium ions and to sodium ions alone. The first studies of Narahashi *et al.* (1960) have been confirmed by other workers (Nakajima *et al.*, 1962; Kao and Nishiyama, 1965b); the contractile system and the excitation–contraction linkage do not appear to be affected (Kao, 1966).

When a nerve–muscle preparation, *in situ* or isolated, is stimulated alternately indirectly (via the nerve) and directly (the muscle) it can be seen that the contractions due to indirect stimulation are usually depressed earlier and to a greater degree than the contractions due to direct stimulation; the more sensitive the preparation the more this is evident, but it varies according to the experimental conditions.

Chronically denervated muscles are usually more sensitive than normally innervated muscles.

(c) *POSTSYNAPTIC MEMBRANE*

The mode of action of these toxins at the end-plate receptor level is

---

to those of Na ions; it can therefore penetrate the sodium pores and channels. In the case of tetrodotoxin and saxitoxin, it would seem that the guanidinium group can enter the pores quite easily, but not the rest of the molecule. In this way the pores become blocked (in much the same way as a champagne cork seals the neck of a bottle) thus preventing the passage of Na ions and blocking the genesis of an action potential. The pores controlling the passage of Na ions into the channels are localized on the external surface of the membrane (Narahashi *et al.*, 1967a).

very debatable, simply because it is difficult to be precise when using a preparation in which the nervous and muscular components are already depressed.

In frog or rat preparations or on the electroplax, most workers agree that the postsynaptic membrane is not affected.* On the other hand, certain nerve–muscle preparations in the cat, which from this point of view are known to resemble that of man, indicate that the sensitivity to acetylcholine by close arterial injection is strongly and rapidly reduced by the action of tetrodotoxin and saxitoxin (Cheymol and Bourillet, 1966; Cheymol *et al.*, 1968).

In conclusion therefore it appears that the paralytic effect of these toxins acts first at the level of the nerve membrane by blocking the action potential all along the motor terminals (perhaps in the case of certain species at the level of the receptors of the synaptic membrane) and secondly and less strongly at the level of the muscle membrane.

8.2.3. DIFFERENCES BETWEEN TETRODOTOXIN AND SAXITOXIN

In spite of the great similarity in the mode of action of these two toxins, some slight differences have been shown (Murtha, 1960; Kao and Nishiyama, 1965a; Cheymol and Bourillet, 1966; Narahashi *et al.*, 1967b; Kao, 1967; Nishiyama, 1967; McFarren, 1967; Evans, 1969).

Saxitoxin is slightly more active than tetrodotoxin but its effect is less prolonged and more easily reversed;

tetrodotoxin, unlike saxitoxin, in subliminal doses produces a small and transient potentiation of the maximal muscular contraction (Cheymol *et al.*, 1961; Ogura, 1963);

the action of saxitoxin on the muscle fiber is more pronounced than that of tetrodotoxin;

the antagonistic action of edrophonium on the paralysis produced by these two toxins is also weaker in the case of saxitoxin than of tetrodotoxin;

saxitoxin is less hypotensive than tetrodotoxin;

* The amplitude of the spontaneous miniature potentials is little or unaffected (Ogura *et al.*, 1964; Kao and Nishiyama, 1965b; Elmquist and Feldman, 1965). Sensitivity to acetylcholine persists even during total paralysis by toxins (Furukawa *et al.*, 1959; Dettbarn *et al.*, 1965; Cheymol and Bourillet, 1966; Nishiyama, 1967; Cheymol *et al.*, 1968). The facilitation of the second postsynaptic potential, usually observed after double stimulation of the nerve terminals, is not affected (Katz and Miledi, 1966, 1967).

saxitoxin sometimes induces a small transient increase in the height of the nerve action potential, which does not occur with tetrodotoxin; saxitoxin is active on the nerves of the newt and *Fugu*, whereas tetrodotoxin is not (Kao and Fuhrman, 1967).

8.3.   OTHER PHARMACOLOGICAL EFFECTS

Apart from the paralytic effect which is the most important symptom of this poisoning, these toxins exert cardiovascular depressor effects, that is to say, hypotension, bradycardia, antiarrhythmia, spasmolytic action on smooth muscle, local anesthetic and ganglioplegic activity. The central depressor actions reported by certain workers are questioned by others (Crawford and Shibata, 1968); only the powerful central emetic effect (trigger zone) seen in certain species is undoubtedly established (Hayama and Ogura, 1963).

No therapeutic use for these toxins is anticipated on account of their extreme toxicity.

8.4.   PREVENTION AND TREATMENT OF POISONING

In effect, there is neither an antidote nor a specific medication available against poisoning by these toxins; treatment being purely symptomatic. It is known that if the patient remains alive longer than 8 hours, the prognosis is favorable.

The following treatment should be undertaken:
1. the poison should be removed using an emetic, accompanied by gastric lavage with a bicarbonate solution (2–5%) or absorbents (charcoal, alumina, resins, . . .);
2. artificial respiration should be applied in conjunction with oxygen therapy, cardiorespiratory analeptics (nikethamide, pentetrazole, lobeline, theophylline, . . .), stimulants (ephedrine, amphetamine), or sedatives (10% calcium gluconate, i.v.).

Atropine or the anticurare drugs neostigmine or edrophonium are almost without effect.

Because the treatment of poisoning is not easy, efforts must be directed towards its prevention. The North American and Japanese food hygiene services have applied strict measures in this context:

regular inspection of fresh shell-fish;

quarantine facilities;

avoiding the consumption of black flesh (hepatopancreas and siphon) of shell-fish, eggs and viscera of *Fugu* (only qualified cooks of the Ministry of Public Hygiene are authorized to prepare *Fugu*);

boiling in an alkaline medium (bicarbonate) aids destruction of the poison but saxitoxin is more resistant than tetrodotoxin, since 30% of the poison still remains after sterilization at 120°.

5. CONCLUSIONS

The studies carried out on the paralytic effect of tetrodotoxin and saxitoxin have been particularly fruitful in a number of different spheres. The following has been shown:

A better understanding of food poisoning caused by *Fugu* and shell-fish, its prevention and treatment.

The discovery of a completely new chemical structure, so far for tetrodotoxin only.

The demonstration also of a new specific pharmacological action: the inhibition of the flux of sodium ions at the level of excitable membranes. These toxins can thus be used as reagents—the "chemical scalpels" of Claude Bernard—particularly valuable for a better understanding, not only of neuromuscular transmission but also from a more general point of view of intrinsic mechanisms underlying the genesis and propagation of action potentials in living tissue.

An hypothesis concerning the biological formation of petrols, the poisonous planktons being responsible for enormous hecatombs of marine animals, the graves of which became transformed little by little into pockets of petrol deposit.

Finally, for everything has its bright and its dark side, the possibility for army secret services to use the incapacitating properties of tetrodotoxin and saxitoxin, which are, in fact, ultimate incapacitating drugs!

REFERENCES

Several general reviews on the subject of these toxins have been published, which give an account and a bibliography virtually complete up to 1966. We therefore only mention certain original articles which are among the most important or the most recent.

CHENG, K. K., LING, Y. L. and WANG, J. C. (1968) The failure of respiration in death by tetrodotoxin. *Quart. J. Exp. Physiol.* **53**: 119–28.

CHEYMOL, J. and BOURILLET, F. (1966) D'une nouvelle classe de substances biologiques: Tétrodotoxine, Saxitoxine, Tarichatoxine. *Actual. Pharmacol.* **19**: 1–61.

CHEYMOL, J., BOURILLET, F., LONG, P. and ROCH-ARVEILLER, M. (1968) Action paralysante neuromusculaire de la saxitoxine. *Arch. Int. Pharmacodyn.* **174**: 393–412.

CHEYMOL, J., BOURILLET, F. and OGURA, Y. (1962a) Influence de la tétrodotoxine cristallisée et de la cocaïne sur la libération d'acetylcholine au niveau des terminaisons nerveuses motrices. *Med. Exp.* **6**: 79–87.

CHEYMOL, J., BOURILLET, F. and OGURA, Y. (1962b) Action de paralysants neuromusculaires sur la libération d'acetylcholine par les terminaisons nerveuses motrices. *Arch. Int. Pharmacodyn.* **139**: 187–97.

CHEYMOL, J., FOULHOUX, P., BOURILLET, F. and SIMON, P. (1962c) Action de la tétrodotoxine sur les phénomènes électriques de la transmission neuromusculaire. *C.R. Soc. Biol.* **156**: 602–6.

CHEYMOL, J., KOBAYASHI, T., BOURILLET, F. and TETREAULT, L. (1961) Action paralysante neuromusculaire de la tetrodotoxine. *Arch. int. Pharmacodyn.* **134**: 28–53.

CHEYMOL, J. and THACH TOAN (1969) Action paralysante de la saxitoxine chez le rat. *Thérapie* **24**: 191–8.

CRAWFORD, M. L. J. and SHIBATA, S. (1968) Tetrodotoxin and the electrocortical response to light. *Brit. J. Pharmacol.* **32**: 25–27.

DEGUCHI, T. (1967) Structure and activity in tetrodotoxin derivatives. *Jap. J. Pharmacol.* **17**: 267–78.

DETTBARN, W. D., HIGMAN, H. B., BARTELS, E. and PODLESKI, T. (1965) Effects of marine toxins on electrical activity and K^+ efflux of excitable membranes. *Biochim. Biophys. Acta* **94**: 472–8.

DETTBARN, W. D., HIGMAN, H. B., ROSENBERG, P. and NACHMANSOHN, D. (1960) Rapid and reversible block of electrical activity by powerful marine biotoxins. *Science* **132**: 300–1.

ELMQUIST, D. and FELDMAN, D. S. (1965) Spontaneous activity at mammalian neuromuscular junction in tetrodotoxin. *Acta Physiol. Scand.* **64**: 475–6.

EVANS, M. H. (1964) Paralytic effects of "paralytic shellfish poison" on frog nerve and muscle. *Brit. J. Pharmacol.* **22**: 478–85.

EVANS, M. H. (1965) Cause of death in experimental paralytic shellfish poisoning. *Brit. J. Exptl. Pathol.* **46**: 245–53.

EVANS, M. H. (1969) Differences between the effects of saxitoxin (paralytic shellfish poison) and tetrodotoxin on the frog neuromuscular junction. *Brit. J. Pharmacol.* **36**: 426–36.

FINGERMAN, M., FORRESTER, R. H. and STOVER J. M. (1953) Action of shellfish poison on peripheral nerve and skeletal muscle. *Proc. Soc. Exptl. Biol. Med.* **84**: 643–6.

FLEISHER, J. M., KILLOS, P. J. and HARRISON, C. S. (1961) Effects of puffer poison on neuromuscular transmission. *J. Pharmacol. Exptl. Therap.* **133**: 98–105.

FURUKAWA, T., SASAOKA, T. and HOSOYA, Y. (1959) Effects of tetrodotoxin on neuromuscular junction. *Jap. J. Physiol.* **9**: 143–52.

HAYAMA, T. and OGURA, Y. (1963) Emetic action of tetrodotoxin. *J. Pharmacol. Exptl. Therap.* **139**: 94–96.

HIGMAN, H. B. and BARTELS, E. (1961) The competitive nature of action of acetylcholine and local anesthetics. *Biochim. Biophys. Acta* **54**: 543–54.

HILLE, B. (1968) Pharmacological modifications of the sodium channels of the frog nerve. *J. Gen. Physiol.* **51**: 199–219.

ISHIHARA, F. (1918) Über die physiologischen Wirkungen des Fugutoxins. *Mitteil. Med. Fak. Tokio Univ.* **20**: 375–426.

ITOKAWA, Y. and COOPER, J. R. (1969) Thiamine release from nerve membrane by tetrodotoxin. *Science* **166**: 759–61.

KAO, C. Y. (1966) Tetrodotoxin, saxitoxin and their significance in the study of excitation phenomena. *Pharmacol. Rev.* **18**: 997–1049.

KAO, C. Y. (1967) Comparison of the biological actions of tetrodotoxin and saxitoxin, In: *Animal Toxins*, pp. 109–14. Russell, F. E. and Saunders, P. R. (eds.). Pergamon Press.

KAO, C. Y. and FUHRMAN, F. A. (1963) Pharmacological studies on Tarichatoxin, a potent neurotoxin. *J. Pharmacol. Exptl. Therap.* **140**: 31–39.

KAO, C. Y. and FUHRMAN, F. A. (1967) Differentiation of the actions of tetrodotoxin, and saxitoxin. *Toxicon* **5**: 25–34.

KAO, C. Y. and NISHIYAMA, A. (1965a) Similarity of the actions of tetrodotoxin and saxitoxin on the excitable membrane. *Fed. Proc.* **24**: 649.

KAO, C. Y. and NISHIYAMA, A. (1965b) Actions of saxitoxin on peripheral neuromuscular systems. *J. Physiol.* **180**: 50–66.

KATZ, B. and MILEDI, R. (1966) The production of end-plate potentials in muscles paralysed by tetrodotoxin. *J. Physiol.* **185**: 5P–6P.

KATZ, B. and MILEDI, R. (1967) Tetrodotoxin and neuromuscular transmission. *Proc. Roy. Soc.*, Ser. B, **167**: 8–22.

MCFARREN, E. F. (1967) Differentiation of poisons of fish, shellfish and plankton. In: *Animal Toxins*, pp. 85–90. Russell, F. E. and Saunders, P. R. (eds.). Pergamon Press.

MOLD, J. D., BOWDEN, P. J., STANGER, D. W., MAURER, J. E., LYNCH, J. M., WYLER, R. S., SCHANTZ, E. J. and RIEGEL, B. (1957) Paralytic shellfish poison. VII. Evidence for the purity of the poison isolated from toxic clams and mussels. *J. Amer. Chem. Soc.* **79**: 5235–8.

MOORE, J. W. (1965) Voltage clamp studies on internally perfused axons. *J. Gen. Physiol.* **48**: 11–17.

MOORE, J. W., ANDERSON, N. and NARAHASHI, T. (1966) Tetrodotoxin blocking early conductance channel or sodium? *Fed. Proc.* **25**: 569.

MOSHER, H. S., FUHRMAN, F. A., BUCHWALD, H. D. and FISCHER, H. G. (1964) Tarichatoxin–Tetrodotoxin: a potent neurotoxin. *Science* **144**: 1100–10.

MURTHA, E. F. (1960) Pharmacological study of poisons from shellfish and pufferfish. *Ann. N.Y. Acad. Sci.* **90**: 820–36.

NAKAJIMA, S., IWASAKI, S. and OBATA, K. (1962) Delayed rectification and anomalous rectification in frog's skeletal muscle membrane. *J. Gen. Physiol.* **46**: 97–115.

NAKAMURA, Y., NAKAJIMA, S. and GRUNDFEST, H. (1964) Selective block of Na-activation in voltage-clamped squid giant and eel electroplaque by tetrodotoxin. *Biol. Bull.* **127**: 382.

NAKAMURA, Y., NAKAJIMA, S. and GRUNDFEST, H. (1965) The action of tetrodotoxin on electrogenic components of squid giant axons. *J. Gen. Physiol.* **48**: 985–96.

NARAHASHI, T., ANDERSON, N. C. and MOORE, J. W. (1967a) Comparison of tetrodotoxin and procaine in internally perfused squid giant axons. *J. Gen. Physiol.* **50**: 1413–28.

NARAHASHI, T., DEGUCHI, T., URAKAWA, N. and OHKUBO, Y. (1960) Stabilization and rectification of muscle fibre membrane by tetrodotoxin. *Amer. J. Physiol.* **198**: 934–8.

NARAHASHI, T., HAAS, H. G. and THERRIEN, E. F. (1967b) Saxitoxin and tetrodotoxin: comparison of nerve blocking mechanism. *Science* **157**: 1441–2.

NARAHASHI, T., MOORE, J. W. and POSTON, R. N. (1967c) Tetrodotoxin derivatives: chemical structure and blockage of nerve membrane conductance. *Science* **156**: 976–9.

NARAHASHI, T., MOORE, J. W. and SCOTT, W. (1964) Tetrodotoxin blockage of sodium conductance increase in lobster giant axons. *J. Gen. Physiol.* **47**: 965–74.

NISHIYAMA, A. (1967) Effect of saxitoxin on the end plate of frog muscle. *Nature* **215**: 201–2.

NISHIYAMA, A. (1968) Effect of saxitoxin on spontaneous release of acetylcholine from the frog's motor nerve endings. *Tohoku J. Exp. Med.* **95**: 201–2.

OGURA, Y. (1963) Analyse du phénomène de potentialisation de la contraction maximale provoquée par de faibles doses de tétrodotoxine. *Annu. Rept. Inst. Food Microbiol. (Chiba)* **15**: 97–100.

OGURA, Y. and MORI, Y. (1968) Mechanism of local anesthetic action of crystalline tetrodotoxin and its derivatives. *Europ. J. Pharmacol.* **3**: 58–67.

OGURA, Y., WATANABE, Y. and MORI, Y. (1964) Effects of crystalline tetrodotoxin on spontaneous miniature end plate potentials in frog muscle and on spontaneous miniature synaptic potentials in cray-fish abdominal ganglion. *Ann. Rept. Inst. Food Microbiol.* (Chiba) **17**: 61–71.

RANNEY, B. K., FUHRMAN, F. A., SCHMIEGEL, J. L. and MOSHER, H. S. (1968) The pharmacological actions of some guanidine esters and their relationship to tetrodotoxin. *Arch. Int. Pharmacodyn.* **175**: 193–211.

RAPOPORT, H., BROWN, M. S. OESTERLIN, R. and SCHUETT, W. (1964) Saxitoxin. *Proc. 147th national meeting of the Amer. Chem. Soc.* (Philadelphia.).

RUSSEL, F. E. (1965) Marine toxins and venomous and poisonous marine animals. *Adv. Marine Biol.* **3**: 255–383.

SCHANTZ, E. J. (1960) Biochemical studies on paralytic shellfish poisons. *Ann. N.Y. Acad. Sci.* **90**: 843–55.

SCHANTZ, E. J. (1961) Some chemical and physical properties of paralytic shellfish poison. *J. Med. Pharm. Chem.* **4**: 459–68.

SCHANTZ, E. J. (1967) Biochemical studies on purified *Gonyaulax catenella* poison. In: *Animal Toxins*, pp. 91–95. Russell, F. E. and Saunders, P. R. (eds.). Pergamon Press.

SCHANTZ, E. J., LYNCH, J. M., VAYVADA, G., MATSUMOTO, K. and RAPOPORT, H. (1966) The purification and characterization of the poison produced by *Gonyaulax catenella* in axenic culture. *Biochem.* **5**: 1191–5.

SCHANTZ, E. J., MOLD, J. D., STANGER, D. W., SHAVEL, J., RIEL, F. J., BOWDEN, J. P., LYNCH, J. M., WYLER, R. S., RIEGEL, B. and SOMMER, H. (1957) Paralytic shellfish poison. VI. A procedure for the isolation and purification of the poison from toxic clam and mussel tissue. *J. Amer. Chem. Soc.* **79**: 5230–5.

SCHUETT, W. and RAPOPORT, H. (1962) Saxitoxin, the paralytic shell-fish poison. Degradation to a pyrrolopyrimidine. *J. Amer. Chem. Soc.* **84**: 2266–7.

SOMMER, H., WHEDON, W. F., KOFOID, C. A. and STOHLER, R. (1937) Relation of paralytic shellfish poison to certain plankton organism of the genus *Gonyaulax*. *A.M.A. Arch. Pathol.* **24**: 537–59.

SUYAMA, M. and UNO, Y. (1957) Puffer toxin during the embryonic development of puffer. *Bull. J. Soc. Sci. Fish.* **23**: 438.

SUYEHIRO, Y. (1948) On the physiological action of balloonfish poison. *Suisan Gakkai Hô* **10**: 12.

TAKATA, M., MOORE, J. W., KAO, C. Y. and FUHRMAN, F. A. (1966) Blockage by tarichatoxin of sodium conductance change in excitation. *J. Gen. Physiol.* **49**: 967–88.

TAWARA, Y. (1910) Über das Tetrodon Gift. *Biochem. Zeitsch.* **30**: 255–75.

TSUDA, K., IKUMA, S., KAWAMURA, M., TACHIKAWA, R., SAKAI, K., TAMURA, C. and AMAKASU, O. (1964) Tetrodotoxin. VII. The structures of tetrodotoxin and its derivatives, *Chem. Pharm. Bull.* **12**: 1357–74.

TSUDA, K. and KAWAMURA, M. (1952) The constituents of the ovaries of globefish. VII. Purification of tetrodotoxin by chromatography. *J. Pharm. Soc. Japan* **72**: 771–2.

WATANABE, M. (1958) The effect of tetrodotoxin on the afferent impulses from the sensory nerves. *Igaku Kenkyu* **28**: 876–84.

WOODWARD, R. B., cited by MCFARREN, E. F. *et al.* (1961) Public health significance of paralytic shellfish poison. *Adv. Food Res.* **10**: 135–79.

WOODWARD, R. B. (1964) The structure of tetrodotoxin. *Pure Appl. Chem.* **9**: 49–74.

YOKOO, A. (1950) Toxic substance of a globefish, *Spheroïdes rubripes*. III. Isolation of spheroïdin. *J. Pharm. Soc. Japan* **71**: 590–2.

CHAPTER 9

HISTORY OF CURARE

A. R. McIntyre

Omaha, Nebraska

9.1. THE ROMANTIC LEGENDS

With the possible exception of hashish there is no drug whose history contains more romantic folk-lore than curare. The stories of the early adventurers to the New World and the fables told by others, some of whom had never crossed the "ocean sea", have been retold many times. Of these fantastic stories three have become firmly embedded in the historical literature and were formerly widely believed and are well known but now discredited. They are the fable of the old women who were shut up in huts to make the poison and "should they escape death were severely beaten" (Gomara, 1552) for not making the poison sufficiently potent. Another story, widely quoted, recounts the death of a small child who died from the poisoned arrow which wounded only the mother (Hartsinck, 1770), and lastly, the horrendous story of a slow poison causing "death in three days, the victims dying with horrifying facial convulsions too dreadful to chronicle" (de la Vega, 1609). Today it seems clear that several types of poison were used on spears and arrows, some of which were undoubtedly curares in the modern pharmacological sense and others were certainly poisons of an entirely different nature. Infected wounds likely resulted in tetanus and the violent symptoms and subsequent death were undoubtedly at times falsely attributed to poisoned weapons. Three types of poisoned weapons are described: arrows, spears and darts. According to Stirling (1938), who made extensive studies of the blow-gun and darts of the Jibaros, the earliest reference to the blow-gun is by Saabedra written in 1620, and Stirling found that the use of this type of weapon is not mentioned in the earlier literature. He writes:

> ... the remarkable parallel between this weapon [i.e. the blow-gun] and its accessories as manufactured in Indonesia and in South America has been a frequent subject of comment by Ethnographers. ... The amazing similarity in the methods of manufacture and materials used would seem to make it extremely unlikely that this highly specialized complex could have developed independently in the two areas.

Stirling continues:

> It seems to the writer much more probably that the use of the blow-gun and its equipment was brought to South America by Southeastern Asiatics, possibly from the Philippines, who were carried across the Pacific on one or more of the many Spanish galleons which followed this route in the sixteenth century.

Nevertheless, as early as 1516, Peter Martyr (1516) described how the voyagers, venturing to "Hispaniola", were attacked by poisonous *darts*, and in the Archeological Institute of Mexico is an illustration, which probably antedates the writing of Saabedra, which clearly depicts the blow-gun in use against birds. Furthermore, the pharmacological actions of the poisons used in Asia and South America are entirely different. The former is a cardiac poison and not a curare (Schebesta, 1941). However, the Asiatic origins of the original inhabitants of the Americas is commonly acknowledged and it is conceivable that the blow-gun is a pre-Columbian Asiatic importation.

9.2. NOMENCLATURE

The word "curare" appears to have first been used by Robertson (1778) more than two and a half centuries after the first written account of the poisoned weapons of the New World. This first account, from Peter Martyr's *De Orbo Novo*, described the death of a Galician from an arrow shot by a woman and "it was discovered that the tip of the arrow broke off and poison oozed into the wound from the broken tip". In the intervening years the literature contains more than thirty different names referring to poison used on arrows and darts; of these approximately twenty belong to the "curare" group. Some of these are: uirary, ourary, urali, urare, wourari, worari, woraru, wourali, worali, woorara, uvari, avara, kurari, curara, curari, curarayae. There are, however, a half-dozen or more other names that seem unrelated to the "curare" group, they are: Lama, Lamisto, Pishuicayno, Kamarua, Caruchi, Tuguakino, Kaytena and Ticunas and of these "Ticunas" is the most widely known and was used in the upper regions of the Amazon by the Indians of Peru and Ecuador. These words bear no resemblance to the curare family of words. Ticunas is said to mean "ticu", a liquid, and "una", black. Curiously one of the earliest careful studies made upon the action of "curare" was performed by Fontana (1781) on a sample of "Ticunas" and the poison studied by Fontana was undoubtedly a curare in the modern sense.

9.3. THE WEAPONS AND THE INGREDIENTS USED AND THE PREPARATION OF CURARE

The natives who prepared arrow poison were as a rule very secretive and attempted to hide the true sources of their materials and made much mystery concerning the manufacturing of the curare. The first table of ingredients used in the preparation of curare is to be found in Edward Bancroft's (1769) *Essay*. Bancroft was not a scientist and while his book published in 1789 entitled "An essay on the natural history of Guiana and South America" is delightful it, like the accounts of Herndon (1854), Hillhouse (1868), Osculati (1850) and Tschudi (1846), contains little exact scientific information. It is noteworthy that Bancroft's recipe contains the bark of five botanically unidentified plants.

> Take of the Bark of the Root of
> Woorara, six parts;
> Of the bark of Warracobba coura, two parts;
> Of the Bark of the Roots of Coura-
> napi, Baketi, and Hatchybaly,
> of each one part:

All these are to be finely scraped, and put into an *Indian* pot, and covered with water. The pot is then to be placed over a slow fire, that the water may simmer for a quarter of an hour; after which the juice is to be expressed from the Bark by the hands, taking care that the skin is unbroken; this being done, the Bark is to be thrown away, and the juice evaporated over a moderate fire to the consistence of tar, when it is to be removed, the flat pieces of the wood of Cokarito are dipped therein, to which the poison, when cold, adheres, appearing like gum of a brown reddish colour. The pieces of wood are then put into large hollow canes, closed at the ends with skins, and in this manner the poison is preserved until it is wanted to envenom the point of an arrow dipped in the solution; or the wood to which it adheres is held over the fire until it melts, and the points of arrows are then smeared with it. The smallest quantity of this poison conveyed by a wound into the red blood vessels of an animal, causes it to expire in less than a minute, without much apparent pain or uneasiness; though slight convulsions are sometimes seen near the instant of expiration (Bancroft, 1769).

9.4. BOTANY

Naturally the eighteenth century's eye-witness accounts of the darts and arrows and of the ingredients and preparation of curare excited much curiosity among scientifically trained botanists, chemists and physicians.

The weapons were vividly described by Waterton (1879) and more exact identifications of the botanical specimens used in curare manufacture were first made by Humboldt and Bonpland (1807), Martius (1830) and the Schomburgks (1841). It is noteworthy that at this early date it was recognized that some varieties of curare were prepared from species of *menispermacea* in addition to those prepared from members of the genus *Strychnos* and indeed it is now known that some varieties of curare contain both. Humboldt was the first scientific observer to see the actual preparation of curare. It was he who first carefully distinguished between the toxic ingredients and those added to confer the right consistency to the product. He writes:

> The concentrated juice of the *mavacure* is not thick enough to attach to arrows. Therefore, to give body to the poison, another, very glutinous vegetable concentrate, drawn from a large, leafy tree called *Kiracaguera*, is mixed with it. This tree grows at a great distance from Esmeralda and was at that period destitute of flowers and fruits like the *bejuco de mavacure*, and we could not identify it botanically.

Martius, a well trained botanist, described five different varieties of poison. They were: the curare of the Orinoco which he believed identical with the "woorali" of Guiana and whose preparation was described by Humboldt; the poison prepared on the upper Amazon, similar to that described earlier by De la Condamine and which was said to contain thirty ingredients; a third poison which has not yet been investigated and which caused numbness of the hands during its preparation; a fourth and particularly deadly poison from the sap of *bejuco de ambihuasca*; and a fifth similar to that mentioned by Garcilasso de la Vega which caused a slow death.

Robert Schomburgk (1848) made every effort to see the curare plants actually collected and to witness the preparation of curare; in this he was only partly successful:

> Our path was over "hill and dale," mostly in a N.N.W. and N.W. direction. It became every moment wilder: we had to cross several mount-streams, which flowed in deep beds, precipitating at their banks a ferruginous matter; underbrush became scarce; it appeared as if Nature here delighted only in gigantic forms. Our Indians thought they had mistaken the track; but as we arrived at a stream which ran rapidly over the sloping ground, exhibiting granitic shelves, we observed that several paths united; and crossing the brook our guides stopped, and pointing to a ligneous twiner which wound itself snake-like from tree to tree, they called out "Urari," the name of the plant in the tongue of our guides.
>
> My wish was thus realized; and that plant which Baron de Humboldt was prevented from seeing, and which was one of the chief objects of Mr. Waterton's "Wanderings," but without success, I now saw before me. Baron de Humboldt, with his usual sagacity, observes, "The danger of the Curare, as of most other

190

Strychneae (for we continue to believe that the Mavacure belongs to a neighbouring family), results only from the action of the poison on the vascular system."

Though I did not find the plant in flower, it was bearing fruit, and their inspection assured me that, as von Humboldt suspected, the plant belongs to the genus *Strychnos*. . . .

However, Richard Schomburgk (1879), brother to Robert, was more fortunate and he writes:

At last my long cherished wish to witness the preparation of the *urari*, of which so many fables had been told (as there always will be about anything enveloped in a certain mystery), was to be fulfilled, and I found the process, except a few unimportant ceremonies, as simple as possible. The small hut, which on my arrival in the village I supposed to be the laboratory of the chemist, was really the *urari* house. The Indian began first to take the bark from the *Strychnos* which we had brought from the Ilamickipang, then produced the other ingredients, which it seemed he had in store, and separated the required quantities. I am sorry to say that from the barks he used besides the *Strychnos*, I could not ascertain the botanical names of these plants, which he called Tarireng, Wakarimo, and Tararemu; but to all appearances they also belonged to a species of *Strychnos*. When I asked him where they grew, he answered, far, far away in the mountains; it would take him five days to get there. The preparation of the several ingredients would be according to the weight, as follows: Bark of *Strychnos toxifera*, 2 lbs., from Yakki (*Strychnos Schomburgkii*), 1/4 lb; Arimaru (*Strychnos cogens*), 1/4 lb; Wakarimo, 1/4 lb; the root of Tarireng, 1/2 oz.; the root of Tararemu, 1/2 oz; the fleshy root of Muramu (*Cissus spec.*); four small pieces of wood of a tree of the species of *Xanthoxylaea* called Manuca. Having finished the preparations, he went to his hut and returned with a new earthen pot, holding about four quarts, and two smaller ones, also quite new, formed like flat pans. He then went into the *urari* house and put down the vessels. In the first the poison was to be boiled, in the others it was to be exposed to the sun for condensation. The great strainer or funnel, made out of palm leaves, was cleaned, and fresh silk-grass put into it to strain the fluid; the great block of wood dug into the ground to serve as a mortar, was cleaned, and in it the several ingredients were crushed. The *urari* preparer, after having arranged everything, built a hearth with three stones, and laid the wood ready to light the fire, and went away to fetch (as I was afterwards informed, for I had not exchanged a single word with the preparer of the poison, and got all the information from my companions) the utensils to light the fire, though there was a large fire burning close to us, but which was of no use, being lighted by profane hands. Neither dare he use any water except that brought in the pot to be used for the operation; in fact no other implement could be used but such as has been made by the cook; neither would he have assistance from any of the inhabitants. Any transgression of the sacred rules would nullify the operation of the poison. In addition to the fleshy root of the Muramu, he crushed the several different kinds of bark, but each one singly, in the mortar, lighted the carefully piled-up wood, and then threw first into the pot—which holds about seven quarts, and which was filled with water—the bark of the *Strychnos toxifera*. As soon as the water began to boil the Indian added at certain intervals a handful of the other ingredients except the Muramu root. In doing so he bent his head over the pot, strongly blowing into the mixture, which he said afterwards was adding considerably to the strength of the poison. During the process he only kept as much fire as was necessary for slow boiling, carefully skimming the foam collecting on the extract.

Within the next twenty-four hours the old man left the fire only for one moment—

keeping the mixture at an equal heat. After the lapse of twenty-four hours the extract became thick, and was reduced by the boiling to about a quart, and had assumed the color of a strong decoction of coffee. The old cook then took the extract from the fire, and poured it into the strainer above mentioned; the extract trickling slowly into another flat vessel, left the remainder in the silk-grass. After exposing the strained extract to the sun for about three hours, he added the slimy juice pressed out of the root of Muramu, which had previously been soaked for a short time in the boiling poison, and then had been pressed out. The poison immediately exhibited a remarkable alteration, curdling to a jelly-like substance. After this peculiar process, he poured the poison into earthen vessels, flatter than those before mentioned, for the purpose of bringing the poison to a consistence equal to that of thick treacle by exposing it to the sun. Afterwards the poison was poured into the peculiar small calabashes or small half-round three earthen vessels, manufactured only for that purpose, where it ultimately changed to a hard substance. On the third day the poison was ready; when the cook, satisfied with the product, tried the strength of the poison in my presence, for which purpose he caught some lizards. He dipped the point of a pin which I gave him into the black treacle-like substance, let the poison get dry, and wounded one of the lizards in one of the toes of the hind foot, and then let it run. After the lapse of nine minutes the peculiar symptoms of the poison made their appearance, and one minute after that the slightly wounded animal was dead. A second and third were wounded on the tails, when the poison operated in the same time. He had chosen the lizards for the trial, maintaining that the operation of the *urari* with a warm-blooded animal takes only half the time which is required for a cold-blooded animal. A rat caught by a boy confirmed that assertion, and died in the fourth minute; a fowl which I had bought for my dinner, died in the third minute. Each of these animals was but slightly wounded. The Indians maintain that the poison, even if kept well, and especially dry, will retain its life-destroying power only two years. Should the poison lose its power, they restore it by adding a little juice of the poisonous manihot root (*Manihot utillissima*). After pouring some of the manihot juice into a calabash containing the *urari*, they dig it into the ground, covering it with earth, and let it remain there for a day and a half. The manihot juice is then mixed with the poison, when it regains its former strength. The truth that after a certain lapse of time the poison would need a longer time to take effect, I have seen confirmed by my own experiences with the *urari* manufactured in my presence.

It is not possible to describe fully the many botanical investigations of the last two centuries or even list the names of all the workers in this field. However, no history would be complete without mentioning Schreber (1783) who was among the first to compile a botanical account of the curare plants, and De la Condamine who was the first scientist to descend the Amazon. Many lost their lives at the hands of Indians, among these was D'Osery, a member of De Castelnau's (1851) exploration group, and Crevaux (1882), the intrepid French naval surgeon who crossed the continent from Cayenne to the Amazon which river he ascended and at length arrived at Quito. He subsequently lost his life when he fell among cannibalistic tribes along the Pilcomayo River. The invaluable contributions made by Aublet, Jobert, Schwacke, Baillon, Candolle, Planchon, Couty and Lacerda in the nineteenth century and by Barbosa Rodrigues,

Sandwith, Krukoff, Moldenke, Diels and others in the twentieth century are described in detail in the author's monograph (1947).

9.5. EARLY ATTEMPTS TO ISOLATE THE "PRINCIPLE" FROM CURARE

The early days of the nineteenth century saw the isolation of a number of alkaloids from the crude Galenical preparations then in common use and no doubt encouraged by this successful work attempts were made by Boussingault and Roulin (1828), who travelled to South America at the invitation of Bolivar to establish a scientific institution at Bogotá, to obtain a "pure" principle, but they were only partially successful. The extremely hygroscopic nature of the evaporated alcoholic extract—its tendency to become yellow and syrupy in air—were difficulties unresolved until today's chromatographic and counter-current methods became available. Following the work of Boussingault many attempts were made in the nineteenth century to obtain a "pure" active principle from various potent South American arrow poisons. It was by this time well known that species of strychnine were used as an ingredient and, because strychnine had already been isolated by Pelletier *et al.* (1819) from *Nux vomica*, many attempts were made to demonstrate the presence of strychnine in these arrow poisons. Thus Pedroni (1844) believed strychnine to be present but Boussingault, Heintz (1847), Oberdorfer (1859) and others were convinced that strychnine was absent. Buchner (1862) described a color reaction in his refined extract somewhat resembling strychnine. Preyer (1865) who, by vigorously removing water from his alcohol, appears to have succeeded in obtaining platinum chloride-curare crystals, came nearest to success but it was not until the work of Boehm (1886) that a highly purified curare was available for precise pharmacological work.

It was Boehm who divided curares into three groups according to their containers as Pot, Tube, and Calabash curares. The "pure" principles from these three types of curares he named respectively Protocurarine, Tubocurarine, and Curarine—all of which behaved like quaternary bases. In addition a number of tertiary bases were also obtained and they were subsequently shown to have marked effects upon the autonomic system and these were termed "curines". Boehm's curarines were largely used in experimentation until the work of King (1935) in England and Wintersteiner and Dutcher (1943) in the United States. It was King who clarified the confusion regarding the bebeerines and their relationship to the curare alkaloids and the botanical origins of *Radix pareirae* and its connection

193

with the menisperm *Chondodendron* tomentosum*. This established the fact that potent curareform alkaloids could be obtained from plants other than *Strychnos*. The work of Wintersteiner and Dutcher resulted in large quantities of the menisperm alkaloid *d*-tubocurarine becoming available for both laboratory experiments and clinical trial, and most of the investigative and clinical work during the last 20 years has been performed with *d*-tubocurarine. However, it is known that the "toxiferin" alkaloids are in some instances many times more potent than those from menispermaceae and the further work of King (1940) and more especially by Wieland and coworkers (1937, 1938, 1941, 1947, 1952, 1953, 1954), Karrer and Schmid (1946, 1955) and Marini-Bettòlo and coworkers (1954, 1955, 1956, 1957), Penna *et al.* (1957), Pimenta *et al.* (1954) and others have resulted in the isolation of some fifty additional alkaloids from various species of *Strychnos*. It is now known that *Strychnos* from the New World contains no strychnine and that curare-form alkaloids are absent or rare from the Asiatic varieties.

9.6. SYNTHETIC SUBSTITUTES FOR THE NATURAL CURARES

The difficulties and uncertainties in obtaining authentic supplies of the naturally occurring vines for the extraction of pure curare alkaloids and the growing clinical usage of *d*-tubocurarine inevitably stimulated interest in the synthesis of curareform compounds. By a curious set of circumstances one of the most important of the synthetic clinical substitutes for curare remained unrecognized for more than 40 years after its initial pharmacological trial. In 1906 Hunt and Taveau (1911) (of acetylcholine fame) experimented with succinylcholine on *curarized* dogs and consequently did not recognize its curaremimetic action. Interest in the quaternary ammonium compounds was aroused by the work of Ing (1936) who reviewed the literature. Ing and Barlow (1948) and Paton and Zaimis (1949) almost simultaneously described the curareform actions of decamethylene-bis-trimethyl ammonium bromide (syncurine) and Tammelin (1953) described a method for the preparation of succinyl choline chloride (anectine) which has gained pre-eminence as a short-acting curaremimetic agent. Many more complex quaternary compounds and in particular [*p*-phenyl oxyethylene]-tri [triethyl-ammonium iodide] were investigated by Bovet (1946) and somewhat later the complex benzoquinonium

---

* The alternative spelling "Chondrodendron" is preferred by some authors including King.

compound myotolon was developed by Cavalito, Soria and Hoppe (1950); both these compounds have been used clinically.

9.7. EARLY EXPERIMENTS WITH ARROW POISONS

A specimen of poison was given to Fontana (1781) by Heberden, the celebrated eighteenth-century London physician. It was part of a collection of South American poisons and was brought from the River Amazon by Don Pedro Maldonado of Ecuador, who was acquainted with De la Condamine. Previous to Fontana's experiments with "Ticunas" De la Condamine's (1813) experiments and those of Herrisant (1751–2), Humboldt and Bonpland (1821), Brodie (1812), Waterton (1879) and many others were little more than demonstrations of the fact that the arrow poisons proved fatal when the poisons were absorbed into the blood stream and that very large doses administered by mouth may also prove fatal. However, one is struck by the extreme variations in potency exhibited by these several "curares". For example, in De la Condamine's experiments in Cayenne a poulet survived for half an hour whereas Waterton reported that an ass poisoned with "wourali" died within 12 minutes. Another animal was saved from death by artificial respiration:

> A she-ass received the wourali poison in the shoulder, and died apparently in ten minutes. An incision was then made in its windpipe, and through it the lungs were regularly inflated for two hours with a pair of bellows. Suspended animation returned. The ass held up her head, and looked around; but the inflating being discontinued, she sank once more in apparent death. The artificial breathing was immediately recommenced, and continued without intermission for two hours. This saved the ass from final dissolution; she rose up, and walked about; she seemed neither in agitation nor pain. The wound, through which the poison entered, was healed without difficulty. Her constitution, however, was so severely affected that it was long a doubt if ever she would be well again. She looked lean and sickly for above a year, and began to mend the spring after, and by Midsummer became fat and frisky.

This was the first demonstration of the effectiveness of artificial respiration in curare poisoning. A close reading of these very early and uncritical experiments leaves the impression that some of the preparations used must have contained alkaloids having considerably greater potency than that of *d*-tubocurarine. The more careful experiments conducted by Fontana on "Ticunas" were well controlled and established the important fact that the poison attacks the irritability of the muscles but not that of the heart, he says: "L'on ne sauroit douter non plus, que le poison Ticunas n'attaque le Principe de l'irratibilité [l'irritabilité] des muscles, quoiqu'il ne touche pas à l'irritabilité du coeur." Fontana also disposed of the "fable of the old women" by demonstrating that the inhalation of fumes from heated curare was not toxic to pigeons and confirmed the observation of Cleaby* (1754) that large amounts of crude curare *per os* may be fatal and that neither salt nor sugar were effective antidotes. The early days of the nineteenth century saw the isolation of a number of alkaloids from the crude Galenical preparations then in common use and a leader in the investigation of these new and relatively pure pharmacological substances was Magendie who successfully demonstrated the locus of action of the alkaloid from *Nux Vomica* isolated by Pelletier *et al.* (1819). Magendie did not have the opportunity to investigate the active "principle" of curare because many years were to elapse before the various "curarines" became available but he frequently made use of curare to immobilize his experimental animals and his famous pupil Claude Bernard became much interested in this potent drug. Bernard's classical experiments by which he determined the locus of action of curare are so well known they hardly require description and are best summarized by repeating Bernard's own words (1857, 1850, 1851): "Quand on empoisonne une grenouille par le curare, nous avons vu que l'irritabilité nerveuse disparaît tout de suite. Il n'en est pas de même de la contractilité musculaire: vous venez de le voir; je dois ajouter que, dans ce cas, les muscles conservent pendant un temps plus long la propriété de se contracter."

The discovery that curare interferes with the effectiveness of a motor nerve impulse to cause muscle-contraction resulted in intensive investigations of the structure and function of the neuromyal junction which, today, more than a century later are still in progress. In fact Bernard's experiments lead directly to the work of Kühne (1887) on the junctional tissue and which in turn, after the work of Loewi (1921) and the discovery of "Vagustoffe", and the subsequent founding of the "Dale School" of Pharmacologists, has brought about a revolution in physiological thinking. Quite naturally Bernard's work on curare aroused the keenest interest and for nearly 30 years numerous experiments confirming and extending Bernard's work ensued. Unfortunately, until the work of Boehm crude or chemically impure preparations of curare were employed and consequently little further advance in knowledge was made. Boehm's monograph on curare marks the beginning of a new era and while his curarine differed chemically from the *d*-tubocurarine of King nevertheless his work established a new milestone in the investigation of the drug and

* Cited in: Fontana, Felix, *Traité sur le vénin de la vipère et sur les poisons américains* (Florence, 1781), **2**: 89.

for the first time a relatively pure curareform substance was available. Most of the best experimental work during the last decade of the nineteenth century and the first 35 years of this century was conducted with Boehm's curarine which appears to have been closely related to Toxiferin. Since the work of King (1936) and Wintersteiner and Dutcher (1943) *d*-tubo-curarine and the synthetic curamimetic substances have been employed in almost all the more exact investigative work on the neuromyal blocking mechanism. However, the history of this subject would not be complete without mention of the work of Louis and Marcelle Lapicque and their theory of Isochronism of motor nerve and muscle. Today with the universal acceptance of the chemical mediator theory of nerve to muscle transmission the theory of isochronism enunciated by these distinguished workers it is almost forgotten and with it the importance with which the concept of chronaxie was formerly held. It was largely out of the contro-versy that arose between the protagonists for the Lapicque ideas and those opposing them that many of the exact experimental techniques on muscle and nerve were developed. The basic concept of chronaxie is best presented in Lapicque's original words:

> Un muscle lisse qui reste inerte sous un choc d'induction violent se contracte sous l'influence d'un courant de pile assez faible durant quelques seconds; ce courant de pile ne perd rien de son efficacité s'il s'établit graduellement, même si sa période d'établissement dure une seconde et davantage. Au contraire, un gastrocnémien de grenouille, qui réagira vivement à un choc d'induction, comme à un courant de pile débutant brusquement, ne sera plus excité par un courant de pile même beaucoup plus intense lorsque ce courant mettra quelques dixièmes de seconde à s'établir.
>
> Pourra-t-on dire que l'un de ces muscles est *plus* ou *moins* excitable que l'autre, sans indiquer de quelle espèce d'excitation il s'agit? Ce *plus* ou *moins* change de signe avec l'excitation considérée; il est donc insuffisant pour caractériser l'excit-abilité même relative. (1909, 1926, 1929.)

The following comment appeared in 1947:

> These historic paragraphs in their beautiful simplicity, state the problem of irritability, long pondered by many. It is unnecessary to reiterate the attempts by others to express the same concept. This has been done by Lapicque himself, who has traced the development of his principal thesis. But it is necessary to emphasize the importance of the paragraphs quoted because, paradoxically, much that is contained in this chapter appears to refute Lapicque's work; in spite of this, the concept of chronaxie and the theory of isochronism have enormously stimulated investigation of muscles and their motor nerves. If today our knowledge of curariza-tion is not complete, it has been immensely enhanced as a consequence of Lapique's efforts (McIntyre, 1947).

And today nearly 20 years later there is no reason why this opinion has to be modified. It was Rushton, one of the chief antagonists of the theory of

197

chronaxie, who was largely responsible for questioning the validity of the fundamental theory. In retrospect it is easy to see that the question involved the locus of action of curare. The protagonists of Lapicque's theory maintained that curare altered the irritability of muscle *per se* to direct stimulation. Rushton (1932) and his group denied any effect of curare on the *direct* excitability of muscle. This stimulating the prolonged dispute and the work arising from the dispute did much to enhance our knowledge of the mechanisms of muscle excitability. Ultimately the views of Lapicque did not prevail but they were nevertheless responsible for stimulating investigations upon which most of today's knowledge of nerve and muscle is based.

It is now 10 years since the International Meeting on Curare was held under the auspices of UNESCO National Research Council of Brazil and the Brazilian Academy of Sciences. As a result of this meeting under the editorial direction of Bovet, Bovet-Nitti and Marini-Bethòlo, there appeared a new comprehensive monograph on curare. But there still remain many questions concerning the precise mechanism of curarization to be answered. Thus the important findings of Estable (1959) on the innervation of the iris muscle in birds in which he reported that cholinergic nerves divide and innervate both radial and circular muscles in the iris has far-reaching implications. Furthermore, the findings by Abdon (1945) concerning the acetylcholine content of denervated muscle and the demonstration by McIntyre *et al.* (1950) of the effect of *d*-tubocurarine on denervated muscles and the work of Hayes and Riker (1963) are strong indications that the classical theory of the role of acetylcholine in neuromyal transmission and curarization may require modification. A study of the history of curare reveals many keys that may open doors to knowledge in the future, and without curare our knowledge of the physiological mechanisms involved in the motor control of muscles would undoubtedly have failed to progress.

9.8. CLINICAL

Historically there are two periods of clinical trial and usage of curare. The earlier period begins during the first few years of the nineteenth century when Brodie (1812) suggested to Flourens that curare could be used to control "spasmodic convulsive disorders". Brodie had shown that curarized animals could be resuscitated by means of artificial respiration. The second period begins shortly after the availability of standardized and uniform preparations of curare became available around 1940 although

King's pure *d*-tubocurarine was used by West in 1935. The early period saw curare used to control the convulsions of tetanus and Travers (1835) reported the successful treatment of equine tetanus by Sewell who obtained his curare from Robert Schomburgk. In 1858 Sayres (1858) of New York reported the use of curare in tetanus but it is hardly surprising that his local application of the curare to the site of injury was unsuccessful. Vella (1859) reported the use of curare on three of the wounded after the battle of Magenta, only one survived posttraumatic onset of tetanus. Similar inconclusive reports were made by Manec (1859), Chassaignac (1859), Follin (1859) and Gintrac (1859). Attempts to treat epilepsy were reported by Thiercelin (1860) and by Benedict (1866) and by Beigel (1868), who incidently used the semicrystalline preparation "urarin" of Preyer. Beigel's work has clinical importance because he accurately described the early signs of curarization in man including the ocular ptoses, change in the voice, difficulty in swallowing and weakness of the neck muscles which of course is the basis of the rabbit head-drop assay.* In 1878 Drummond reported the use of curare in chorea and in this century there were reports of favorable effects of curare in this disease by Tsocankis (1923) and by Papez *et al.* (1942), who used intocostrin. Simpson (1878), in a letter to the *Lancet*, indicates that curare had been used in rabies.

The second period of clinical trial of curare resulted in the successful use of standardized preparations and begins with the work of Bennett (1941) and the control of convulsions in shock therapy. In 1942 Griffith and Johnson and Griffith (1944, 1945) published their first paper on the use of curare as an adjuvant in anesthesia, and 3 years later Griffith reported upon the use of curare in 300 cases where curare was used for obtaining more complete relaxation. As a result of this achievement the Accademia Nazionale Dei Lincei awarded the Antonio Feltrenelli prize to Johnson and Griffith for their successful introduction of curare to anesthesia and to the author for his pharmacological study of the drug.

There are few topics whose history is as rewarding of study as curare. Knowledge of this drug embraces Geographic adventures and exploration, Botany, Chemistry, Physiology and Therapeutics—in a word it epitomizes the most exacting of all biological sciences—Pharmacology.

* The Rabbit "Head Drop" Assay method was originated by Mr. H. A. Holaday of the Squibb Biological Institute, New Brunswick, about 1945.

REFERENCES

ABDON, N. O. (1945) *Acta Pharm. Tox. Kbh.* **1**: 325.

ANGHERA, P. M. D' (1516) *De Orbe Novo.* Trans. Francis MacNutt (1912). G. P. Putnum's Sons, New York, 1st volume, pp. 75 ff.

BANCROFT, E. (1769) *An Essay on the Natural History of Guiana and South America.* T. Beckel & P. A. DeHont, London, pp. 286 ff.

BARBOSA RODRIGUES, J. (1903) *L'uiraêry ou curare.* Brussels.

BEIGEL, H. (1868) Versuchemit Curare und Curarin. *Berl. klin. Wchnschr.* **5**: 73, 98.

BENEDICT, M. (1866) Positive Resultate zur Curare-Therapie. *Wien. med. Presse.* **7**: 791.

BENNET, A. E. (1941) Clinical investigations with curare in organic neurological disorders. *Amer. J. M. Sci.* **202**: 102–12.

BERNARD, C. and PELOUZE, T. J. (1850) Recherches sur le curare. *Compt. Rend. Acad. Sci.* **31**: 533–537.

BERNARD, C. (1850) Action de curare et de la nicotine sur le système nerveux et sur le système musculaire. *Compt. Rend. Soc. Biol.* **2**: 195.

BERNARD, C. (1857) *Leçons sur les effets des substances toxiques.* Paris, pp. 316 ff.

BOEHM, R. (1886) *Chemische Studien über das Curare.* Leipzig, pp. 176 ff.

BOEHM, R. (1897) *Über Curare und Curare Alkaloide.* Leipzig, pp. 84 ff.

BOEHM, R. (1920) In: *Handbuch der Experimentellen Pharmakologie.* Heffter, A. (ed.). Julius Springer Press, Berlin.

BOUSSINGAULT and ROULIN (1828) Examen chimique du curare. *Ann. Chim. Phys.* **39**: 29.

BOVET, D. (1946) Rapports entre constitution chimique et activité pharmacoynamique dans quelques séries de curares de synthèse. In: *Curare and Curare-like Agents,* pp. 252–87. Bovet, D., Bovet-Nitti, F. and Marini-Bettòlo, G. B. (eds). Elsevier, Amsterdam.

BRODIE, Sir B. (1812) *Phil. Trans. Roy. Soc.* **102**: 378.

BUCHNER (1862) In: *Handbuch der Toxikologie,* Huseman, pp. 528 ff.

CASTELNAU, F. DE (1851) *Expédition de l'Amérique du sud.* Paris.

CHASSAIGNAC (1859) Use of curare in man: a communication to the Soc. de chir. *Gaz. Hebd. Méd.* **6**: 643.

CONDAMINE, DE LA (1813) In: *Voyagers and Travels.* Pinkerton, J. (ed.). Longman, Hurst, Rees Press, London, pp. 255 ff.

CREVAUX, J. (1882) Explorations des fleuves, Yary, Parou, Iça et Yapura, 1878–1879. *Bull. Soc. Geog.* **7**: 674–92.

DIEU, A. (1863) *Histoire du Curare.* Strasbourg.

DRUMMOND, D. (1878) A case of chorea treated by the subcutaneous injections of curara. *Brit. Med. J.* **1**: 857.

FOLLIN (1859) Curare in tetanus. *M. Times & Gaz.* **19**: 563 and *Bull. de Thérap.* **57**: 422.

FONTANA, F. (1781) *Traité sur le vénin de la vipère sur les poisons américains.* Florence, **2**: 89.

GARCILLASO DE LA VEGA (1609) Quoted in: *The Royal Commentaries of the Yncas.* Lisbon. Trans. C. R. Markham (1869). Hakluyt Society, London, 1st volume, pp. 59 ff.

GINTRAC, H. (1859) Observation de tétanos traumatique traité sans succés par le curare. *Gaz. Hop.* **32**: 554.

GOMARA, L. DE (1552) *Historia general des Indias.* Traduit en français par le S. de Genillé Mart. Fumée (1604), Paris, pp. 256 ff.

GRIFFITH, H. R. (1944) The use of curare in anaesthesia and for other clinical purposes. *Canad. Med. Ass. J.* **50**: 144–7.

GRIFFITH, H. R. (1945a) Curare in anesthesia. *J.A.M.A.* **127**: 642–4 and *Lancet* **2**: 74–75.

GRIFFITH, H. R. (1945b) Curare in anesthesia (reply). *J.A.M.A.* **127**: 644.

GRIFFITH, H. R. (1945c) Curare—a new tool for the anaesthetist. *Canad. Med. Ass. J.* **42**: 391–4.

GRIFFITH, H. R. and JOHNSON, G. E. (1942) The use of curare in general anesthesia. *Anesthesiology* **3**: 418–20.

HARTSINCK, J. VAN (1770) Part I, chapter iii, *Beschryving van Guiana*. Amsterdam, pp. 13 ff.

HAYES, A. H. and RIKER, W. F. (1963) Acetylcholine release at the neuromuscular junction. *J. Pharm. & Exper. Therap.* **142**: 200–5.

HEINTZ (1847) In: *Reisen in British Guiana*. Schomburgk, R. (ed.). pp. 452 ff.

HERISSANT (1751–1752) Experiments made on a great number of living animals, with the poison of Lamas, and of Ticunas. Trans. Thomas Slack, *Phil. Trans. Roy. Soc.* **47**: 75–92.

HERNDON, Lieut. W. L. (1854) *Exploration of the valley of the Amazon*. Washington, pp. 135 ff.

HILLHOUS (1868) In: *Anat. & Physiol.*, vol. 2. Biegel, H. J. (ed.). pp. 330 ff.

HUMBOLDT, A. VON and BONPLAND, A. (1807) *Voyage aux régions équinoxiales du nouveau continent*, vol. 5.

HUMBOLDT, A. VON and BONPLAND, A. (1821) *Personal Narratives*. Trans. Helen M. Williams. Longman, Hurst, Rees Press, London, pp. 527 ff.

HUNT, R. and TAVEAU, R. DE M. (1911) U.S. Public Health and Marine Hosp. Serv. *Hyg. Lab. Bull.* no. 73.

ING, H. R. (1936) Curariform action of onium salts. *Physiol. Rev.* **16**: 527–44.

ING, H. R. and BARLOW, R. B. (1948) Curare-like action of polymethylene bis-quaternary ammonium salts. *Brit. J. Pharm. Chemother.* **3**: 298–304.

KARRER, P. and SCHMID, H. (1946) *Helv. Chim. Acta* **29**: 1953.

KARRER, P. and SCHMID, H. (1955) *Angew. Chem.* **67**: 361.

KING, H. (1935a) Curare alkaloids. I. Tubocurarine. *J. Chem. Soc.* pp. 1381–9.

KING, H. (1935b) Curare. *Nature* **135**: 469.

KING, H. (1935c) Correspondence—Tubocurarine. *J. Soc. Chem. Indust.* **13**: 739.

KÜHNE, W. (1887) Neue Untersuchungen über motorische Nervenendigungen. *Ztschr. f. Biol.* **5**: 91.

LAPICQUE, L. (1909) Définition expérimentale de l'excitabilité. *Compt. Rend. Soc. Biol.* **67**: 280–2.

LAPICQUE, L. (1926) *L'excitabilité en fonction du temps la chronaxie*. Presses universitaires de France, Paris.

LAPICQUE, L. and LAPICQUE, M. (1929) Action du curare sur la fatigue musculaire. *Compt. Rend. Soc. Biol.* **101**: 915–17.

LOEWI, O. (1921) Über humorali. *Pflüger's Arch. des Phyiol.* **189**: 239–42.

MCINTYRE, A. R. (1947) *Curare: Its History, Nature, and Clinical Use*. University of Chicago Press, Chicago.

MCINTYRE, A. R. (1947) Theories of Curarization. In: *Curare: Its History, Nature, and Clinical Use*, pp. 102–25. The University of Chicago Press, Chicago.

MCINTYRE, A. R., KING, R. E. and DUNN, A. L. (1945) Electrical activity of denervated mammalian skeletal muscle as influenced by d-tubocurarine. *J. Neurophysiol.* **8**: 297–308.

MANEC (1859) Tétanos traumatique traité sans succès par le curare: lettre de M. Manec. *Gaz. Hebd. Méd.* **6**: 604.

MARINI-BETTÒLO, G. B., IORIO, M. A., LEDERER, M. and PIMENTA, A. (1954a). *Gazz. Chim. Ital.* **84**: 1155.

MARINI-BETTÒLO, G. B., IORIO, M. A., PIMENTA, A., DUCKE, A. and BOVET, D. (1954) *Gazz. Chim. Ital.* **84**: 1161.

MARINI-BETTÒLO, G. B. and IORIO, M. A. (1955) *Résumés Trav. XIVe Congr. Intern. Chim. Pure et Appl.* Zurich, pp. 152 ff.

MARINI-BETTÒLO, G. B., BERREDO CARNEIRO, P. DE and CASINOVI, G. C. (1956) *Gazz. Chim. Ital.* **86**: 1148.

MARINI-BETTÒLO, G. B. and IORIO, M. A. (1956) *Gazz. Chim. Ital.* **86**: 1305.

MARINI-BETTÒLO, G. B. and BOVET, D. (1956) *Selected Sci. Papers Ist. super. Sanità.* **1**: 26.

MARINI-BETTÒLO, G. B. (1957) *Festschrift Arthur Stoll.* Birkhauser, Basel, pp. 257 ff.

MARTIUS, C. F. VON (1830) Ueber die Bereitung des Pfeilgiftes Urari bei den Indianern Juris am Rio Japura in Nordbrasilien. In: *Buchner, Repertorium für die Pharmacie*, vol. 36, pp. 340–9. J. Johann Leonhard Schrag, Nuremberg.

OBERDORFER, A. (1859) Ueber das Urari. *Wittstein Vierteljahrschr. f. Prakt. Pharm.*, pp. 568–9.

OSCULATI, G. (1850) *Esplorazione delle Regioni Equatoriali.* Milan, pp. 108 ff.

PAPEZ, J. W., BENNETT, A. E. and CASH, P. T. (1942) Huntington's chorea. *Arch. Neurol. Psychiat.* **47**: 667–76.

PATON, W. D. M. and ZAIMIS, E. J. (1949) The pharmacological actions of polymethylene bistrimethylammonium salts. *Brit. J. Pharm. Chemother.* **4**: 381–400.

PEDRONI, J. (1844) Analyses du poison qu'emploient les Indiens des environs de Caracas. *J. Pharm. Chim.* **5**: 321–2.

PELLETIER, J., CAVENTOU, J. and BIENAIMÉ, J. (1819) *Ann. de Chim. Phys.* **12**: 113.

PENNA, A., IORIO, M. A., CHIAVERELLI, S. and MARINI-BETTÒLO, G. B. (1957) *Gazz. Chim. Ital.* **87**: 1163.

PERROT, E. and VOGT, E. (1911) *Poisons de Flèches et Poisons d'Eprouve.* Paris.

PIMENTA, A., IORIO, M. A., ADANK, K. and MARINI-BETTÒLO, G. B. (1954) *Gazz. Chim. Ital.* **84**: 1147.

PREYER, N. W. (1865) Ueber das wirksame Princip des Curare. *Ztschr. f. Chemie* **1**: 381–4.

ROBERTSON (1778) History of America. In: *Oxford Dictionary*, pp. 19 ff.

RUSHTON, W. A. H. (1932) The identification of Lucas's α excitability. *J. Physiol.* **75**: 445–70.

SAABEDRA, C. DE (1620) In: *Historical and Ethnographical Material on the Jivaro Indians.* Stirling, M. W. (ed.) Smithsonian Institute, Bulletin 117, Washington, D.C., pp. 136 ff.

SAYRES, L. A. (1858) Two cases of traumatic tetanus. *N. Y. J. Med.* **4**: 250.

SCHEBESTA, P. (1941) The arrow poisons of the Bambubi Pygmies. *Ciba Symposia* **3**: 1010.

SCHOMBURGK, R. (1841) On the Urari. *Ann. & Mag. Nat. Hist.*, 7th vol., pp. 409 ff.

SCHOMBURGK, R. (1848) *Ralegh's Discovery of Guiana.* Hakluyt Society, London, pp. 71 ff.

SCHOMBURGK, R. (1879) *On the Urari: the deadly arrow poison of the Macusis, an Indian tribe in British Guiana.* Adelaide, Australia, pp. 7 ff.

SCHREBER, J. C. D. VON (1783) Ueber das Pfeilgift der Amerikaner in Guiana, und die Gewächse aus denen es bereitet wird. *Naturforsch.* **19**: 129–58.

SIMSON, A. (1878) Curara (letter to the editor). *Lancet* **1**: 776.

STIRLING, M. W. (1938) *Historical and Ethnographical Material on the Jivaro Indians.* Smithsonian Institute, Bulletin 117, Washington, D.C., pp. 1 ff.

TAMMELIN, L. E. (1953) Succinylcholine iodide (Celocurine): a synthetic drug with a curare-like effect. *Acta Chem. Scand.* **7.1**: 185–95.

THIERCELIN, L. (1860) Note sur l'emploi du curare dans le traitement des névroses convulsives et en particulier dans celui de l'épilepsie. *Compt. Rend. Acad. Sci.* **51**: 716.

TRAVERS, B. (1835) *A Further Inquiry Concerning Constitutional Irritation.* Longman, Hurst, Rees Press, London, pp. 308 ff.

Tschudi, J. J. von (1847) *Travels in Peru*. Trans. Thomasina Ross (Eng. Ed.), London, pp. 407 ff.

Tsocankis, G. (1923) *De l'Action Thérapeutique du Bromhydrate de Cicutine et du Curare dans les États Spasmodiques*. Paris, pp. 64 ff.

Vella, M. (1859) Use of woorara as a remedy in traumatic tetanus. *M. Times & Gaz.* **19**: 343–4.

Vulpian, A. (1881) *Leçons sur l'Action Physiologiques des Substances Toxique et Médicamenteuses*. Paris.

Waterton, C. (1879) *Wanderings in South America*. Macmillan & Co., London, pp. 133 ff.

West, R. (1932) Curare in man. *Proc. Roy. Soc. Med.* **25**: 1107–16.

West, R. (1935) Pharmacology and therapeutics of curare. *Brit. Med. J.* **1**: 125–6.

Wieland, H., Konz, W. and Sonderhoff, R. (1937) *Ann.* **527**: 160.

Wieland, H. and Pistor, H. J. (1938) *Ann.* **536**: 68.

Wieland, H. and Pistor, H. J. (1940) Curare Alkaloids. Ger. 695–066.

Wieland, H., Pistor, H. J. and Bähr, K. (1941a) *Ann.* **547**: 140.

Wieland, H., Bähr, K. and Witkop, B. (1941b) *Ann.* **547**: 156.

Wieland, H., Witkop, B. and Bähr, K. (1947) *Ann.* **558**: 144.

Wieland, T. and Merz, H. (1952) *Ber.* **85**: 731.

Wieland, T. and Merz, H. (1953) *Ann.* **580**: 204.

Wieland, T., Fritz, H., and Hasspacker, K. (1954) *Ann.* **588**: 1.

Wintersteiner, O. and Dutcher, J. D. (1943) Curare alkaloids from *Chondodendron tomentosum*. *Science* **97**: 467–70.

CHAPTER 10

CHEMISTRY AND PHARMACOLOGY OF NATURAL CURARE COMPOUNDS

P. G. Waser

Zürich

10.1 INTRODUCTION

Since the discovery of the Americas in the sixteenth century the Old World knows about the existence of very potent arrow poisons known as "curare". This interest-rousing and feared material—the only new secret weapon the Aztecs, Toltecs, Incas and other native inhabitants of Central and South America were able to use against the armory and horses of the Spanish conquistadores—was very soon investigated by science-minded padres and educated followers of the invaders. The most interesting and colorful descriptions of the famous explorers (Sir Walter Raleigh, La Condamine, Alexander von Humboldt, the Schomburgk brothers and others) are today well known. They wrote about the mysterious preparation of the aqueous extracts of many unknown plants and animals, the concentrating procedures, the testing of curare activity on animals and sometimes men, and finally the use in hunting or war (Boehm, 1897, 1920; Lewin, 1923; McIntyre, 1947; Craig, 1948; Cheymol, 1949; Waser, 1953). Only in the last 20 to 30 years have modern chemistry and pharmacology cleared the field from fantastic tales to sober scientific statements. With the powerful analytical methods of our time the most important problems in this field have been solved and new drugs for widespread practical use in anesthesiology, surgery and other clinical fields of medicine have evolved.

It is my task to describe the most important details of this story and to give the facts to the pharmacologists for a better understanding of the most selective curare action of some important natural curare compounds. My starting point as a reviewer will be the chemistry of these drugs, but for a fruitful synopsis of knowledge on curare action I will have to mention pharmacological data and to discuss relations of chemical structure to biological activity.

Curare and curare-activity are phenomenological terms describing neuromuscular block of impulse transmission at the end-plate. The result is complete paralysis of the skeletal or striated muscle apparatus. The selection of many curarizing compounds was done from substances following this definition and with important practical application. Therefore some derivatives of natural alkaloids with marked curariform activity and used in anesthesiology will also be mentioned.

10.2. THE CLASSICAL CURARE COMPOUNDS OF BOTANICAL ORIGIN

The large amount of information on curare accumulated before 1900 is only of historical interest today. The variation of the composition and the complexity of the mixtures investigated prevented accurate and repeatable scientific investigation. The old terminology introduced by Boehm (1920) and Lewin (1923) is still used. They distinguished different types of curare preparations by the container in which they were packed:

(a) Tubo-, bamboo- or para-curare, packed in bamboo tubes. They originate mostly from the lower Amazonas region. The plants used by the natives for the preparation of a light-brown powder are mainly Menispermaceae.

(b) Pot-curare, which is contained in small earthenware pots and may have a quite different botanical origin (Menispermaceae or Logani-aceae), as we found alkaloids of the genus Strychnos in pots from the central part of the Amazon basin.

(c) Calabash-curare, the most active type, is packed in small gourds or calabashes, often the hollow fruits of some Strychnos species. This curare is mainly produced in the region of the great rivers Orinoko and Amazonas from different species of Strychnos.

(d) Lewin described curare put in little twisted bags by the Ticuna tribe and having similar properties as calabash curare.

Plants of different Erythrina species are not used in preparation of arrow-poisons. The extracts of seeds show marked paralytic action in animals, and some alkaloids were used in the clinic for similar purposes as tubocurarine and the calabash alkaloids.

The calabashes and pots collected in the same region, shown in Fig. 1, contained on paper chromatograms nearly the same different alkaloids

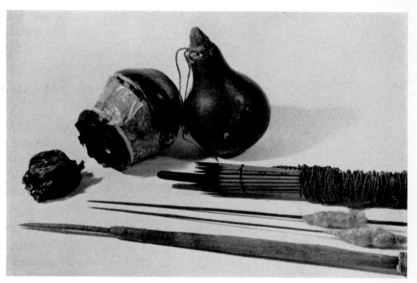

FIG. 1. Original calabash and pot containing black material from which calabash curare alkaloids were extracted. Darts with cotton plug for blow-pipes carry the crude curare at their tips.

in similar amounts. This proves the term tubo-, pot- or calabash-curare to be mainly phenomenological and not to depend on its content.

10.3. ALKALOIDS OF MENISPERMACEAE

Menispermaceous plants contain different types of alkaloids:

(a) Those containing a single nitrogen in a dibenzoquinolizine ring-system (berberine, columbamine, coptisine and others).

(b) Those with *l*-benzyl-tetrahydroisoquinoline ring-systems (coclaurine and isococlaurine).

(c) Bisbenzyltetrahydroisoquinoline alkaloids in which two *l*-benzyl-tetrahydroisoquinoline types are joined through ether linkages (the curines, chondodendrines, tetrandrine, danricine, etc.).

(d) The quaternary alkaloids of bisbenzyltetrahydroisoquinoline type with two quaternary nitrogens. The most important is *d-tubo-*

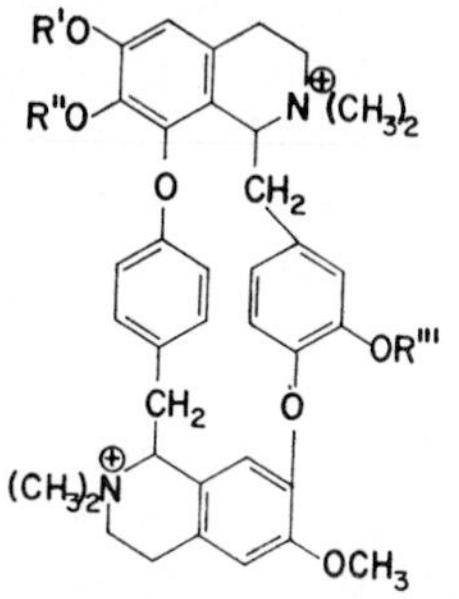

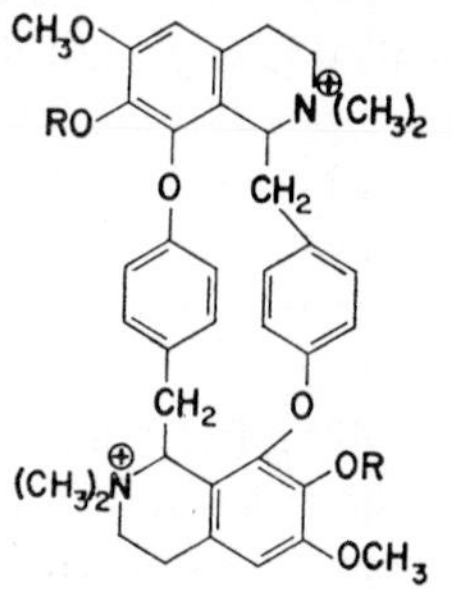

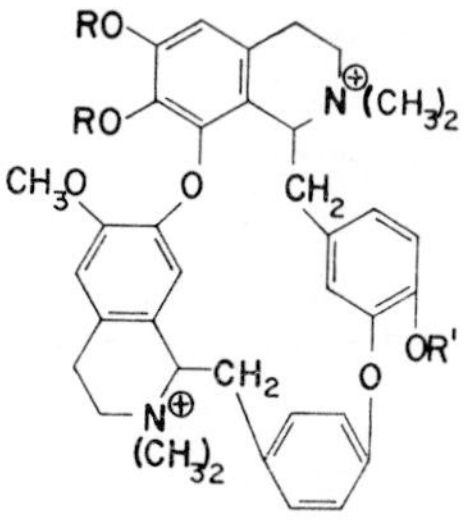

Fig. 2. Different types of natural bisbenzylisoquinoline alkaloids found in tubocurare.

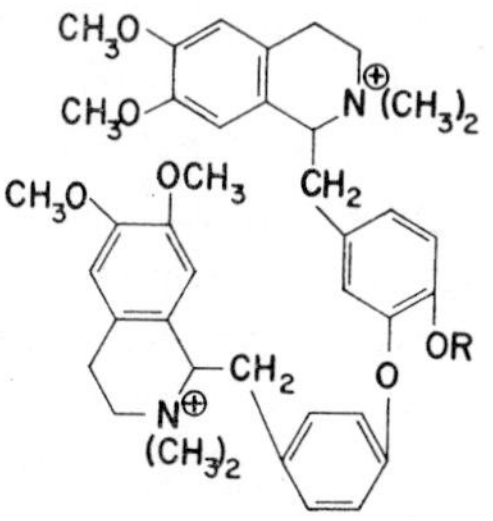

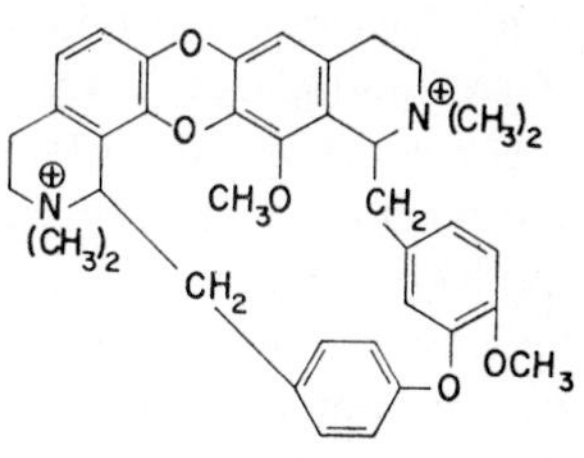

207

curarine, as principle ingredient of tubocurare and later isolated from a single menispermaceous plant species (*Chondodendron tomentosum*, Ruiz and Pavon). Other quaternary alkaloids which have been isolated from this plant are *l*-tubocurarine (levorotatory enantiomorph of *d*-tubocurarine), *d*-chondocurarine, *l*-tomentocurarine and others. They and the quaternary derivatives of other bisbenzyltetrahydroisoquinoline alkaloids are potent curarizing agents. All of the other alkaloids have little or no curariform activity, even when the single nitrogen atoms in the molecules are converted to quaternary salts.

The bisbenzylisoquinoline alkaloids are of several types (I–V), differing in the manner in which the benzylisoquinoline moieties are joined by ether linkages (Fig. 2).

Chondodendron alkaloids

Most Chondodendron alkaloids are diacidic bisbenzyltetrahydroisoquinoline bases in which the two halves of the molecule are joined together in the so-called head-to-tail/head-to-tail fashion. An exception is isococlaurine (VI), a secondary base of the monobenzyltetrahydroisoquinoline type from pareira brava. It is the structure isomer of *d*-coclaurine (VII) which occurs in the Asiatic menisperm *Cocculus laurifolius*, and where only the *O*-methyl group and the phenolic hydroxyl at positions 6 and 7 are exchanged (Fig. 3).

In the isochondodendrin group the two benzyltetrahydroisoquinoline or coclaurine units are joined by the two connecting ether bridges in such a way that a centrosymmetric system results. The group furthermore includes two tertiary bases *D*-protocuridine (VIII) and i-neoprotocuridine (IX) which have been encountered so far only in pot curare. They are isomers of isochondodendrine (X).

The pharmacologist Boehm (1920) isolated from tubocurare the tertiary base curine in crystallized form which was hardly curare-active. Later Späth (1928) showed *l*-curine (XI) to be the optical antipode of *D*-bebeerine. *Radix pareirae bravae* from Brazil or Mexico contained both depending on the content of *Chondodendron platiphyllum* (*l*-curine) or *Ch. microphyllum* (*D*-bebeerine). Finally King (1935) proved Boehm's *d*-tubocurarine to be the diastereomer of curine-chlormethylate, and Wintersteiner and Dutcher (1943) isolated directly *d*-tubocurarine chloride from *Ch. tomentosum*. In addition the extracts yielded *l*-curine, *d*-isochondodendrine and its dimethyl ether, and *d*-chondocurine. Later,

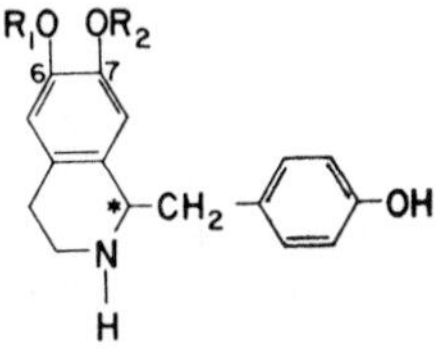

$$R_1O \quad OR_2$$

VI   d-Isococlaurine: $R_1=H, R_2=CH_3$
VII   d-Coclaurine: $R_1=CH_3, R_2=H$

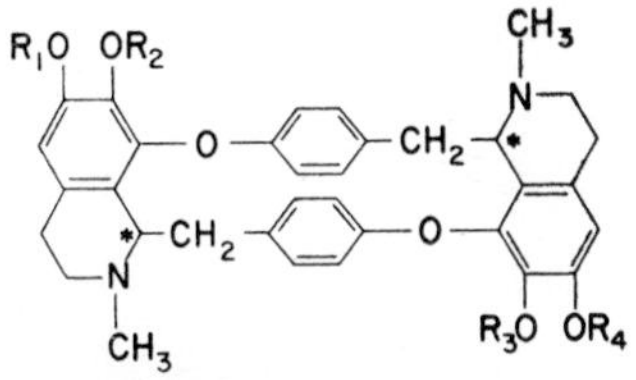

		R_1	R_2	R_3	R_4
VIII	d-Protocuridine:	CH_3	H	CH_3	H
IX	i-Neoprotocuridine:	H	CH_3	CH_3	H
X	d-Isochondodendrine:	CH_3	H	H	CH_3

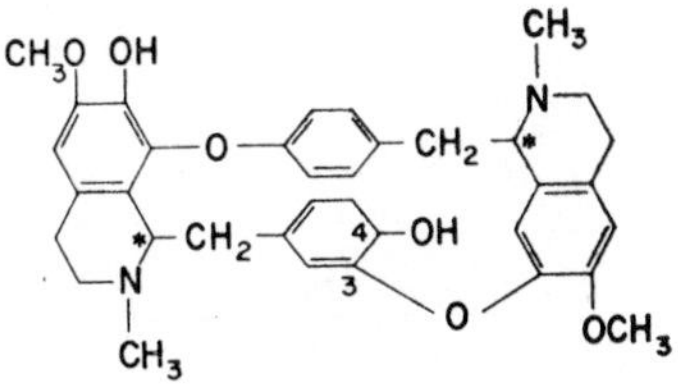

XI   d and l-Curine

Fig. 3. Structural formulae of chondodendron alkaloids.

Dutcher (1951) showed that a substantial part of the activity of such extracts was due to a second quaternary base, *d*-chondocurarine, which is present in only a small amount in the alkaloid mixture.

For reasons of space the degradative and synthetic routes by which the structure of chondodendron alkaloids was established are only discussed in short. Boehm (1897) proposed for curine (XI) the formula $C_{18}H_{19}O_3N$, but Faltis *et al.* (1932), King (1939) and Späth and Kuffner (1934) suggested

209

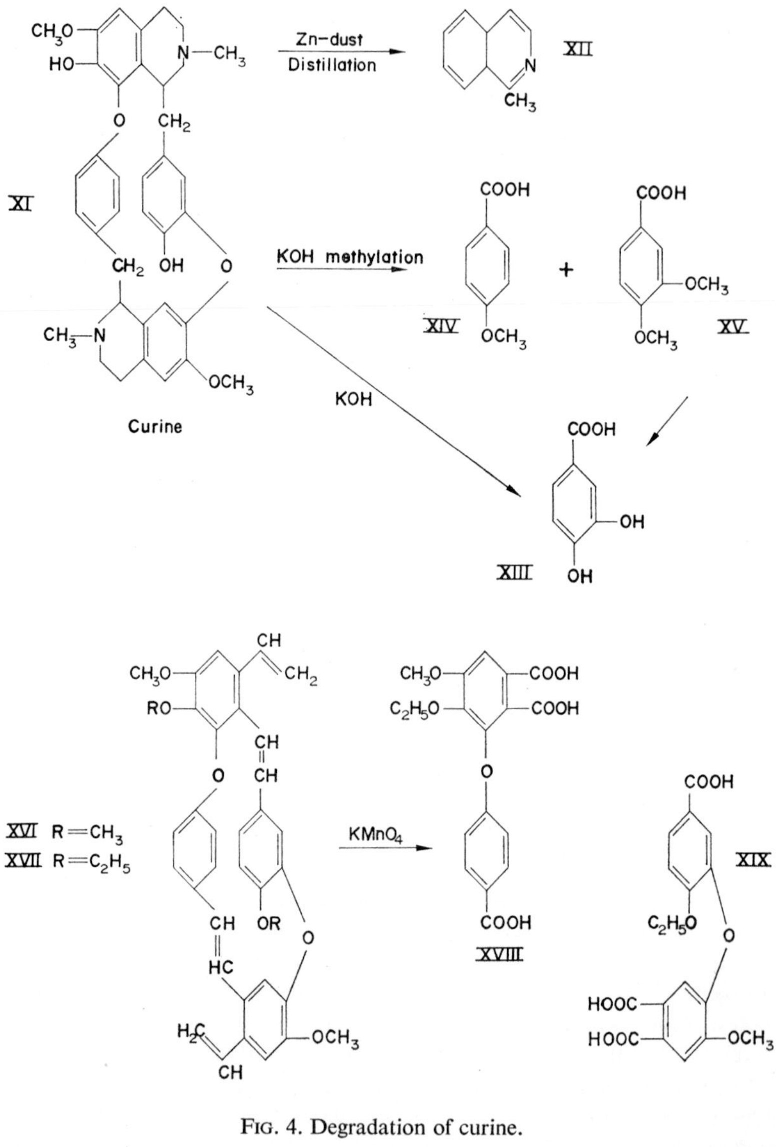

FIG. 4. Degradation of curine.

210

for different reasons the doubling to $C_{36}H_{38}O_6N_2$. For instance, partial methylation led to an ether with one free phenolic hydroxyl group, but in the $C_{18}H_{19}O_3N$ formula two of the three oxygens were already determined as one methoxy and one ether group. King's structural formula of curine (Fig. 4) was based on the following evidence:

Distillation with zinc dust gave *l*-methyl-isoquinoline (XII), melting of demethylated bebeerine with potassium hydroxide gave degradation products as protocatechinic acid (XIII), or after methylation anisic (XIV) or veratric acid (XV). Hofmann degradation of the quaternary *O*-methyl-curinechlormethylate and *O*-methyltubocurarine-chloride gave the same *N*-free product *O*-methylbebeerylen (XVI). King (1936) determined the position of the free hydroxy group of Hofmann-degradation of the ethyl-ated-compounds (XVII) to *O*-ethyl-bebeerylen and $KMnO_4$-oxydation to two isomeric acids (XVIII, XIX). Their constitution was proved by synthesis.

Curine differs from isochondodendrine in that one inner hydroxyl function supplies an ether link to position 3' of the opposed benzyl group, baring a free phenolic hydroxyl in position 4' of this group. In the isomeric *d*-chondocurine from *Ch. tomentosum* the benzylic hydroxyl group is likewise free, while the positions of the vicinal free and methylated hy-droxyl groups in the other aromatic ring might be reversed. This early structure is now contested by Everett *et al.* (1970) who believe chondocurine to be synonymous with tubocurine with no difference in the relative posi-tions of methoxy- and phenolic groups.

Quaternary bases

Tubocurarine occurs in nature in both enantiomorphic modifications. Although the distribution of free and methylated groups is the same as that in curine, they differ in diastereoisomerism. *D*-tubocurarine (XX) and *d*-chondocurarine yield on methylation of their hydroxyl groups an identical dimethyl ether. This shows that the two alkaloids have the same stereochemistry but differ structurally (Fig. 5). Recently Everett *et al.* (1970) have proved by using nuclear magnetic resonance spectroscopy and by methylation and cleaving studies that *d*-tubocurarine has only three *N*-methyl groups instead of four. Tubocurarine surprisingly is monoquaternary, but the second tertiary nitrogen is easily protonized.

D-chondocurarine chloride is the dimethochloride of *d*-tubocurine differing from *d*-tubocurarine only in the degree of quaternization and not in the location of methyl ether residue.

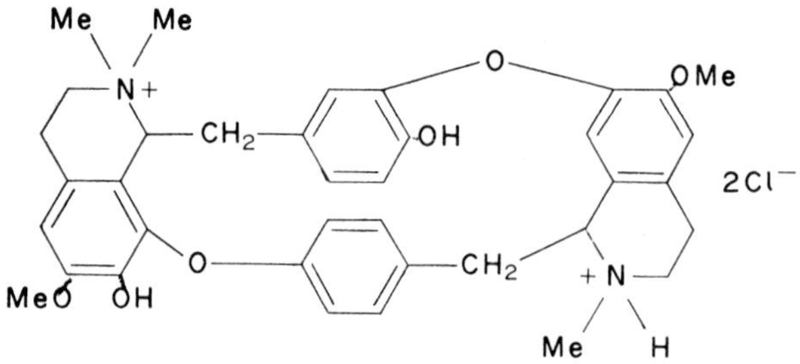

(XX)

FIG. 5. New structure of (+)-tubocurarine chloride. The quaternary nitrogen is located in the tetrahydroisoquinoline ring bearing the free phenolic group.

TABLE 1. COMPARATIVE POTENCIES OF QUATERNARY ALKALOIDS IN HOLADAY RABBIT HEAD-DROP ASSAY

(O. Wintersteiner, 1959)

Compound	Potency d-TC cation$=1$	Remarks
d-Tubocurarine (d-TC)	1.00	HD 50 rabbit: 0.125 mg/kg, dog: 0.16, man: 0.15
O-Dimethyl-d-TC	8.7	Dog: 9.4; monkey, 6.6; human, 1.5–3; mouse, 1.1
O-Diethyl-d-TC	1.9	
O-Di-n-butyl-d-TC	0.09	
O-Dibenzyl-d-TC	0.07	
l-Tubocurarine	0.05–0.1	0.03–0.06 in rat-diaphragm test
d-Chondocurarine	2.5	Ethers identical with those of d-TC
N-Diethyl-d-chondocurine	0.9	Half duration of head-drop
N-Dibenzyl-d-chondocurine	0.17	
N-Dimethyl-d-curine	3.5	
O-Dimethyl-N-dimethyl-d-curine	1.3	
N-Dimethyl-l-curine	1.3	
O-Dimethyl-N-dimethyl-l-curine	3.3	
N-Dimethyl-d-isochondo-dendrine	0.05	
O-Dimethyl-N-dimethyl-d-isochondodendrine	0.26	

Pharmacological potencies of quaternary alkaloids

In this group only the quaternary alkaloids have curare activity in different tests. Therefore different tertiary bases were quaternized and free hydroxyl groups were alkylated. As standard method mainly Holaday's head-drop of rabbits (Varney *et al.*, 1949) was used. The potency is calculated on the weight bases of the weight of the cations, the potency of *d*-tubocurarine serving as unit (Table 1). Attempts to correlate chemical structure with the activity of bisquaternary alkaloids base on the facts given in Table 1.

Surprisingly, *O*-methylation of *d*-tubocurarine raises its potency 9 times, *O*-ethylation twice. However, this high ratio is obtained only in the rabbit and the dog; in the monkey it falls to 6, in the human to 2 and in the mouse to equipotency. Larger substituting groups held in ether linkage diminish the activity to less than one-tenth. The enantiomorph *l*-tubocurarine is much less active, which emphasizes the importance of steric factors for activity or interaction with specific and non-specific receptors. *D*-chondocurarine is 3 times more active than *d*-tubocurarine. All other than *N*-methyl-derivatives are less active. *N*-dimethyl-*d*-curine is also 3.5 times more active than *d*-tubocurarine. The enantiomorph quaternary base derived from *l*-curine is less active, but its *O*-dimethyl-derivative shows again the amplifying effect of activity.

The symmetrical *N*-methyl-derivative of *d*-isochondodendrine has very low activity enhanced only by *O*-methylation. Asymmetry of the curarizing quaternary molecule seems to be of some importance. *D*-tubocurarine is the classical example of non-depolarizing muscle relaxant.

The presence of two quaternary nitrogens in a single molecule is responsible for the high activity. The distance between the two nitrogens is about 14 Å, which is about the same distance for maximal curare activity of synthetic compounds. But as the stereospecificity of *d*-tubocurarine demonstrates, not only the size but also the shape of the molecule plays an important part in the mechanism of action (Loewe and Harvey, 1952).

In different animals (rat, cat, dog, rabbit) and man secondary effects were carefully investigated by Marsh and Herring (1950). Generally speaking, side effects such as salivation, lacrimation, vomiting, defecation and urination were more pronounced in compounds of types I and IV and almost non-existent in types III and V (Fig. 2). Type I (as *d*-tubocurarine) always produced some fall in blood pressure in barbitalized cats by action on autonomous transmission. This effect on blood pressure was very strong in compounds of types II and IV, but much less of types III and V.

213

D-tubocurarine produces some bronchoconstriction, hypotension and lowering of blood pressure which are attributed to liberation of histamine.

The doses required to produce minimal surgical relaxation in a 70 kg unanesthetized man is 9.5 mg *d*-tubocurarine and 4.0 mg *O,O*-dimethyl-*d*-tubocurarine. The grip strength is reduced by 90–95%, the vital capacity by 30%. Grip strength recovered to 75% of the original value in 25 minutes. The neuromuscular effect of *d*-tubocurarine and dimethyl-tubocurarine is markedly potentiated by ether and cyclopropane and it is antagonized by physostigmine, neostigmine and edrophonium. Combination with halothane leads to severe hypotension. With up to 14 mg of *d*-tubocurarine side-effects such as throbbing headache, bronchoconstriction, cold sweat, vertigo, fall in blood pressure, salivation and flushing of extremities have been occasionally reported. No central stimulant, depressant or analgesic actions were observed in a volunteer even after 2.5 times the paralysing dose. Dimethyl-tubocurarine has a shorter action and relatively fewer side-effects than tubocurarine (Foldes, 1957).

10.4. THE CURARIZING ALKALOIDS OF ERYTHRINA SPECIES

The seeds of different Erythrina species growing all over the world in subtropical and tropical zones contain alkaloids with curarizing activity. Altamirano and Dominguez (1876 and 1886) first described in Mexico the curarizing effect of extracts from seeds of *E. americana* (Lehman, 1937). In Argentina extracts from parts of *E. crista galli* (leaves, barks, flowers and especially seeds) were pharmacologically active (Cicardo and Hug, 1937). Folkers and Unna (1938; 1939) investigated many other species (*E. eggersii*, *E. coralloides*, *E. macrophylla*, *E. buchii*, etc.) from different parts of the world and found that all of them gave extracts with curare-like action.

10.4.1. CHEMISTRY OF ERYTHRINA ALKALOIDS

Erythrina seeds contain different bases. In all species so far studied, *hypaphorine* (XXI), the betaine of tryptophane, has been found (Table 2). Besides this alkaloid of no special pharmacological interest, Folkers and Major (1937) isolated the first crystalline active base erythroidine (XXII) from *E. americana*. The most interesting fact about this and other active alkaloids was their tertiary basic nature, not being quaternary bases like the curarizing alkaloids from Chondodendron or Strychnos.

TABLE 2. BASES FROM ERYTHRINA SEEDS (Deulofeu, 1959)

XXI

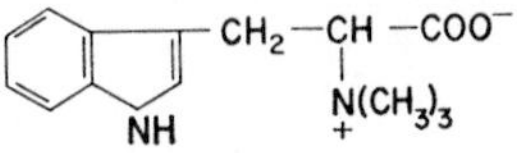

$$CH_2-CH-COO^-$$

$$N(CH_3)_3^+$$

NH

Hypaphorine

Aromatic alkaloids

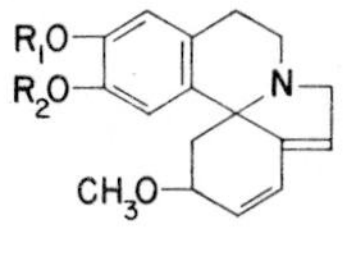

	Free		Liberated	
XXV	$R_1 + R_2 = CH_2$ Erythraline	$R_1 = R_2 = H$	Erysopine	
	Erythramine = Dihydro-erythraline	R_1 or $R_2 = H$ R_2 or $R_1 = CH_3$	Erysodine	
		R_2 or $R_1 = CH_3$ R_1 or $R_2 = H$	Erysovine	

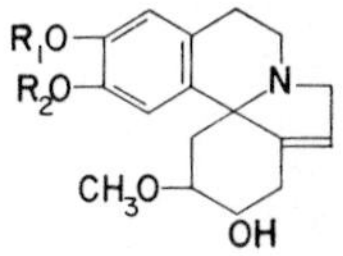

R_1O-
R_2O-
CH_3O-
N

$R_1 + R_2 = CH_2$ Erythratine
$R_1 = R_2 = CH_3$ Erythratidine

R_1O-
R_2O-
CH_3O-
OH
N

Lactone alkaloids

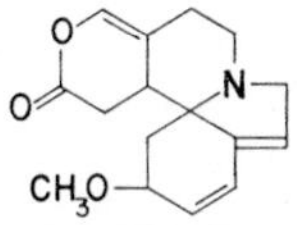

O
O
CH$_3$O-
N

XXII α-Erythroidine

O
O
CH$_3$O-
N

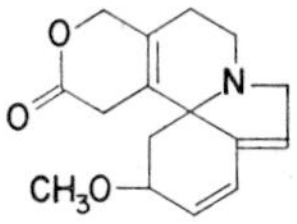

XXII β-Erythroidine

The Erythrina alkaloids may be divided into two groups: aromatic and lactone alkaloids (Table 2). Some of the aromatic, the so-called free alkaloids, can be extracted directly with solvents from the alkalinized water extracts of seeds. Others exist in conjugated complexes and must first be liberated by acid hydrolysis before extraction. They may be linked to sulfoacetic acid (erysothiovine and erysothiopine) (Folkers *et al.*, 1944) or conjugated with *D*-glucose.

The free alkaloids are rather difficult to separate in pure form (Deulofeu *et al.*, 1959), but bound bases can easily be extracted and crystallized after acid hydrolysis.

Folkers and his group started work on the structure of Erythrina alkaloids, which was later continued mainly by Boekelheide and Prelog (1955). Erysothrine (XXIII) ($C_{19}H_{23}NO_3$) is oxidized to *m*-hemipinic acid (XXIV), erythraline (XXV) in similar ways to hydrastic acid. The methoxy group in allyl position is split off by weak acids and three conjugated double bonds are found with a spectrometer. Concentrated acids lead to

215

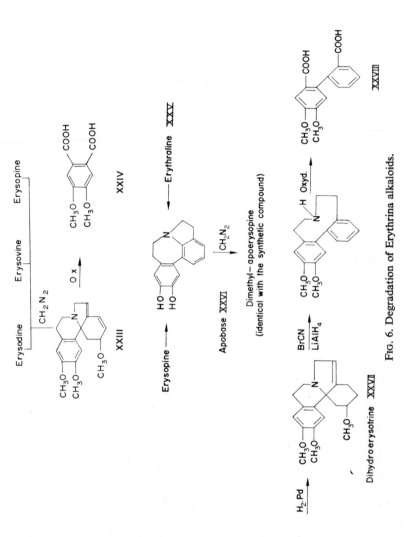

FIG. 6. Degradation of Erythrina alkaloids.

rearrangement of the ring structure to an apobase (XXVI) with an indoline system, which is optically inactive and a weak base (Fig. 6). The spiro structure was suggested by this characteristic rearrangement and was then proved by degradation of the dihydroerysothrine (XXVII) with cyanobromide followed by reduction with lithium aluminum hydride. Final oxydation gave dimethoxy-diphenyl-dicarbonic acid (XXVIII). The spiro structure was confirmed by X-ray studies and later by synthesis.

10.4.2. PHARMACOLOGY OF ERYTHRINA ALKALOIDS

The Erythrina alkaloids are the first compounds containing a tertiary nitrogen that exhibit a pronounced curariform action. In most cases the conversion of a tertiary base which has a curare action to a quaternary compound greatly enhances the action. This is not true with the Erythrina alkaloids as β-erythroidine (XXII) (Table 2) is reduced in effectiveness by a factor of about 20 on conversion to the methiodide. This is also true to a lesser extent with erythraline, erythramine and erythratine. Another important difference to quaternary curare alkaloids is their high oral activity, which is in animals often greater than after subcutaneous administration.

β-Erythroidine paralyses frogs in doses of 3–8 mg/kg as compared to doses of 0.5 mg/kg *d*-tubocurarine chloride. It is claimed to be more than 7 times less toxic than tubocurare (Burman, 1940). Dihydro-β-erythroidine is 5–10 times more effective than β-erythroidine itself. The β-tetrahydro-β-erythroidine also has an action greater than that of the unsaturated alkaloid, but the α-isomer (Table 2) is very much less effective. Erysothiopine and erysothiovine are 3–4 times as effective as erysopine and erysovine, and differ from them only by the presence of a sulfo-acetic residue in the ring. This indicates that the sulfo-acetic group, attached as a sulfonic ester, enhances curare activity.

In cats and rabbits the muscles recover very quickly, after intravenous injections of erythroidines. The action is antagonized by physostigmine and other anticholinesterases. The oral administration is reported to have a hypnotic rather than a curare action not seen when given by injection. A second relaxing effect on neural transmission is exerted by action on spinal internuncial neurons. They cause depression of blood pressure and, frequently, respiration in paralysing doses. They do not liberate histamine but are synergistic with certain anesthetics and hypnotics (Burman, 1940). β-Erythroidine and its dihydroderivative have at one time been tried clinically on dystonic and spastic conditions and to mitigate the convulsion treatment of schizophrenia. They are used no longer in the clinic because better curarizing compounds are available.

10.5. CURARIZING ALKALOIDS OF CALABASH CURARE

This curare type comes from the primeval forests of Brazil and its neighboring states Guyana, Venezuela and Columbia. Most of its alkaloids are found in the barks of different Strychnos species, which are used by the natives as starting material for the preparation of the very powerful calabash curare. The same alkaloids were isolated by Wieland and his co-workers (Wieland *et al.*, 1937; 1941), Karrer, Schmid and their group (Karrer and Schmid, 1955; Karrer *et al.*, 1949; 1960), and Battersby and Hodson (1965), and other chemists in various laboratories, from calabashes or extracted from Strychnos barks (*Str. Mitcherlichii, Str. toxifera, Str. Melinoniana, Str. Guianensis, Str. diaboli, Str. macrophylla, Str. trinervis, Str. tomentosa, Str. cogens, Str. Amazonica, Str. Peckii,* etc.). Only ten of the forty isolated alkaloids have an interesting pharmacological activity; a few more are weak curarizing substances. In the clinic, a short-acting derivative of toxiferine (*N,N'*-diallyl-bis-nortoxiferine, alcuronium alloferine[R]) is used in increasing amounts, because of its low incidence of side effects. Twenty-five years after the first isolation of the main alkaloids of calabash curare (the prefix C means isolation from calabash material) (C-curarine, C-toxiferine, C-calebassine, C-dihydrotoxiferine) and intensive scientific research, the clinical usefulness of this compound is firmly established.

10.5.1. CHEMISTRY OF SOME CALABASH ALKALOIDS

The first isolation of alkaloids from methanol water extracts of calabashes was successful by chromatography of the reineckates (Reinecke acid $H[Cr(NH_3)_2(SCN)_4]$) in acetone on Al_2O_3-columns. The use of cellulose powder in large columns by Karrer and Schmid (1955) gave a more powerful separation of the alkaloid chlorides. This method was combined with paper or thin layer chromatography. Cerium (IV) sulfate or iodide-solution was used as coloring reagent. A paper chromatogram shows the separation of 1 mg alkaloid chlorides of a calabash (Fig. 7). The most active compounds being more polar remain near the starting point.

One of the difficulties in the analysis of the content of calabashes is the easy conversion of its alkaloids to new compounds which may not have been present in the original plant. Spectroscopic methods first showed

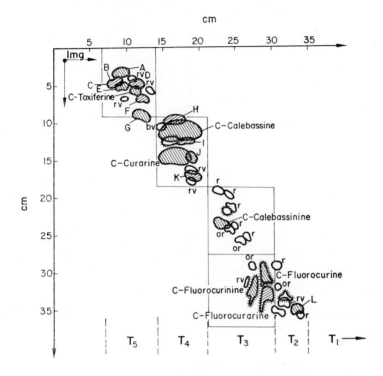

FIG. 7. Paper chromatogram of alkaloid chlorides of a calabash (Schmid, *et al.*, 1952).

that most of these alkaloids are closely related indole derivatives. The indole chromophor is responsible for the color reaction with Cerium sulfate. Beside the indole nitrogen N(a) with weak basic influence there is a second nitrogen group N(b) of strong basic character due to its quaternary methyl group.

The difference in these N-groups was used to demonstrate the active calabash alkaloids to be biquaternary with a high molecular weight (38–42 carbon and 4 nitrogen atoms) instead of only one-half. When the tertiary base norcurarine, derived from the quaternary ammonium salt curarine by demethylation, was partially requaternized by addition of methylchloride in half equivalent acid, three kinds of salts were formed (Fig. 8) (Philipsborn *et al.*, 1956). The first was biquaternary, the second monoquaternary-monoprotonized and the third diprotonized. They were separated by paper chromatography. In the monochloromethylate one

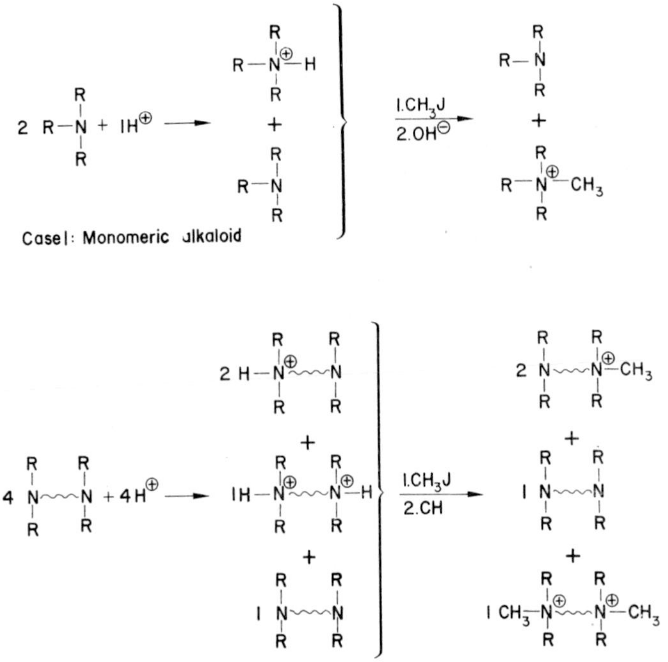

Case I: Monomeric alkaloid

Case 2. Dimeric alkaloid

FIG. 8. Partial quaternization of a monomeric and a dimeric tertiary base, using half equivalent acid. With norcurarine three different methylated compounds are formed.

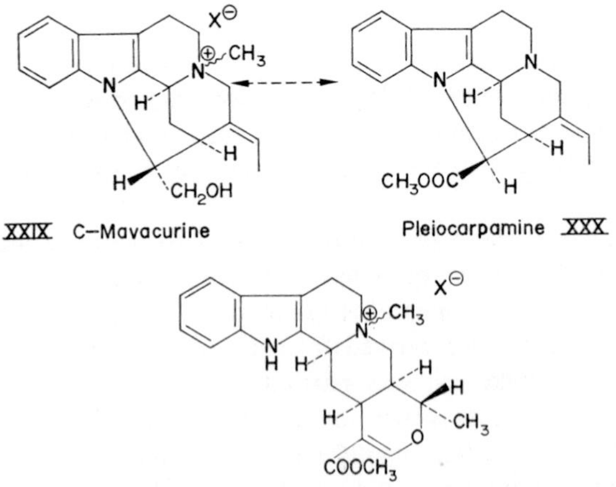

XXIX C—Mavacurine

Pleiocarpamine XXX

XXXI   Melinonine A

FIG. 9. Monomeric calabash alkaloids of α-type.

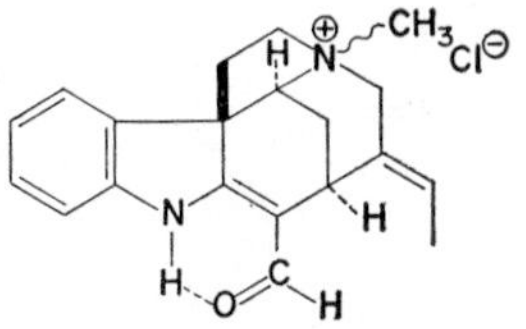

XXXII C—Fluorocurarine

FIG. 10. Monomeric calabash alkaloids of β-type.

mole of CH_3Cl corresponded to four atoms of nitrogen and thirty-eight of carbon ($C_{38}H_{38}ON_4.CH_3Cl$). Further methylation converted this compound to curarine dichloride ($C_{38}H_{38}ON_4.2CH_3Cl$).

Those calabash alkaloids containing only nineteen to twenty-one carbon atoms are monoquaternary and have very low curare activity (fluorocurarine, fluorocurine, mavacurine, melinonine A, etc.) (Fig. 9).

The monomeres were especially important for the elucidation of the structure. Correlations to alkaloids from other plant families and spectroscopic methods gave the final clue of their ring structure and microanalytical methods proved the nature of the side groups.

Typical examples of monomer alkaloids of the α-type are C-mavacurine (XXIX) (related to the tertiary alkaloid pleiocarpamine (XXX), from the African *Apocynacea Pleiocarpa mutica*) and melionine A (XXXI). More important for us are the alkaloids of β-type (Fig. 10). Monoquaternary alkaloids such as fluorocurarine (XXXII) and the group of very active biquaternary alkaloids belong to this group.

The most important discovery was the intimate relationship of this β-type alkaloid group to the Wieland–Gumlich aldehyde, a degradation product of strychnine (XXXIII) (Fig. 11) (strychnine is the main alkaloid of African Strychnaceae but is not found in the South American plant family). The aldehyde group forms a hemiacetal with its neighboring hydroxyl group. The quaternary chloromethylate is identical with the N(b)-methocaracurine VII (XXXIV), isolated from calabashes.

When two N(b)-methylated molecules of the Wieland–Gumlich aldehyde are combined by linking twice the basic N(a)-atom of one molecule to the aldehyde group of a second molecule a dimer molecule, toxiferine (XXXV), is formed (Fig. 11). This double condensation reaction is catalized by acid, and leads to a new double unsaturated eight-membered

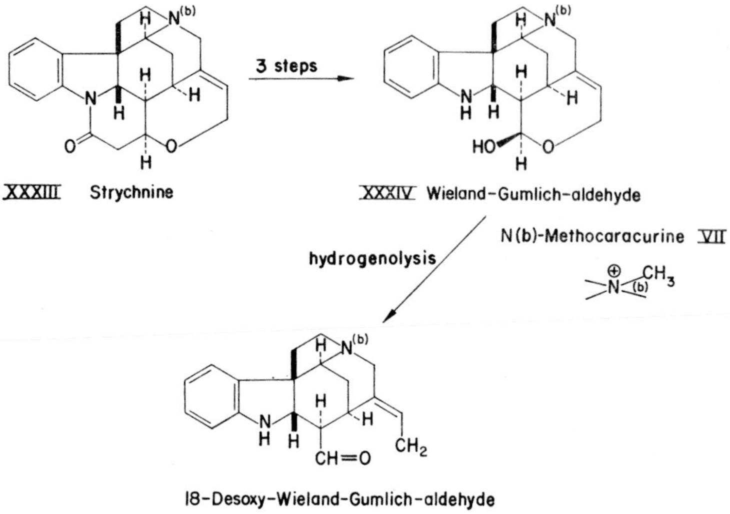

XXXIII Strychnine

XXXIV Wieland–Gumlich–aldehyde

3 steps

hydrogenolysis

N(b)-Methocaracurine VII

18-Desoxy-Wieland-Gumlich-aldehyde

$$2 C_{20}H_{25}O_2N_2^+Cl^- \xrightarrow{H^+} 2 H_2O + C_{40}H_{46}O_2N_4^{++}2Cl^-$$

N(b)-metho-Wieland-
Gumlich–aldehyde

C-toxiferine

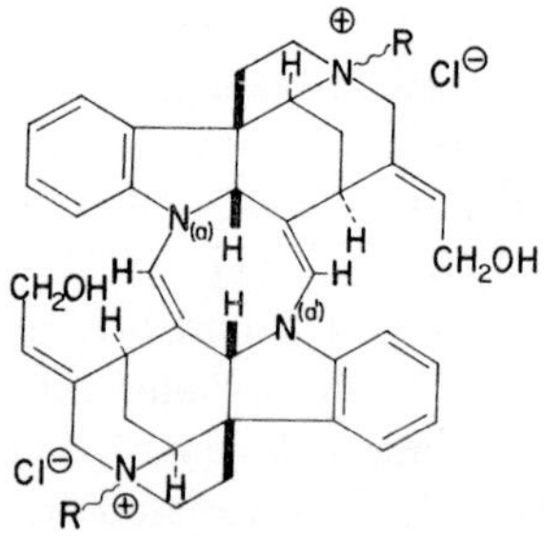

XXXV C-toxiferine: R = –CH₃
alloferine: R = –CH₂–CH=CH₂

C-toxiferine: $R = -CH_3$
alloferine: $R = -CH_2-CH=CH_2$

FIG. 11. Synthesis of toxiferine by condensation of two molecules of N-methylated Wieland–Gumlich aldehyde.

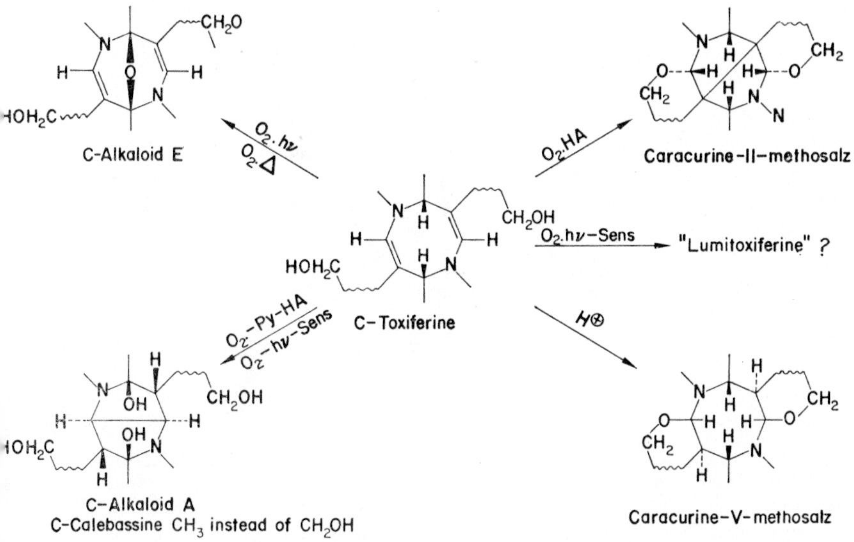

FIG. 12. The central eight-membered ring of some calabash alkaloids.

ring (bis-aza-cyclooctadien) (Fig. 12). When the hydroxyl group of the Wieland–Gumlich aldehyde is replaced by hydrogen, the condensation will give C-dihydrotoxiferine without the two C 18-hydroxyl groups. By light and oxygen two hydroxyl groups are added and a carbon–carbon bridge is formed in the central eight-membered ring (alkaloids of cale-bassine group). An oxygen bridge may be formed by another type of photo reaction (curarine-group).

The C–C bridging of the central ring is again different in the caracurine-II-methocompounds where the hydroxyl groups of the side chains are linked to the saturated central ring system (caracurines XXXVI) (Fig. 13).

The structure of all the biquaternary calabash alkaloids with their eleven to thirteen heterocyclic and aromatic rings is rigid, the volume quite large. The distance between the two quaternary N(b)-atoms is about 14 Å, but in the caracurine-II-metho salt and probably in cale-bassine because of a deformation of the molecule by the C–C bridge in the central ring, only 8.6 Å. Both alkaloids have a low curare activity compared to the extreme toxicity of toxiferine.

By replacement of the two quaternary N(b)-methyl groups in toxiferine different synthetic derivatives were obtained (Boller *et al.*, 1962). Best suited for clinical purposes was *N,N'*-diallyl-bis-nortoxiferine (XXXVII)

223

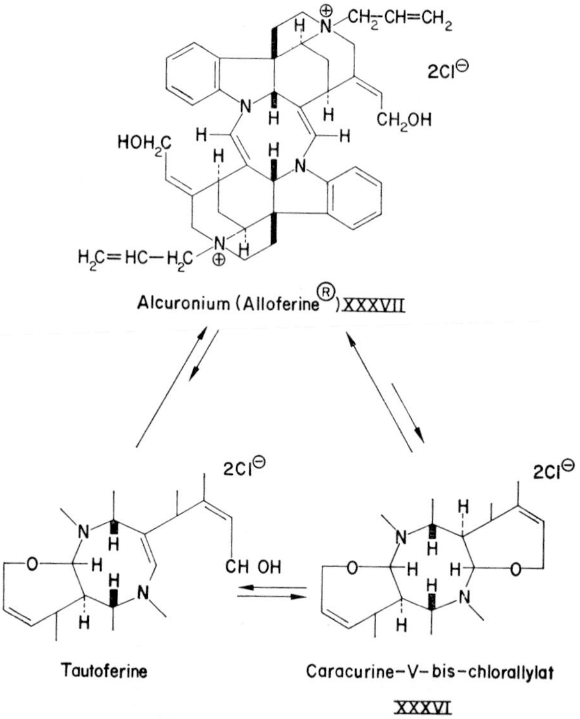

FIG. 13. Structure of synthetic alcuronium (*N,N'*-diallyl-bis-nortoxiferine) and caracurine-V-bis-chlorallylat with two additional ring systems.

(alloferine[R]) which has 4 times less curariform action but of short duration (Waser and Harbeck, 1962) (Fig. 13).

10.5.2. PHARMACOLOGY OF CALABASH CURARE

10.5.2.1. *PARALYTIC ACTIVITY*

It was easy to show that some Strychnos alkaloids have considerably greater paralytic action than any previously known natural or synthetic neuromuscular blocking agent (Waser, 1953). Unfortunately, frogs are not suitable for the evaluation of curare effects because they show seasonal variation toward many drugs. Therefore, a simple test was developed. The alkaloid solutions were injected into the tail-veins of mice and the time

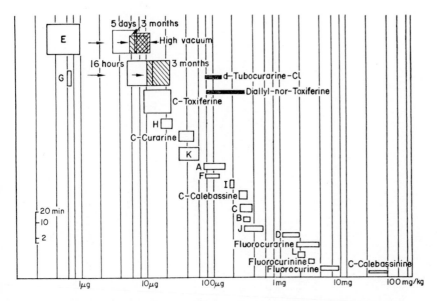

FIG. 14. Action in mouse test of different calabash alkaloids, alcuronium, and
d-tubocurarine (abscissa: dose/kg; ordinate: duration of paralysis).

that elapsed before head-drop, abolition of righting reflexes and death or
recovery was measured. Compared with the rabbit head-drop method
this technique has the great advantage that it requires only small amounts
of the rare alkaloids for each experiment and allows the determination
of at least three distinct end-points. Average values were determined for
each alkaloid in twenty to fifty experiments. The combined activities of
all the isolated alkaloids equalled 99.6% of the original curare activity
of the calabash, indicating the great accuracy of the test method used.

There is a wide variation in the paralytic activity of calabash alkaloids.
In Fig. 14 the corners of the different areas on the abscissa represent the
head-drop and the minimal lethal dose for mice; the ordinate indicates
the duration of paralysis caused by an intermediate dose (logarithmic
scale). Seven alkaloids were found to be more active than tubocurarine;
of these toxiferine was very potent. The lethal doses of two alkaloids, G
and E, were less than 1 mcg/kg, indicating that their potency is 100 times
greater than that of tubocurarine.

It was surprising that the activities of these alkaloids, determined by the
dose-activity relation for head-drop, diminished appreciably within hours

225

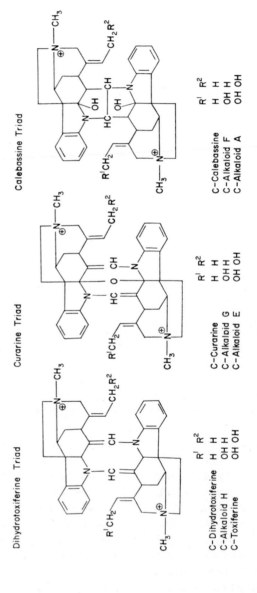

Fig. 15. The three alkaloid triads investigated for their structure/activity relationship.

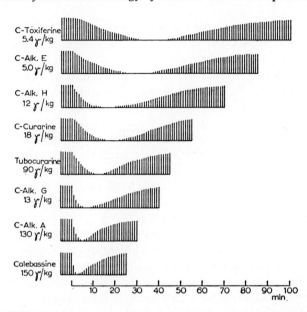

FIG. 16. Duration of paralysis (paralytic dose i.v.). Contraction of cat gastro-cnemius by electrically stimulated sciatic nerve (4 × /min).

and became constant only after 1 to 2 months. These alkaloids seem to change their configuration, the stable form having an activity of 10% or less of the original value. This interesting observation might partly explain the discrepancy between the quick and deadly effect of poisoned arrows and the rather slow and often weak action of isolated alkaloids on laboratory animals and man.

In different chemical groups of calabash alkaloids there is a remarkable parallelism between curarizing potency and polarity, as determined by paper chromatography. Slowly diffusing alkaloids (toxiferine group) with greater solubility in the water phase have greater neuromuscular activity than fast-moving alkaloids (fluorocurarine group) (Fig. 7). The differently hydroxylated alkaloids of the three alkaloid triads of dihydrotoxiferine, curarine and calebassine (Fig. 15) show this interesting correlation (Table 3). In all three groups consecutive introduction of hydroxyl groups into the two side chains induces higher curare activity. The most active alkaloids belong to the curarine triad with an ether oxygen in the central eight-membered ring. The stereochemistry of these molecules seems to be even best suited for maximum curarizing action and must be very similar to the toxiferine group.

227

The probable reason for the low activity of the calebassine and the caracurine II groups has already been mentioned. Alkaloids D, C and caracurine-II-metho salt have a very low toxicity in mice of DL: 2000, 380 and 350 mcg respectively. Tetrahydrocurarine, with a completely saturated central ring, has low activity. Caracurine-V-metho compounds with the two allyl hydroxyl groups fixed to the central ring (the only difference to toxiferine) has as well a very low toxicity (DL: 750 mcg/kg).

The rabbit head-drop test indicated that the alkaloids occurring most abundantly in calabash differ in their paralytic properties: 0.004 mg/kg C-toxiferine, 0.025 mg/kg C-curarine I and 0.10 mg/kg C-calebassine (*d*-tubocurarine: 0.15 mg/kg) caused head-drop of 3 minutes duration. This effect was antagonized by small doses of neostigmine, whereas larger doses prolonged the paralytic action.

Figure 16 demonstrates the duration of the neuromuscular block produced by some alkaloids after their administration in doses just sufficient to prevent transmission in the electrically stimulated sciatic-gastrocnemius preparation of cats. Calabash curare contains various alkaloids with a short action and some with an extremely long action. The duration of action of toxiferine is outstanding; it takes nearly 2 hours for the muscle to recover after a slow, progressive onset of paralysis. With a 20-fold paralytic dose total paralysis lasts 8 hours. Alkaloid E shows similar properties and the action of C-curarine I is comparable to that of tubocurarine. Respiration may be paralysed before the gastrocnemius muscle. Neostigmine again immediately antagonized all paralytic symptoms. In comparison to intravenous injection intramuscular injection of curarine was 5 times slower and subcutaneous injection 10 times slower as regards onset of action. An oral dose of 1.35 mg/kg curarine paralysed the animal completely within 1 hour.

With the isolated rectus abdominis preparation of frogs we found the mode of action to be of the curare type. Like *d*-tubocurarine, all the alkaloids investigated antagonized acetylcholine contractions. Alkaloid E and toxiferine were the most active (Fig. 17) (Waser, 1953).

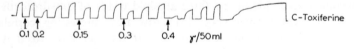

0.1 0.2   0.15   0.3   0.4 γ/50ml   C-Toxiferine

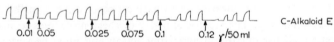

0.01 0.05   0.025   0.075   0.1   0.12 γ/50ml   C-Alkaloid E

Fig. 17. Contractions of isolated muscle rectus abdominis of frog by 25 mcg acetylcholine/50 ml fluid. Antagonism by toxiferine and alkaloid E.

TABLE 3

	R^1	R^2	R_F*	Head-drop dose (mcg/kg mouse i.v.)	Minimum lethal dose (mcg/kg mouse i.v.)	Duration of paralysis (min)
Dihydrotoxiferine-triad						
C-Dihydrotoxiferine	H	H	1.22	30	60	5.5
C-Alkaloid H	OH	H	0.71	16	24	3.7
C-Toxiferine	OH	OH	0.42	9	23	12
Curarine-triad						
C-Curarine	H	H	1.00*	30	50	4
C-Alkaloid G	OH	H	0.65	5	12	7
C-Alkaloid E	OH	OH	0.36	4	8	18
Calebassine-triad						
C-Calebassine	H	H	0.80	240	320	3
C-Alkaloid F	OH	H	0.49	75	120	1.3
C-Alkaloid A	OH	OH	0.23	70	150	2

* Paper chromatogram, R_F curarine = 1.00.
Duration of paralysis with middle dose (between head-drop and lethal dose).

10.5.2.2. SIDE-EFFECTS ON BLOOD PRESSURE AND CARDIAC ACTIVITY

Calabash alkaloids with great curarizing potency had little effect on blood pressure. With artificial respiration paralytic doses of toxiferine and alkaloids H, E, G and K had practically no depressing effect (Fig. 18). Thirty times the paralytic dose of toxiferine caused only a slight depression. C-alkaloid E lowered the blood pressure in the case of a 10-fold paralytic dose and alkaloid H in that of a 4-fold dose.

Like *d*-tubocurarine, alkaloids of the curarine group usually lowered the blood pressure for a short time. The hypotensive effects of the alkaloids of the calebassine group last somewhat longer. Liberation of histamine may play a role in this effect. Alkaloid B, evidently owing to ganglionic block, lowered the blood pressure before any paralysis occurred.

All curarizing substances in high doses will paralyse autonomic synapses. This is the main reason for side-effects, such as lowering of blood pressure, vagus block, changes of the heart rate and frequency of respiration. We therefore investigated ganglionic block in cats by measuring the contraction

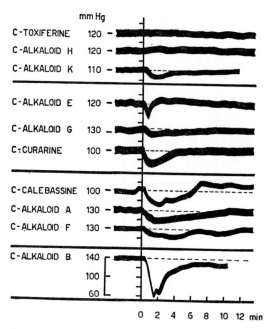

FIG. 18. Blood pressure of cat with artificial respiration after intravenous paralytic doses.

TABLE 4. RATIO OF THE GANGLIONIC AND NEUROMUSCULAR BLOCKING DOSES

Alkaloid		Partial block	Total block
C-Toxiferine	I	80	
C-Alkaloid	E	20	24
C-Alkaloid	G	20	12
C-Alkaloid	H	12	
C-Curarine	I	8	8
C-Alkaloid	A	5	
C-Alkaloid	K	3	3.5
C-Alkaloid	F	3	
Calebassine		2.5	3.3
C-Alkaloid	B	0.3	0.8
d-Tubocurarine		11	10
Alloferine		40	50

230

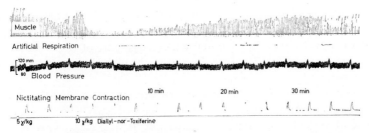

FIG. 19. Paralytic action of 10 mcg/kg alcuronium on cat under artificial respiration. No change of blood pressure and transmission through ganglionic synapses (nictitating membrane contraction).

of the nictitating membrane after preganglionic (ganglion cervicale superius) stimulation of the sympathetic nerve. The ratios of ganglionic and neuromuscular blocking doses are summarized in Table 4.

Blocking of parasympathetic synapses could be demonstrated by the inhibition of the effects of vagal stimulation. The doses required to block parasympathetic transmission were higher than those necessary for sympathetic block. With toxiferine in doses of up to 300 mcg/kg no changes in vagus effects were detected, but higher doses would probably paralyse the entire autonomic nervous system. Alloferine behaved as favorably as toxiferine in animal experiments (Fig. 19).

10.5.2.3. *ABSORPTION, DISTRIBUTION AND ELIMINATION*

The metabolism of calabash curare alkaloids was investigated with ^{14}C-labeled curarine (Waser *et al.*, 1954). ^{14}C or ^{3}H-toxiferine and ^{3}H-N,N'-diallyl-bis-nortoxiferine (Waser, 1953; Waser and Lüthi, 1966; Waser and Reller, 1968). Absorption after intramuscular or subcutaneous injection was found to be rapid. In order to achieve the same degree of paralysis as with intravenous injections, approximately 10 times as much curarine is needed if the drug is applied subcutaneously, and 100 times as much of it is given by stomach tube. In the latter case paralysis persists until the administered drug is completely absorbed. Up to 200 minutes after intravenous injection the largest concentration of alkaloid is found in the liver and the kidneys. The total mass of muscles contains about half as much as the liver and kidney. The blood or muscle curarine concentration required for paralysis are very small (0.02–0.2 mcg/g). The distribution of curarine in different muscles (gastrocnemius, diaphragm, intercostal muscles) is very similar. The peripheral nerves and the ganglia contain larger amounts of the drug than the spinal cord or the brain. Most of the alkaloids (toxiferine, curarine, alkaloids, E, G, H) are eliminated unchanged by the kidneys (in 3 hours 25–30% curarine, in 6 hours 90% toxiferine, in 4 hours 50% alloferine). A large part of these alkaloids is eliminated in the bile (10–15%). Excretion through the intestine is barely detectable.

The short-acting N,N'-diallyl-bis-nortoxiferine was accumulated 15–60 minutes after intravenous injection in different tissues in acid mucopolysaccharides (tendons, cartilage, connective tissue, etc.). This transient binding seems to limit the curare action to a short period of 10–20 minutes. Metabolism of all investigated alkaloids is small, as only traces of radioactive breakdown products are found in the expired air, but small amounts of other non-labeled metabolites may be formed.

One hundred years ago Claude Bernard made his famous experiments with frogs showing curare to block the neuromuscular junction. Now, using a special autoradiographic technique we were able to show for the first time an accumulation of labeled curare molecules at their receptor sites in the end-plates of mouse diaphragms (Figs. 20a, b) (Waser and Lüthi, 1957; Waser, 1967). With densitometric measurements the number of radioactive toxiferine and curarine molecules per end-plate were determined and the kinetics and interactions with cholinergic drug molecules or anticholinesterases were investigated (Waser, 1967). The results are important for the understanding of the molecular action of curarizing and depolarizing molecules on the post-synaptic membrane.

10.5.2.4. CLINICAL USE

Of all investigated calabash alkaloids only curarine, toxiferine and the synthetic N,N'-diallyl-bis-nortoxiferine (alcuronium alloferine[R]) have been used in the clinic (Waser and Harbeck, 1959, 1962). Their advantages compared to other curare compounds are: high selectivity, no depression of blood pressure, no broncho-constriction, no liberation of histamine, long action of toxiferine, and short action of alloferine. Ten to fifteen mg calabash curarine paralyse the artificially respirated man of 70 kg during 20–25 minutes. A second intravenous injection of 5 mg prolongs paralysis to 50–160 minutes. With this dose no side-effects were observed. Toxiferine acts much stronger. Here 2 mg intravenously injected produce paralysis for 50–160 minutes. Side effects of circulation or respiration (broncho-constriction) were never observed. Anticholinesterases such as pyridostigmine (5–10 mg) antagonize the curare action within minutes. Toxiferine is the most active and specific curarizing agent in man, and of longest paralytic

232

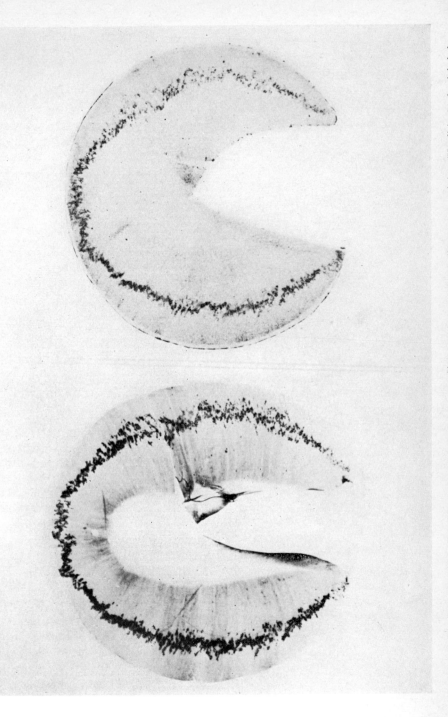

FIG. 20(a). Mouse diaphragm after intravenous injection of ^{14}C-toxiferine. *Left:* cholinesterase staining (Koelle). *Right:* labeled toxiferine concentrated in the end-plates (autoradiography).

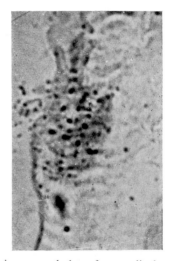

FIG. 20(b). Silver grains over end-plate of mouse diaphragm containing labeled toxiferine (magnification: 1000 ×).

action. It is therefore especially suited for use in surgical operations of long duration and in the treatment of tetanus.

In contrast to this, alloferine may be used for short operations. Initial intravenous doses of 5–10 mg produce paralysis of 15–20 minutes, and repetitive doses of 2–5 mg may be given. No undesired side-effects are described and alloferine is now widely used by anesthetists (Curare Symposium, 1967).

10.6. QUATERNARY DERIVATIVES OF OTHER ALKALOIDS

Quinine has long been known to exert a weak curare-like action. This is reinforced by quaternization. Quinine *N*-methylchloride was found to be effective orally and to produce in cats a sequence of effects similar to that produced by curare (Harvey, 1940). Mono-quaternary derivatives of quininium have been tested as curarizing agents. Maximum activity in rabbits (HD 50: 4.2 mg/kg) and frogs is obtained with the *N*-amyl derivative. The quininium salts are more active than erythroidine in the rabbit head-drop test. The most active of the cinchona alkaloids are *N*-methyl-quinidinium and *N*-methyl-cinchonidinium iodides (HD 50: 2–3 mg/kg),

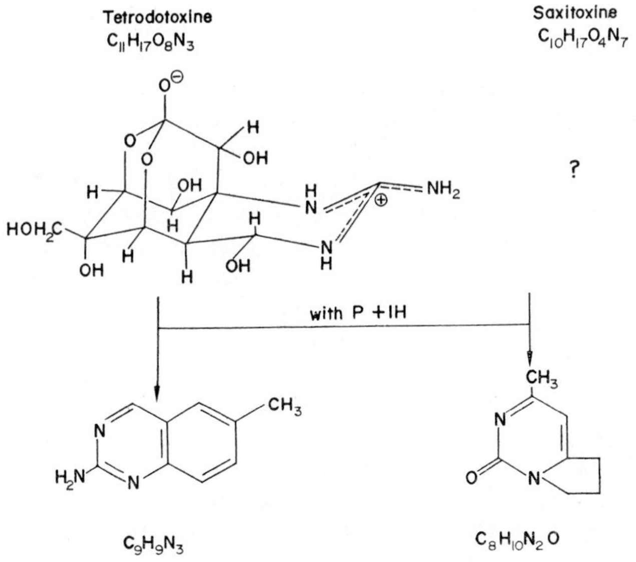

Tetrodotoxine
$C_{11}H_{17}O_8N_3$

Saxitoxine
$C_{10}H_{17}O_4N_7$

with P + IH

$C_9H_9N_3$

$C_8H_{10}N_2O$

Fig. 21. Structure of tetrodotoxin and saxitoxin.

but they are also the most toxic (Marsh and Pelletier, 1948). It is interesting that the biquaternary N,N'-dialkyl-quininium and cinchonium salts have much less activity than the monoalkyl derivatives (Chase and Lehman, 1942). N-methyl-quininium chloride has been used on a limited scale in clinical medicine for the relief of muscle spasms (Paton, 1949).

Of the many other quaternary derivatives of alkaloids only a few more have an interesting curarizing potency. N-methylatropinium is fairly effective, but decamethylene-bis-atropinium diiodide is 140 times as potent as d-tubocurarine (Kimura and Unna, 1950). High activity was found with different N-alkyl-salts of strychnidine and of yohimbine (Waser, 1949; Karrer *et al.*, 1949). It is interesting to note that quaternary salts of some isoquinoline alkaloids (papaverine, canadine, coclaurine) or pyridine alkaloids (coniine, conhydrine, nicotine, etc.) have only slight curare activity compared to the bis-benzyl-isoquinoline type alkaloids in tubocurare (Craig, 1948, 1955). Sometimes the monoquaternary compounds have central activity.

10.7. CURARIZING COMPOUNDS FROM OTHER NATURAL SOURCES

Not only plant alkaloids have curarizing properties. In the last few years many dangerous biological toxins from different animals have been investigated (Russell and Saunders, 1967; Baslow, 1969). Only a few of these will be mentioned or discussed here. The chemical structure of *tetrodotoxin* has been described recently (Fig. 21), whereas that of *saxitoxin* is not fully known (Kao, 1966; Cheymol and Bourillet, 1966). The pharmacological actions of these compounds are very complicated. They have a general paralytic effect on different nervous systems and muscles. The toxins have caused numerous lethal alimentary intoxications in Asia and California. The animals themselves must possess a protection mechanism against their own curarizing toxins.

At this point the powerful effects on muscle of both *Botulinus toxin* and *Cobra toxin*, which are of a proteinous nature, have to be mentioned. The cobra neurotoxin of *Naja naja siamensis* is a potent neuromuscular blocking agent and the toxin was shown to act specifically and irreversibly with the cholinergic receptor of the frog neuromuscular junction (Lester, 1970) and on the extra junctional cholinergic receptors of chronically denervated rat skeletal muscle (Eaker *et al.*, 1971). α-Bungarotoxin is a component of the venom of a Formosan snake (*Bungarus multicinctus*)

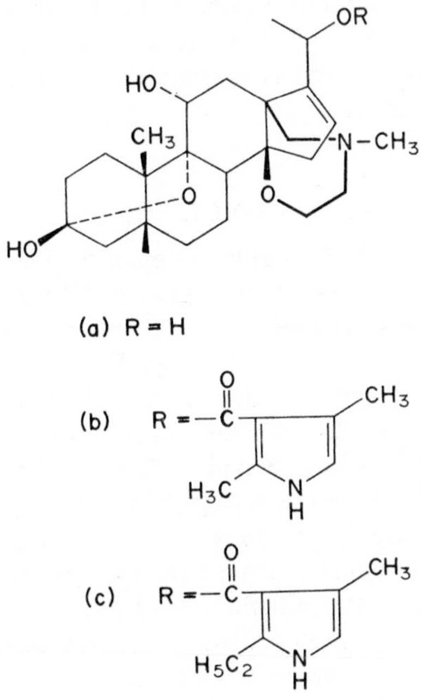

FIG. 22. Structures of (a) batrachotoxinin A; (b) batrachotoxin; (c) homobatrachotoxin.

with a curare-like action (Chang and Lee, 1963) and several proteins from this venom block the action of acetylcholine on neuromuscular junctions or block transmitter release from the motor nerves (Miledi *et al.*, 1971).

The structure of α-bungarotoxin is not known, although its molecular weight is ~8000. It is bound strongly to the postsynaptic membrane, thus blocking the cholinergic receptors.

Batrachotoxin is a steroidal alkaloid (Fig. 22), isolated from the skin of the Columbian poison arrow frog (*Phyllobates aurotaenia*). It is used by Indians of the Choco rain forest to prepare the darts for their blowguns (Märki and Witkop, 1963; Albuquerque *et al.*, 1971).

In the very poisonous venom four major bases were found: batrachotoxin, homobatrachotoxin, pseudobatrachotoxin and batrachotoxinin A. Their structure was elucidated by X-ray analysis, spectral analysis and confirmed by partial synthesis of batrachotoxin (Fig. 22). The pharmacology shows irreversible neuromuscular block and later muscle contracture, various cardiac arrhythmias and death. Most of these complicated peripheral and central actions appear to be due to a selective and irreversible increase in permeability of membranes to sodium ions. On the muscle membrane this action is reversibly antagonized by tetrodotoxin but not by *d*-tubocurarine.

10.8.   CONCLUSIONS

Although several alkaloids of different plant families with extraordinary neuromuscular blocking activity are known only a few animal toxins have this property. The natural alkaloids and their synthetic derivatives are widely used in anesthesiology today. For the pharmacologist the relationship between chemical structure and activity are most interesting. The active molecules are large, voluminous and carry two quaternary ammonium groups (pachy-curare type of Bovet). The only exceptions are the erythrina alkaloids with one tertiary ammonium group. The distance between these two cationic groups is important, being optimal at about 14 Å. Ether oxygen, hydroxyl groups or aliphatic side-chains influence the curare activity and the distribution of the molecules in the body. Highest curare activity is associated with hydrophilic properties. We therefore assume that a limited number of molecules covers the post-synaptic membrane of the end-plate inhibiting ional exchange and depolarization (Waser, 1967). The high structural specificity of curare molecules may be explained by binding at specific receptor sites.

Therefore, the curare group is very suitable for research on structure/activity relationship and more generally on the concept of receptors. In practical medicine the use of some curare alkaloids as an aid to modern surgical technique is firmly established.

REFERENCES

ALBUQUERQUE, E. X., DALY, J. W. and WITKOP, B. (1971) Batrachotoxin: chemistry and pharmacology. *Science* **172**: 995–1002.

ALTAMIRANO and DOMINGUEZ (1876) Estudio comparativo de la Erythrina Americana Tesis. Cited in *Arzac-Behnken*, Universidad nacional autonoma, Mexico, 1934.

BASLOW, M. H. (ed.) (1969) *Marine Pharmacology*. Williams & Wilkinson, Baltimore.

BATTERSBY, A. R. and HODSON, H. F. (1965) Alkaloids of calabash curare and strychnos species. In: *The Alkaloids*, vol. VIII, pp. 515–79. Manske, R. H. F. (ed.). Academic Press, New York/London.

BERNAUER, K. (1959) Alkaloide aus Calebassencurare und südamerikanischen Strychnosarten. *Fortschr. Chem. Organ. Naturstoffe* **17**: 183–247.

BERNAUER, K. (1961) Alkaloide aus Calebassencurare und Strychnosarten. *Planta Medica* **9**: 340.

BOEHM, R. (1897) Ueber Curare und Curarealkaloide. *Arch. Pharm.* **235**: 660–84.

BOEHM, R. (1920) Curare und Curarealkaloide. In: *Handbuch d. Exp. Pharmakol.*, *II/I*, pp. 179–248. Heffter, A. (ed.). Springer, Berlin.

BOEKELHEIDE, V. and PRELOG, V. (1955) Indole alkaloids. *Progress in Organ. Chem.* **3**: 218–66.

BOLLER, A., ELS, H. and FÜRST, F. (1962) Personal communcation by F. Hoffmann-La Roche.

BOVET, D. and BOVET-NITTI, F. (1948) Curare. *Experientia* **4**: 325–48.

BURMAN, M. S. (1940) Clinical experiences with some curare preparations and curare substitutes. *J. Pharmacol.* **69**: 143.

CHANG, C. C. and LEE, C. Y. (1963) Isolation of neurotoxins from the venom of *Bungarus multicinctus* and their modes of neuromuscular blocking action. *Arch. Int. Pharmacodyn.* **144**: 241–57.

CHASE, H. F. and LEHMAN, A. J. (1942) Studies on synthetic curare-like compounds. I. Action of some quinine and other quaternary ammonium derivatives. *J. Pharmacol. Exp. Ther.* **75**: 265–70.

CHEYMOL, J. (1949) Curares naturels et curares de synthèse. *Actualités Pharmacologiques*, pp. 1–52.

CHEYMOL, J. and BOURILLET, F. (1966) D'une nouvelle classe de substances biologiques: tétrodotoxine, saxitoxine, tarichatoxine. *Actualités Pharmacol.* **19**: 1–61.

CICARDO, V. H. and HUG, E. (1937) Action curarisante de l'extrait d'Erythrina crista galli. *Compt. Rend. Soc. Biol.* **126**: 154–6.

CRAIG, L. E. (1948) Curariform activity and chemical structure. *Chem. Rev.* **42**: 285–410.

CRAIG, L. E. (1955) Curare-like effects. In: *The Alkaloids*, vol. V, pp. 265–93. Manske, R. H. F. (ed.). Academic Press, New York.

DEULOFEU, V. (1959) The curarizing alkaloids of erythrina species. In: *Curare and Curare-like Agents*, pp. 163–9. Bovet, D., Bovet-Nitti, F. and Marini-Bettolo, G. B. (eds.). Elsevier Publishing, Amsterdam.

DUTCHER, J. D. (1951) The isolation and identification of additional physiologically active alkaloids in extracts of *Chondodendron tomentosum* Ruiz and Pavon. In: *Curare and Anti-curare agents. Ann. N.Y. Acad. Sci.* **54**: Art. 3, pp. 326–36.

EAKER, D., HARRIS, J. B. and THESLEFF, S. (1971) Action of a cobra neurotoxin on denervated rat skeletal muscle. *Europ. J. Pharm.* **15**: 254–6.

EVERETT, A. J., LOWE, L. A. and WILKINSON, S. (1970) Revision of the structure of (+)-tubocurarine chloride and (+)-chondrocurine. *Chem. Comm.* 1020–1.

FALTIS, F., WRANN, S. and KÜHAS, E. (1932) Ueber die Konstitution des Iso-Chondodendrins. V. *Justus Liebigs Ann. der Chemie* **497**: 69–90.

FOLDES, F. F. (1957) *Muscle Relaxants in Anesthesiology*. Thomas, Springfield.

FOLKERS, K., KONIUSZY, F. and SHAVEL, J. (1944) Erythrina alkaloids. XIV. Isolation and characterization of erysothiovine and erysothiopine, new alkaloids containing sulfer. *J. Amer. Chem. Soc.* **66**: 1083.

FOLKERS, K., and MAJOR, R. T. (1937) Isolation of erythroidine, an alkaloid of curare action, from *Erythrina Americana* Mill. *J. Amer. Chem. Soc.* **59**: 1580.

FOLKERS, K. and UNNA, K. (1938) Erythrina alkaloids. II. A review, and new data on the alkaloids of species of the genus *Erythrina. J. Amer. Pharm. Assoc.* **27**: 693–9.

FOLKERS, K. and UNNA, K. (1939) Erythrina alkaloids. V. Comparative curare-like potencies of species of the genus *Erythrina. J. Amer. Pharm. Assoc.* **28**: 1019–28.

HARVEY, A. M. (1940) Action of quinine methochloride on neuromuscular transmission. *Bull. Johns Hopkins Hosp.* **66**: 52–59.

KAO, C. Y. (1966) Tetrodotoxin, saxitoxin, and their significance in the study of excitation phenomena. *Pharm. Rev.* **18**: 997–1049.

KARRER, P., EUGSTER, C. H. and WASER, P. G. (1949) Ueber Curarewirkung einiger Strychnidin- und Dihydrostrychnidin-chlor-alkylate. *Helv. Chim. Acta* **32**: 2381.

KARRER, P. and SCHMID, H. (1955) Neuere Arbeiten über Curare, insbesondere Cale-bassen-Curare und Alkaloide aus Strychnos-Rinden. *Angew. Chem. (Eng.)* **67**: 361–73.

KARRER, P., SCHMID, H. and WASER, P. G. (1960) Kurzer Ueberblick über die Chemie und Pharmakologie der Calebassencurare Alkaloide. *Il Farmaco* **15**: 126–36.

KIMURA, K. K. and UNNA, K. R. (1950) Curare-like action of decamethylene-bis-(atropinium iodide). *J. Pharmacol. Exp. Ther.* **98**: 286–92.

KING, H. (1935) Curare alkaloids. Part I. Tubocurarine. *J. Chem. Soc.*, pp. 1381–9.

KING, H. (1936) Curare alkaloids. Part II. Tubocurarine and bebeerine. *J. Chem. Soc.*, pp. 1276–9.

KING, H. (1939) Curare alkaloids. Part IV. Bebeerine and tubocurarine. Orientation of phenolic groups. *J. Chem. Soc.*, pp. 1157–64.

KING, H. (1940) Curare alkaloids. Part V. Alkaloids of some chondrodendron species and the origin of *Radix pareirae bravae*. *J. Chem. Soc.*, pp. 737–46.

LEHMAN, A. J. (1937) Actions of *Erythrina americana*, a possible curare substitute. *J. Pharmac. Exp. Therap.* **60**: 69–81.

LESTER, H. A. (1970) Postsynaptic action of cobra toxin at the myoneural junction. *Nature* **227**: 727–8.

LEWIN, L. (1923) *Die Pfeilgifte*. Barth, Leipzig.

LOEWE, S. and HARVEY, S. C. (1952) Equidistance concept and structure-activity relationship of curarizing drugs. *Arch. Exp. Pathol. Pharmakol.* **214**: 214–26.

MÄRKI, F. and WITKOP, B. (1963) The venom of the Columbian arrow poison frog (*Phyllobates bicolor*). *Experientia* **19**: 329–38.

MARSH, D. F. and HERRING, D. A. (1950) The curariform activity of the menisper-maceous alkaloids. *Experientia* **6**: 31–37.

MARSH, D. F. and PELLETIER, M. H. (1948) Curariform activity of quaternary ammonium iodides derived from cinchona alkaloids. *J. Pharmacol. Exp. Ther.* **92**: 127.

McINTYRE, A. R. (1947) *Curare, its History, Nature and Clinical Use*. Univ. of Chicago Press.

MILEDI, R., MOLINOFF, P. and POTTER, L. T. (1971) Isolation of the cholinergic receptor protein of Torpedo electric tissue. *Nature* **229**: 554–7.

PATON, W. D. M. (1949) Pharmacology of curare and curarising substances. *J. Pharm. Pharmacol.* **1**: 273–86.

PHILIPSBORN, W. V., SCHMID, H. and KARRER, P. (1956) Ueber die Bruttoformeln der Curare-Alkaloide aus Calebassen und Strychnos-Arten. *Helv. Chim. Acta* **39**: 913.

RUSSELL, F. E. and SAUNDERS, P. R. (1967) (eds.) *Animal Toxins*. Ed. Pergamon Press, Oxford.

SCHMID, H. (1967) *Schweizerische Akademie der Medizinischen Wissenschaften* 24/25 *Juni* 1966: *Curare Symposium*. Schwabe & Co., Basel, pp. 415–28.

SPÄTH, E. and KUFFNER, F. (1934) Ueber Curare-Alkaloide, II: Zur Konstitution des Curins (Bebeerins). *Ber. d. Deutschen Chem. Gesell.* **67**: 55–59.

SPÄTH, E., LEITHE, W. and LADECK, F. (1928) Ueber Curare-Alkaloide, I: Die Konstitu-tion des Curins. *Ber. d. Deutschen Chem. Gesell.* **61**: 1698–1709.

VARNEY, R. F., LINEGAR, C. R. and HOLADAY, H. A. (1949) The assay of curare by the rabbit "head-drop" method. *J. Pharmacol. Exp. Ther.* **97**: 72–73.

WASER, P. G. (1949) Weitere pharmakologische Eigenschaften einiger curare-aktiver Yohimbinderivate. *Helv. Physiol. Acta* **7**: 493–7.

WASER, P. G. (1953) Calebassen-curare. *Helv. Physiol. Pharmacol. Acta* **11**: Suppl. VIII.

WASER, P. G. (1967) Receptor localization by autoradiographic techniques. *Ann. N.Y. Acad. Sci.* **144**: 737–55.

WASER, P. G. and HARBECK, P. (1959) Erste klinische Anwendung der Calebassen-Alkaloide Toxiferin I und Curarin I. *Anaesthesist* **8**: 193–8.

WASER, P. G. and HARBECK, P. (1962) Pharmakologie und klinische Anwendung des kurzdauernden Muskelrelaxans Diallyl-nor-Toxiferin. *Anaesthesist* **11**: 33–37.

WASER, P. G. and LÜTHI, U. (1957) Autoradiographische Lokalisation von ^{14}C-Calebassen-Curarin I und ^{14}C-Dekamethonium in der motorischen Endplatte. *Arch. Int. Pharmacodyn.* **112**: 272–96.

WASER, P. G. and LÜTHI, U. (1966) Verteilung, Metabolismus und Elimination von ^{3}H-Diallyl-nor-Toxiferin (Alloferin) bei Katzen. *Helv. Physiol. Acta* **24**: 259–73.

WASER, P. G. and RELLER, J. (1968) Verteilung und Metabolismus von radiomarkiertem Toxiferin (in publication).

WASER, P. G., SCHMID H. and SCHMID, K. (1954) Resorption, Verteilug und Ausscheidung von Radiocalebassencurarin bei Katzen. *Arch. Int. Pharmacodyn.* **96**: 386–405.

WIELAND, H., BÄHR, K. and WITKOP, B. (1941). Ueber die Alkaloide aus Calebassen-Curare. IV. *Annalen der Chemie* **547**: 156–79.

WIELAND, H., KONZ, W. and SONDERHOFF, R. (1937) Ueber das Curarin aus Calebassen-Curare. *Annalen der Chemie* **527**: 160–8.

WINTERSTEINER, O. and DUTCHER, J. D. (1943) Curare alkaloids from *Chondodendron tomentosum. Science* **97**: 467–70.

B. SYNTHETIC INHIBITORS

CHAPTER 11

SYNTHETIC INHIBITORS OF NEUROMUSCULAR TRANSMISSION, CHEMICAL STRUCTURES AND STRUCTURE ACTIVITY RELATIONSHIPS

D. Bovet

Rome

11.1. HISTORICAL

The chemical study of the curares represents one of the most complex problems undertaken during the last 50 years. Thus, although the alkaloids have been known since 1850, it is only relatively recently that their chemical structures have been elucidated.

11.1.1. IDENTIFICATION OF THE ACTIVE CONSTITUENTS OF SOUTH AMERICAN CURARES

The first chemical studies on preparations containing native curares were carried out in 1829 by Roulin and Boussingault, who managed to isolate a syrupy mass to which they gave the name *curine*.

Buchner (1861), Preyer (1865), Sachs (1878), and Boehm (1897) characterized different amorphous alkaloids. Among these they distinguished between the pharmacologically active quaternary bases and the inactive tertiary bases (cf. general revue of Boehm, 1923; Craig, 1948).

As has already been pointed out (see "Naturally occurring inhibitors of neuromuscular transmission"), two groups of alkaloids are responsible for the toxicity of the curares prepared by the South American natives. These are:

(i) Bis-benzylquinoline alkaloids, present in various species of the menispermaceous family. The prototype is *d*-tubocurarine isolated from *Chondodendron tomentosum* (Ruiz and Pavon), a constituent of "crude tubocurare".

(ii) Indole alkaloid dimers with forty carbon atoms. These come from various South American species of Strychnos (*Strychnos toxifera* Schomburgk). The main examples here are C-toxiferine I and C-dihydrotoxiferin.

A first attempt to establish the chemical formula of *d*-tubocurarine was made by King in 1935 who proposed a model containing two quaternary ammonium groups. Such a structure was generally accepted until 1970 when further investigations by Everett, Lowe and Wilkinson brought the evidence that actually only one center has a quaternary nitrogen, the other being a tertiary nitrogen.

The chemical structure of toxiferine whose molecule contains two quaternary ammonium centers was established in 1958 by Karrer, Schmidt and their collaborators.

11.1.2. QUATERNARY DERIVATIVES OF ALKALOIDS

In parallel with studies aimed at the isolation of the active principle of the natural product, other workers showed the existence of "curarizing" properties in synthetic *N*-alkyl derivatives of naturally occurring alkaloids.

Thus, in 1869 Crum-Brown and Fraser described the curare-like properties of quaternary derivatives of three alkaloids:

(i) strychnine methylsulfate, a compound already studied in 1859 by Stahlschmidt;
(ii) brucine methylsulfate; and
(iii) thebain methylsulfate.

More recently several workers have studied the quaternary derivatives of quinine. For example, quinine ethylchloride antagonizes pentylenetotrazol (Leptazol)-induced convulsions (Chase *et al.*, 1942, 1944; Lehman *et al.*, 1942). Studies with quaternary derivatives of strychnine, on the other hand, have always led to disappointing results.

11.1.3. QUATERNARY AMMONIUM COMPOUNDS

The pharmacological activities of tetra-alkylammonium compounds and of many others in which a quaternary ammonium group was attached to an aromatic or heterocyclic structure(s) were subsequently studied by numerous workers including Rabuteau (1873), Brunton and Cash (1884), Santesson and Koraen (1900).

The rule of Crum-Brown and Fraser (1869), named after the authors who first enunciated the generalization, states: "The pharmacological activities of the quaternary ammonium derivatives of the various bases show greater similarity with each other than each one does with its corresponding tertiary amine."

Thus, the introduction of a quaternary ammonium group in a molecule containing an amino function is accompanied by a number of characteristic pharmacological properties.

The affinity of numerous quaternary ammonium compounds for different cholinergic receptors can, according to present concepts of chemical mediators of synaptic transmission, explain the varied actions of such compounds on the autonomic nervous system, and the neuromuscular junction.

The extensive literature on mono-quaternary compounds has been reviewed by Trendelenburg (1923), Kulz (1923), Oswald (1924), Gasser (1930), Pfankuch (1930), Bovet and Bovet-Nitti (1948). Ing (1936) and Craig (1948) have analyzed their actions on neuromuscular transmission.

The first attempts to make clinical use of the muscle relaxant properties of mono-quaternary ammonium compounds were those by West (1935) with trimethylhexylammonium iodide (1a) and by Burman (1939) and Huguenard (1950) with trimethyloctylammonium iodide (1b). In both cases the results were unsatisfactory due largely to the prominence of the side effects.

$$CH_3(CH_2)_{12} N^+Me_3 . I_2 \qquad\qquad (1)$$

(1a)   n = 5   trimethylhexylammonium iodide,
(1b)   n = 7   trimethyloctylammonium iodide (curaryl).

11.1.4. BIS-QUATERNARY AMMONIUM DERIVATIVES

It is interesting to note that even in 1907 Willstaetter and Heubner reported the curarizing properties of tetramethylene-bis-trimethylammonium diiodide (2). However, 40 years were to elapse before studies were made on the really active members of the series of polymethylene-bis-trimethylammonium salts.

$$Me_3 N^+(CH_2)_4 N^+Me_3 . 2I^- \qquad\qquad (2)$$

tetramethylene-bis(trimethylammonium iodide).

245

The studies of West (1935) in England, of Bennett (1941) in the United States, and of Griffith and Johnson (1942) in Canada, not only attracted attention to the possible uses of curare-like drugs in anesthesia, but also stimulated the chemical synthesis of other compounds in this group (McIntyre, 1947).

Taking into consideration the structure activity data from the previous literature and the tentative bis-quaternary formula proposed by King (1937) which was the only one known at that time, Bovet *et al.* (1946) introduced the bis-quinoleinic derivative (3) pentamethylenedioxy-bis-8 (1-ethylquinolinium), the first synthetic compound with an inhibitory action on neuromuscular transmission comparable to that of the naturally occurring curares.

Strangely enough, even if originally based on an erroneous formulation of the structure of the natural alkaloid, the concept of the particular activity of the molecules containing two quaternary ammonium centers had to prove to be, for more than 20 years, very useful during the subsequent researches on synthetic substitute analogs of tubocurarine.

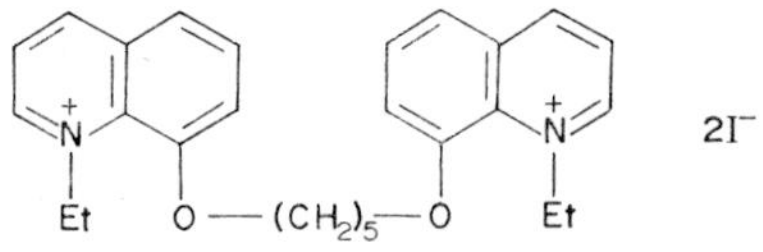

$$2I^-$$

$$(3)$$

Pentamethylene dioxy bis-8
[1-ethylquinolinium iodide] (3381 R.P.)

At the present time, numerous inhibitors of neuromuscular transmission have been synthesized based on the model of *d*-tubocurarine.

These studies have rather paradoxically moved from rather complex chemical structures to simple molecules. This is reminiscent of synthetic work on analgesics and local anesthetics where, starting from the complex structures of cocaine and morphine, relatively simple molecules were developed.

In this field the major advances were the introduction of: succinylcholine chloride in 1949; benzoquinonium chloride in 1950; gallamine triethiodide in 1947; decamethonium in 1948; hexacarbacholine bromide in 1952; paramioniodide in 1952 and diplacine bromide in 1952; as well as the semi-synthetic dimethyl tubocurarine iodide in 1943 and diallyl-nor-toxiferine chloride in 1966.

The synthesis and study of new inhibitors of neuromuscular transmission affords important information from the theoretical standpoint on the mechanism of synaptic transmission at the neuromuscular junction and on the associated role of cholinergic elements.

The common elements between the molecule of acetylcholine (4) and the functional groups in inhibitors of neuromuscular transmission are particularly clearly seen in the structure of succinylcholine (Bovet *et al.*, 1949) (5). The latter molecule resembles a "doubled acetylcholine".

$$CH_3COO . CH_2CH_2N^+Me_3 . Cl^-$$
Acetylcholine $\hspace{6cm}$ (4)

$$CH_2COO . CH_2CH_2N^+Me_3$$
$$| \hspace{3cm} . 2Cl^-$$
$$CH_2COO . CH_2CH_2N^+Me_3$$
Succinylcholine $\hspace{6cm}$ (5)

Furthermore, studies on compounds of this group have led not only to synthetic substitute of *d*-tubocurarine, but also to new types of pharmacological agents.

Thus some compounds have been synthesized which act as depolarizing, rather than as competitive, inhibitors at the neuromuscular junction (Paton and Zaimis, 1948), and there is also the hemicholinium group with an action which is primarily presynaptic.

11.1.5. AMINE DERIVATIVES (NON-QUATERNARY)

In contrast with the quaternary ammonium compounds, molecules containing primary, secondary or tertiary amino groups have, in general, only a weak action on neuromuscular transmission.

The main and important exceptions to this are the alkaloids of *Erythrina* species; β-erythroidine (6a) and its dihydroderivative (6b). Their pharmacological properties have certain similarities with those of curare, in spite of their chemical dissimilarity (Unna *et al.*, 1944).

It has recently been suggested (Lüllmann *et al.*, 1967) that their action on neuromuscular transmission is related to the presence of the *N*-alkyl-octahydro-indole moiety.

Some early experiments carried out on the frog led to the classification of some simple tertiary bases such as pyridine and quinoleine as well as some alkaloids as varied as nicotine, conidine, veratrine, aconitine and delphinine as "curarizing poisons" (Santesson, 1920). In point of fact, none of these compounds has an inhibitory action sufficiently potent or specific to justify their being called inhibitors of neuromuscular transmission.

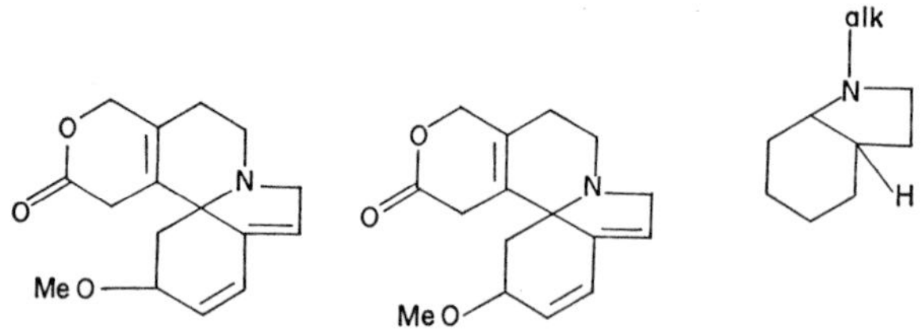

(6)

(a) β erythroidine   (b) dihydro−b−erythroidine   (c) N alkyl−octahydro indole

Amongst the non-quaternary amine derivatives which recent studies have shown to have fairly specific neuromuscular blocking properties, one should mention the following:

bis-(2-heptyl) amine (Phillippot, 1952), aminoalkylamirobzieoquin-ones derivatives (Cavallito *et al.*, 1950), 3562 eT (7) (Jacob *et al.*, 1950), chloroguanide (8) (Dallemagne and Phillippot, 1955) and other *N,N*-disubstituted guanidine [derivatives] (Barzaghi *et al.*, 1965).

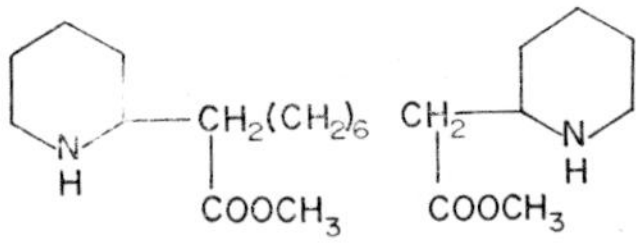

(7)

3562 eT

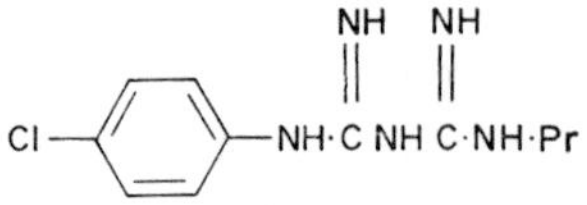

(8)

Chloroguanide

11.2. RELATIONSHIP BETWEEN STRUCTURE AND ACTIVITY IN THE BIS-QUATERNARY AMMONIUM SERIES

The relative simplicity of the molecules, the ease and precision of their biological assay and their possible usefulness in anesthesiology has led to a large number of studies on inhibitors of neuromuscular transmission.

The data at present available, particularly those concerning bis-quaternary ammonium compounds, are sufficiently complete to give a fairly clear picture of the relationships between chemical structure and pharmacological activity. In the study of this topic, the experimenters have the advantage that the majority of the compounds are quite stable and not metabolized in the body. Furthermore, the experiments carried out in the whole animal can easily be confirmed by experiments on isolated organ preparations.

A more detailed analysis of the results, however, raises a number of difficulties. These are due partly to the plurality of the physiological functions of acetylcholine as a neural mediator, partly to the complexity of the interaction between the "inhibitor" and the "receptor", and in general to our ignorance of the ultimate nature of the "cholinergic receptors".

It is generally accepted that inhibitors of neuromuscular transmission exert their principal action:

  (i) presynaptically, by inhibition of the synthesis of acetylcholine (by an effect on the liberation of acetylcholine at the presynaptic level, or by an effect on the presynaptic membrane (Riker *et al.*, 1959; Schueler, 1960));

 (ii) postsynaptically, by combination with the postsynaptic receptor (competition), by modification of the chemically excitable post-synaptic membrane (depolarization) (Paton and Zaimis, 1948) or by other forms of non-competitive and non-depolarizing antagonism (Cheymol and Bourillet, 1960; Bowman, 1962; Thesleff and Quastel, 1965).

Although it appears desirable, experience shows that it is often difficult to assign to a particular group of pharmacological agents a precise mechanism of action. In the case of inhibitors of neuromuscular transmission, the mechanism of action is sometimes not clearly established and appears complex, the same drug being able to act by a number of mechanisms.

For this reason, the relationships to be considered here between structure and activity will take into account the overall activity.

Nevertheless, a distinction will be made between the *acetylcholine-competitive* action of the curare-like drugs, pachycurares or non-depolarizing inhibitors, and the *acetylcholine-mimetic* action of the leptocurares or depolarizing inhibitors.

11.2.1. METHYL-*d*-TUBOCURARINE AND DECAMETHONIUM.
SIMILARITIES AND DIFFERENCES IN THE TYPE OF ACTION

It has already been indicated how studies with synthetic curare-like agents began from the structure of *d*-tubocurarine and proceeded by progressive simplification of the molecule to the discovery of the properties of decamethonium.

From both the point of view of chemical structure and mode of action, these two molecules show a number of common characteristics and also important differences.

A comparison can be established between the properties of *d*-tubocurarine (9b) or of methyl-*d*-tubocurarine (9a, b, c, d), a semisynthetic derivative of the natural alkaloid and decamethonium (9a) based on the fact that the chemical structures of both are characterized by the presence of two basic groups approximately 14 Å apart and joined by a chain of ten carbon atoms.

The linear structure of decamethonium contrasts with the rather massive structure of the molecule of the methyl-*d*-tubocurarine. From the pharmacological standpoint, the two drugs have the common property of producing in mammals, and particularly in the rabbit and the dog, an inhibition of neuromuscular transmission which is apparent at low doses and which is completely reversible.

With regard to the differences between the pharmacological properties of methyl-*d*-tubocurarine and decamethonium, these concern primarily:

    (a) the stimulant action (muscular fasciculations, augmentation of the potential changes accompanying repetitive discharge) which accompanies the initial phase of action of decamethonium, particularly in the cat;

    (b) the depolarization of the motor end-plate by decamethonium;

    (c) the fact that inhibitors of cholinesterase (e.g. eserine) do not have the same characteristic action on inhibition produced by decamethonium as they do on inhibition produced by methyl-*d*-tubocurarine;

    (d) a mutual antagonism between the two agents;

    (e) the contracture produced by decamethonium in avian muscle.

These observed differences have led to the recognition of two groups of inhibitors of neuromuscular transmission:

    (i) Drugs which compete with acetylcholine, such as *d*-tubocurarine. These are also called "true curares", curaremimetics, or pachycurares (competitive inhibitors).

    (ii) Drugs which mimic the action of acetylcholine, such as decamethonium. These are also called leptocurares or depolarizing inhibitors.

The similarity of the neuromuscular inhibitory properties shown by *d*-tubocurarine or methyltubocurarine, and other structurally related compounds, such as cyclo-octadecane-1,10-bis(trimethylammonium) (9c) and laudexium (9d), has been shown by d'Arcy and Taylor (1962).

In the analysis of the relationships between chemical structure and pharmacological action we will frequently have the opportunity to indi-

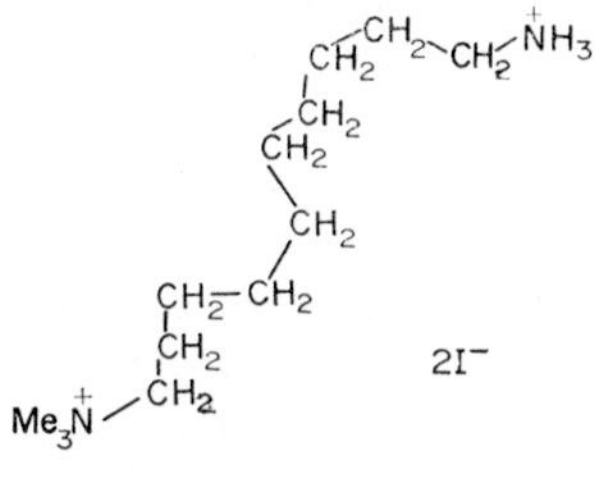

(a) Decamethonium iodide
HDD = 0.1 mg/kg

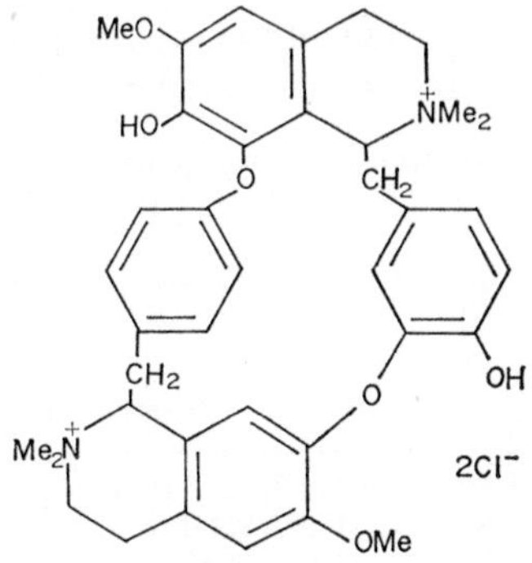

(b) *d*-tubocurarine chloride
HDD = 0.15 mg/kg

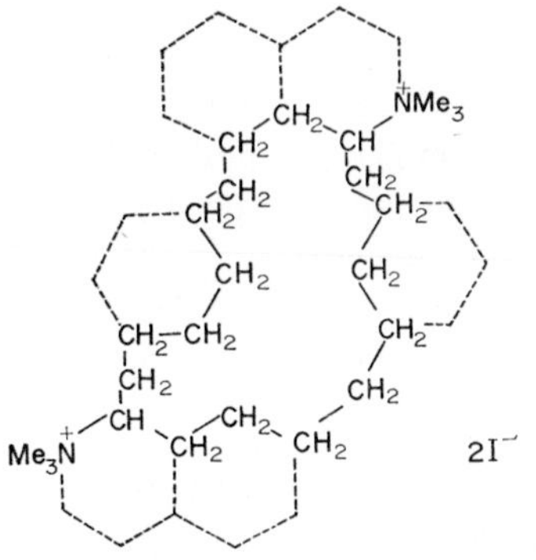

(c) Cyclo-octadecane-1.10-bis-trimethylammonium diiodide
HDD = 0.13 mg/kg

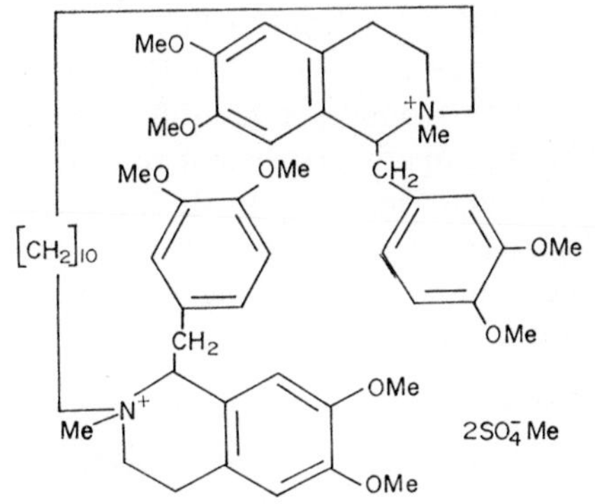

(d) Laudexium methylsulfate
HDD = 0.03 mg/kg

cate to which of these two classes a particular compound belongs. In addition, there are those which have a mixed action corresponding to a transition between the two classes.

11.2.2. NUMBER OF QUATERNARY AMMONIUM CENTERS

Pharmacological studies with synthetic neuromuscular blocking agents have generally shown that the presence of two quaternary ammonium groups in a molecule leads both to an augmentation of the potency of the compound as an inhibitor of neuromuscular transmission and to a decrease in the muscarinic and nicotinic properties present in numerous mono-quaternary ammonium compounds.

251

Concordant observations have been made in an aliphatic series with derivatives of decamethonium and of succinylcholine (Table 1).

TABLE 1. NEUROMUSCULAR BLOCKING ACTIVITY OF SOME ALIPHATIC MONO- AND BIS-QUATERNARY AMMONIUM COMPOUNDS
(After Bovet, 1959)

Compound	Head-drop dose (rabbit) (mg/kg i.v.)
(a) $Me_3 N^+(CH_2)_{10} N Me_3$ (decamethonium)	0.1
$Me_3 N^+ (CH_2)_{10} NH_2$	>0.1 (less active)
$Me_3 N^+ (CH_2)_9 CH_3$	5.0
(b) $Me_3 N^+ CH_2 CH_2OCOCH_2CH_2CH_2COOCH_2CH_2N^+Me_3$ (succinylcholine)	−0.2
$Me_3 N^+ CH_2 CH_2OCOCH_2CH_2 COOH$	5.0
(c) $Me_3 N^+ (CH_2)_5 COOCH_2CH_2N^+ Me_3$	0.2
$Me_3N^+ (CH_2)_5 COOCH_2CH_2 N Me_2$	7.0
$Me_3 N^+ (CH_2)_5 COOEt$	5.0

In an aromatic series, different ethers of mono-, di- and triphenols have been compared for their actions on arterial pressure, respiration and neuromuscular transmission. It was found that an increase in the number of quaternary ammonium groups was accompanied by an increase in the neuromuscular blocking activity and a decrease in their action on the autonomic nervous system (Table 2).

TABLE 2. NEUROMUSCULAR BLOCKING ACTIVITY OF SOME PHENOLIC ETHERS OF ETHOCHOLINE
HDD = head-drop dose
(Rabbit mg/kg i.v.)
(After Bovet, 1951)

(2 triethyl ammonium ethoxy) benzene iodide
HDD. = 20mg/kg

1,2 – bis (2 triethyl ammonium ethoxy) benzene diiodide
HDD. = 1·5 mg

Gallamine triethiodide
1,2,3 – tris (2 – triethyl ammonium ethoxy) benzene triiodide
HDD. = 0·5 mg

11.2.3. DISTANCE BETWEEN TWO QUATERNARY AMMONIUM GROUPS

Comparative studies on the neuromuscular blocking activity of members of a homologous series have shown that the separation of the two quaternary ammonium centers is one of the factors influencing the pharmacological activity.

The first studies in this direction were carried out with aliphatic compounds. In the course of the studies which led to decamethonium, Paton and Zaimis (1948) and Barlow and Ing (1948) found that there was considerable difference in the potency of various members of the series of methonium compounds (Table 3).

TABLE 3. NEUROMUSCULAR BLOCKING
ACTIVITY OF POLYMETHYLENE-BIS-
TRIMETHYLAMMONIUM DERIVATIVES

Head-drop doses
[Rabbit (given mg/kg i.v.)]
(After Barlow and Ing, 1948)

$Me_3 N^+ (CH_2)_n N^+ Me_3$

n=	HDD
2	—
3	—
4	—
5 (pentamethonium bromide)	80
6 (hexamethonium chloride)	30
7	13
8	0.9
9	0.3
10 (decamethonium bromide)	0.1
11	0.5
12	0.6
13	0.9

They developed the attractive hypothesis that the optimum biological activity was related to a chain length of about 14 Å, corresponding to ten carbon atoms between the two quaternary nitrogen atoms.

Although the studies carried out since 1949 with other straight-chain aliphatic compounds have not led to the rejection of the hypothesis of Paton and Zaimis, they have, however, undermined its universal applicability.

Derivatives of penta- and hexamethonium

Let us consider first the members of the methonium series in which the quaternary ammonium groups are relatively close.

It has been known for some time that those compounds in which the quaternary ammonium groups are close together have only weak cholinergic activity. A reduction in the number of methylene groups in the molecule of decamethonium leads to a reduction in the neuromuscular blocking potency and a change in the mechanism of action. Thus, in contrast to the potent neuromuscular blocking activity of decamethonium acting by a depolarizing mechanism, there is the weak activity of pentamethonium and hexamethonium; these act by a competitive mechanism.

The weak inhibitory effect of penta- or hexamethonium on neuromuscular transmission can be considerably increased by replacing the methyl groups attached to the quaternary nitrogen atom by a larger radical. Thus, pentamethylene bis(N-quinoleinium)-dibromide (Bovet *et al.*, 1949) (10a) and pentamethylene bis(N-atropinium)-diiodide (Kimura *et al.*, 1949) (10b) show characteristic curaromimetic properties.

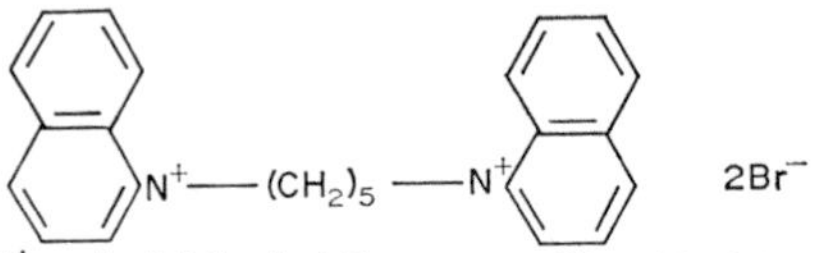

(10a)

bis–(N,N'–quinoleinium)–1,5–pentane dibromide HDD = 1·0 mg

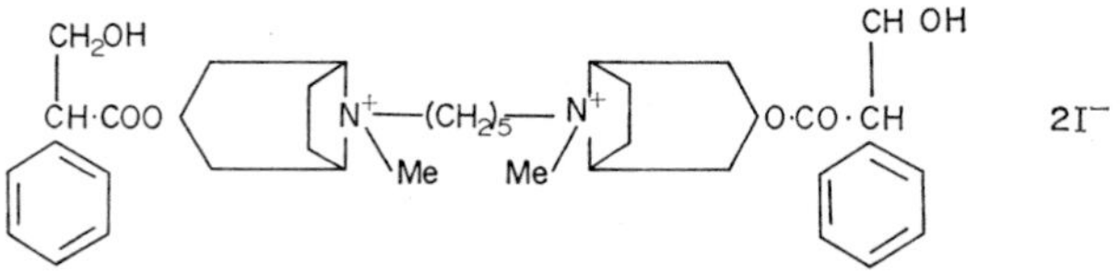

bis–(N,N'–atropinium)–1,5–pentane diiodide HDD =0·35 mg/kg

(10b)

A comparison of the properties of hexamethonium (11a) with those of its N-benzyl (11b) and its N-p-nitrobenzyl derivatives show that the introduction of an aromatic substituent increases the activity by a factor of 40 and 60 respectively (Alexandrova, 1966).

$$RMe\ N^+(CH_2)_6N^+Me_2R$$

R=Me	(11a)
R=CH$_2$Ph	(11b)
R=p-NO$_2$CH$_2$Ph	(11c)

(11d) R =

(11e)
R =

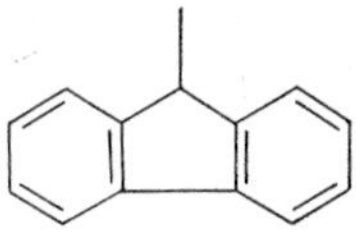

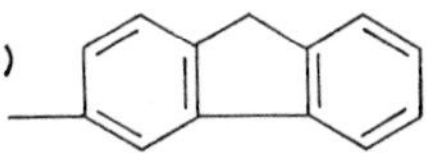

The replacement of one of the methyl groups by 9-fluorenyl (11d) increases the potency by a factor of 200–300. By contrast, the 2-fluorenyl isomer is quite inactive (11e).

Hexamethylene bis(9-fluorenyl-dimethylammonium bromide) (hexa-fluorenium bromide) (11d) has been introduced into clinical practice and has a competitive mechanism of action. Its effective rabbit head-drop dose is 0.08 mg/kg intravenously (Cavallito *et al.*, 1954; Macri, 1954).

A series of asymmetric bis-quaternary pyridinium derivatives deserves special mention. The C$_3$ member (12) (Cavallito, 1968) has potent neuro-muscular blocking properties

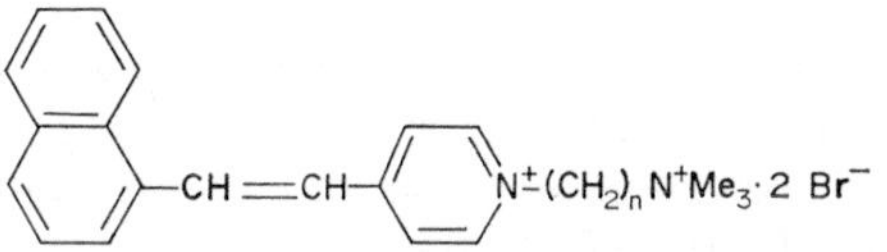

(12)

$$-CH=CH- \quad N^\pm(CH_2)_n N^+Me_3 \cdot 2\ Br^-$$

a) n=3	Effective dose in the dog =0.05–0.1mg
b) n=6	Effective dose in the dog =0.01–0.015

Long-chain derivatives

At the opposite end of the scale, a high degree of neuromuscular blocking activity has been found in a number of compounds in which the two quaternary ammonium groups are separated by a chain with more than ten carbon atoms. Barlow and Zoller (1964) studied members of the methonium series on the cat sciatic-tibialis preparation and the isolated rat phrenic nerve-diaphragm preparation. They found that there were two points of maximum activity corresponding to 9–10 and to 14–18 methylene groups respectively (Fig. 1).

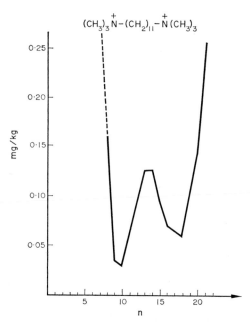

FIG. 1. Curarizing dose in the series of polymethylene-bis-trimethylammonium compounds. Cat, m. tibialis. From the data of Barlow and Ing (1948) and of Barlow and Zoller (1964). (After Khromov-Borison and Michelson, 1966.)

The C_{16} derivative is rather less potent than decamethonium (0.4/1) on the cat sciatic-tibialis preparation, but it is some ten times more potent than decamethonium on the isolated rat phrenic nerve-diaphragm preparation. On avian muscle, the predominantly competitive mode of action of the C_{16} compound contrasts with the contracture characteristic of decamethonium. It will be seen later that studies with series of aliphatic esters, ethers, amides, and carbamides largely confirm the conclusions reached from a study of the methonium series.

The higher members of the methonium series (C_{12}–C_{19}) also show high activity. When this series is compared with the methonium series it is seen (Fig. 2) that the neuromuscular activity ranges over a larger number of members (Barlow and Zoller, 1964). This fact, taken in conjunction with the data from the polymethylene-bis-quinoleinium series (Collier, 1952) and the polymethylene-bis-atropinium series (Haining *et al.*, 1960), leads to the conclusion that the distance between this quaternary nitrogen centers where these contain large radicals is a less important factor determining pharmacological activity than in the methonium series (Figs. 3 and 4).

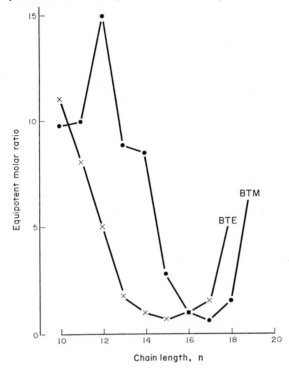

FIG. 2. Neuromuscular blocking activity on the rat diaphragm. Graph of equipotent molar ratios (all relative to BTE 16) against chain length. The ratios for the members of the BTM series were all calculated relative to BTM 16 but this has been found to have the same activity as BTE 16. (After Barlow and Zoller, 1969.)

11.2.4. ANALOGS OF DECAMETHONIUM

It would seem that as a general rule ten carbon atoms represent the upper limit for compounds with highly branched chains and the lower limit for activity in the methonium series.

Decamethonium iodide

The inhibitory action of decamethonium iodide (Table 1, b) on neuromuscular transmission was first described in 1948 independently by Barlow and Ing and by Paton and Zaimis.

These two groups of workers studied the activity of members of the series of polymethylene-bis-trimethylammonium. The muscle relaxant effect of the C_{10} member is some five times greater than that of *d*-tubocurarine in man.

257

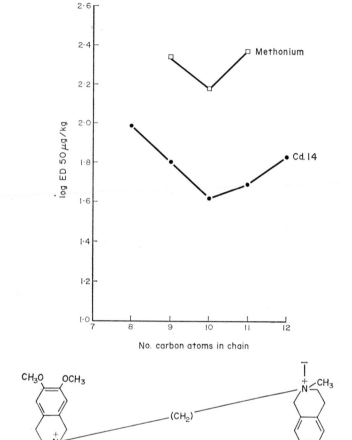

FIG. 3. Relation of neuromuscular blocking potency in rabbit to chain-length in two series of polymethylene-bis-quaternary ammonium salts (methonium figures from Paton and Zaimis, 1949). (After Collier, 1952.)

Decamethonium differs from other neuromuscular blocking agents known up to that time in that it is the prototype of drugs acting by a depolarizing (leptocurare) mechanism of action; like other depolarizing agents, its action is not reversed by anticholinesterases.

Two examples will show the effects of increasing the size of the substituents (1) on the onium centers and (ii) on the chain which joins the onium centers.

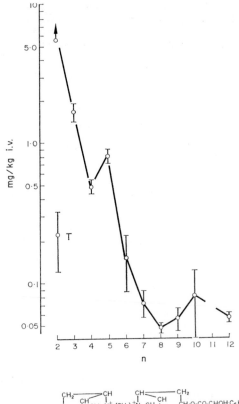

FIG. 4. Effect of chain length (n) on the neuromuscular and ganglionic blocking activity of mandelic acid esters of polymethylene-bis(tropinium halides). T = tubocurarine, o = mean head-drop dose in rabbits by intravenous infusion with s.d. (After Haining, Johnston and Smith, 1960.)

Compounds (9c) and (9d) (d'Arcy and Taylor, 1962) illustrate the structures which may be considered intermediate between those of decamethonium and of d-tubocurarine.

Laudexium methylsulfate (Collier and Taylor, 1949; Taylor and Collier, 1950, 1951) (9d) and cyclo-octadecane-1,10-bis-trimethylammonium diodide (Luttringhaus *et al.*, 1957) (9c) both inhibit neuromuscular transmission by a competitive mechanism of action and have potencies of the same order as d-tubocurarine (9b) and decamethonium (9a).

259

TABLE 4. THE EFFECT OF ALKYL, HETEROCYCLIC OR ARYLAROMATIC
SUBSTITUTION ON THE QUATERNARY AMMONIUM GROUPS OF DECAME-
THONIUM ON THE TYPE OF NEUROMUSCULAR BLOCKADE
Data from Thesleff and Unna (1954)

$R^+N(CH_2)_{10}N^+R$	Paralyzing dose (mol/kg)		Mechanism of block
	Mouse	Chicken	
Me$_3$ (decamethonium)	1.4	0.01	Depolarizing
Me$_2$Et	4.5	0.05	Depolarizing
MeEt$_2$	—	0.5	Mixed
Et$_3$	—	0.9	Competitive
Me$_2$*Iso*propyl	2.0	0.08	Depolarizing
Butyl$_3$	202	0.5	Competitive
Pyridyl	8.3	0.2	Depolarizing
Me Pyrrolidine	1.9	0.03	Depolarizing
Me$_2$Benzyl	7.1	0.8	Competitive
Me$_2$Nitrobenzyl	0.5	0.2	Competitive

Effect of increasing the size of the groups fixed to the two quaternary ammonium centers of decamethonium

Systematic studies have been carried out on the effect of substitutions in the quaternary ammonium centers. The effect depends to some extent on the distance between the two quaternary centers.

The replacement by ethyl of the methyl groups attached to the nitrogen atoms in decamethonium reduces or abolishes the depolarizing action of the drug. The resulting compounds are competitive neuromuscular blockers, i.e. pachycurares (Barlow, 1955; Thesleff and Unna, 1954) (Table 4).

In the case of decamethylene bis-[triethylammonium] bromide the reduction in activity appears to be due to steric hindrance (Cavallito, 1959). Comparative studies of members of the decamethylenebis (tri-alkylammonium) series on the frog rectus abdominis preparation have shown that an increase in the size of the radical attached to the quaternary nitrogen atom leads to a modification in the type of cholinergic activity. Three properties are present in different members of the series

$$R.(CH_2)_{10}.R \tag{13}$$

(a) Depolarizing or acetylcholinomimetic action.
EXAMPLE: $R = N^+Me_3$ (decamethonium); $R = -N^+Me_2Et$
(Fig. 5).

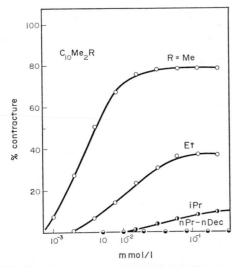

FIG. 5. Cumulative log concentration–response curves for the $C_{10}Me_2R$ series. Note that with elongation of the alkyl chain R there is a progressive decrease of the intrinsic activity shown as a decline in the slope and a decrease of maximal height. Consequently there is a gradual change from agonist ($C_{10}Me_3$) to competitive antagonist ($C_{10}Me_2Pr$). (After van Rossum and Ariens, 1959.)

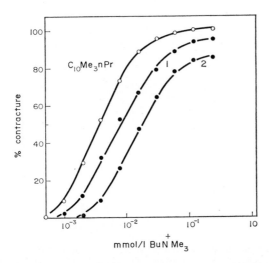

FIG. 6. Cumulative log concentration–response curves for $BuNMe_3$. Effect of a competitive antagonist ($C_{10}Me_2Pr$). (After van Rossum and Ariens, 1959.)

261

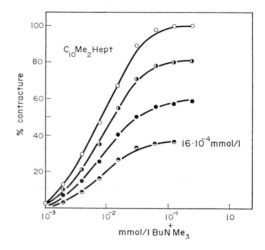

FIG. 7. Cumulative log concentration–response curves for BuNMe₃. With elongation of the alkyl chain R in the $C_{10}Me_2R$ series there is a progressive decrease of the competitive–non-competitive affinity ratio. Thus the higher homologue $C_{10}Me_2$Hept. is practically a pure non-competitive antagonist. (After van Rossum and Ariens, 1959.)

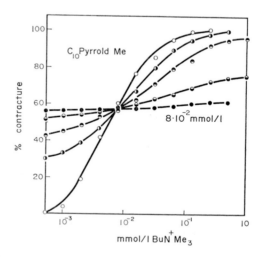

FIG. 8. Cumulative log concentration–response curves for BuNMe₃ in the presence of constant concentrations of C_{10}Pyrrolol Me intrinsic activity. Note agonistic, competitive antagonistic and non-competitive antagonistic properties. (After van Rossum and Ariens, 1959.)

TABLE 5. DECAMETHYLENE-BIS-AMMONIUM DERIVATIVES

$Me_3 N -$			Rabbit head-drop dose (mg/kg i.v.)	References
			0.1 10.0	Collier and Taylor (1949)
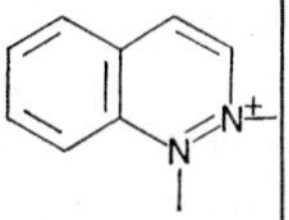	a	non-substituted	4.5	
	b	6-methoxy	4.4	Taylor and Collier
	c	8-methoxy	0.2	(1950)
	d	6,7-dimethoxy	0.15	
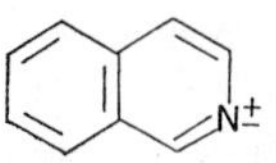	e	non-substituted	4.0	
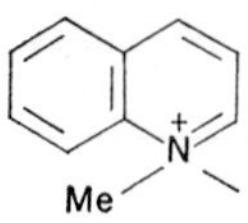	f	non-substituted	0.75	
	g	6-methoxy	0.2	
	h	8-methoxy	0.1	
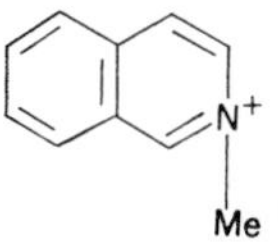	i	non-substituted	1.5	
	j	6-methoxy	0.2	
	k	6,7-dimethoxy	0.05	
	l	6,7,8-trimethoxy	0.02	
		Laudexium methosulfate		
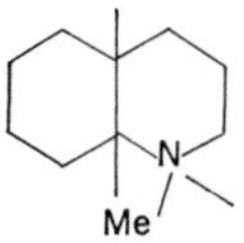	m	cis-	0.12	
	n	trans-	0.1	
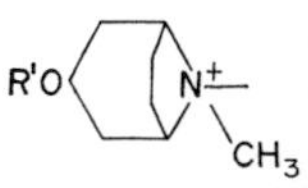	o	R = H	10.0	
	p	COC_6H_5	0.2	
	q	$COCHOH_6C_5H$	0.08	Haining and Johnston
	r	$COCH_2C_6H_5$	0.19	(1962)

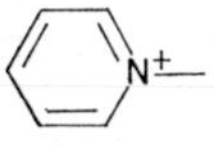

(b) Competitive or curarimetic action.

EXAMPLE: $R = N^+Et_3$ (decamethonium); $—N^+Pr_3$; $—N^+Bu_3$; $—N^+Me_2Pr$; $—N^+Me_2Bu$; $—N^+Me_2Benz$; $—N^+Me_2$ $p\text{-}NO_2Ph$ (Fig. 6).

263

(c) Non-competitive antagonism.

EXAMPLE: R = —N$^+$Me$_2$Hept.   (Fig. 7).

The derivative R = N$^+$Me$_2$isoPr (Fig. 8) is particularly suggestive, since it possesses both depolarizing and stimulant properties at low doses and a competitive curarizing action at high doses (van Rossum and Ariens, 1959).

The incorporation of the onium group into a heterocyclic-substituent which is not incorporated into the inter-onium structure tends to alter the activity which becomes competitive (Table 5).

In the case of more complex molecules, such as tetrahydroquinoleine or tropeine derivatives, the presence of an additional active center or of a center capable of binding with other receptors may increase the total binding of the molecule to the postsynaptic membrane (Taylor and Collier, 1950; Collier and Taylor, 1949, 1952; Haining and Johnston, 1962).

Laudexium methylsulfate (Laudolissin, 13) (Taylor, 1952; Collier, 1952) 2,2′-decamethylenebis (1,2,3,-4-tetrahydro-6,7-demethoxy-2-methyl-1-vere-trylisoquinoleinium methylsulfate) (see Table 5) which is used clinically as a long-acting muscle relaxant may be considered as the prototype of this group of drugs.

(13′)

Effect of increasing the size of the hydrocarbon chain joining the two quaternary ammonium centers

The difference in the activity of some aliphatic and aromatic derivatives of decamethonium compared with parent molecule may be attributed to branching of the hydrocarbon chain joining the two quaternary ammonium centers.

Whilst keeping constant the distance between the two quaternary centers and also keeping methyl groups as the substituents on the quaternary nitrogen atoms, it has been possible to synthesize various cyclic and aromatic compounds with properties similar to those of decamethonium (Table 6a). This is the case for the phenylhexane derivative (Table 6b), the 4-stilbazoline derivative (Table 6c) and the 2- or 4-piperidine derivatives (Table 6d, e).

In other cases, branching of the chain was followed by a reversal of the mechanism of action which becomes typically competitive, as in the bis-cyclohexylethane derivative (Table 6g) and for the polymethylene bis-(2-pyridinium) (Table 6h) and cyclo-octodecane bis(trimethylammonium) compounds (Table 6i). A dual mechanism of action, both depolarizing and competitive, was reported for diphenyl methane derivative (Table 6f) (Thesleff and Unna 1954).

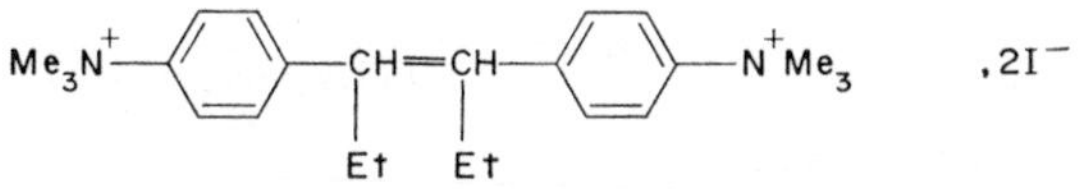

$$\text{Me}_3\text{N}^+ \!-\!\!\langle\rangle\!\!-\!\!\underset{\underset{\text{Et}}{|}}{\text{CH}}\!\!=\!\!\underset{\underset{\text{Et}}{|}}{\text{CH}}\!\!-\!\!\langle\rangle\!\!-\!\text{N}^+\text{Me}_3 \qquad , 2\text{I}^- \qquad (14)$$

Paramion diiodide meso-3,4-bis(*p*-dimethyl amino phenyl) hexane dimethyliodide. HDD = 0.07 mg/kg intravenously.

Paramion diiodide (14), which is widely used in the U.S.S.R., is one of the most active members of this group (Torf *et al.*, 1952). The mesomeric compound, consisting of a double molecule whose two halves have different optical activity, is ten times more active than the racemic mixture of L- and D-isomers.

11.2.5 DERIVATIVES OF SUCCINYLCHOLINE

The importance of the ester grouping in acetylcholine in relation to its physiological activity justifies the interest attached to the presence of a carbonyl group in many synthetic neuromuscular blocking agents.

The chemical structure of succinylcholine (Suxamethonium, diacetyl-choline) bis(2-dimethyleminoethyl) succinate bis(methochloride) (5), is closely related to that of acetylcholine (4) and decamethonium (Table 7).

Succinylcholine possesses neither the muscarinic nor the ganglion blocking properties of acetylcholine; like decamethonium, however, it

TABLE 6. MECHANISM OF NEUROMUSCULAR BLOCKADE PRODUCED BY
SOME COMPOUNDS RELATED TO DECAMETHONIUM IODIDE
HDD = head-drop dose (rabbit, i.v.). ED = effective dose in
leptocurares—depolarizing drugs
(After Bovet, 1959)

Leptocurares – Depolarizing

a) I $Me_3N^+(CH_2)_{10}N^+Me_3$ HDD 0.1 mg

b) II $Me_3N^+(CH_2)_6$—⟨⟩—N^+Me_3 ED (cat) = d-tubocurarine

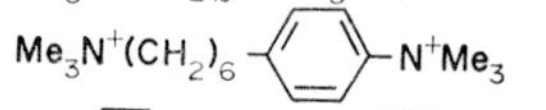

c) III Me_2N^+⟨⟩—$(CH_2)_2$—⟨⟩—N^+Me_3 HDD = 0.125

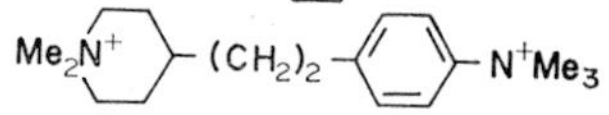

d) IV Me_2N^+⟨⟩—$(CH_2)_6$—⟨⟩N^+Me_2 HDD = approx $\frac{1}{2}$ d-tubocurarine

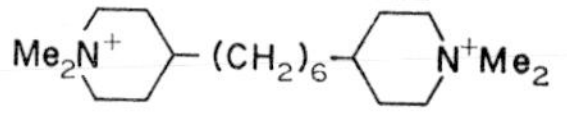

e) V $Me_2N^\pm$⟨⟩—$(CH_2)_8$—⟨⟩N^+Me_2 ED (bird) = 0.12 mg

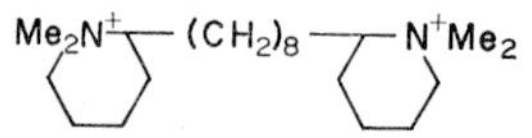

Partially Leptocurares – Mixed

f) VI $Me_3N^\pm$⟨⟩—$(CH_2)_2$—⟨⟩—N^+Me_3 LD_{50} (mouse) = 0.7 gm

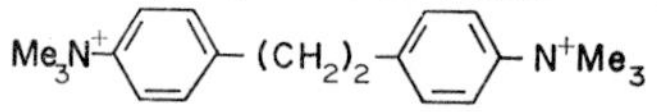

Pachycurares – Competitive

g) VII $Me_3N^\pm$⟨⟩—$(CH_2)_2$—⟨⟩—N^+Me_3 LD_{50} (mouse) = 0.6 gm

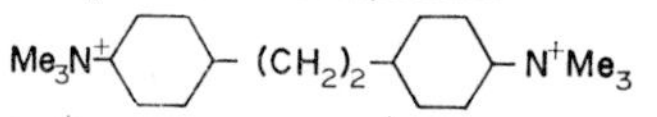

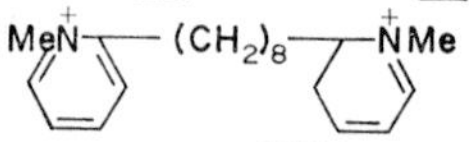

h) VIII MeN⟨⟩—$(CH_2)_8$—⟨⟩$N\,Me$ ED (bird) = 0.74 mg

i) IX Me_3N^+—CH $\overset{(CH_2)_8}{\underset{(CH_2)_8}{\diagdown\diagup}}$ CH —N^+Me_3 HDD approx. 2 × d-tubocurarine

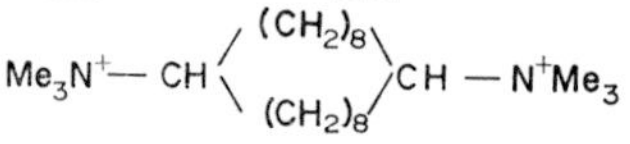

inhibits neuromuscular transmission by a depolarizing mechanism (acetyl-cholinomimetic).

Without a doubt, succinylcholine represents the most significant advance in the field of synthetic neuromuscular blocking agents.

Although the compound was synthetized many years previously (Hunt and de M. Taveau, 1911), its neuromuscular blocking properties were not observed until 1949 (Bovet *et al.*, 1949; Fusco *et al.*, 1949). The compound still represents the typical short-acting muscle relaxant. The short duration of the neuromuscular blocks produced by the drug is due largely to its rapid hydrolysis by cholinesterases in the blood and tissues. Anticholinesterase drugs potentiate its action.

According to d'Arcy and Taylor (1962) "practically every conceivable modification of the suxamethonium molecule has been made, but as often occurs in this field, optimal activity still remains with the parent compound".

The overall conclusions reached from the study of members of the poly-methylene-bis-onium series are in general applicable to the aliphatic ester derivatives of succinylcholine.

(a) *Number and position of ester group.* Activity comparable with that of decamethonium (Table 7) has been found for a mono-ester (Table 7b), and for a di-ester (Table 7a); for the ester of an aminoalcohol with a dicar-boxylic acid (Table 7a) and for the ester of an aminoacid with a glycol (Table 7c). Irrespective of the interonium distance, compounds in which the ester function is brought closer to (Table 7d, e, f) or further from (Table 7g) the trimethylammonium center are considerably less potent than the parent molecule (Fusco *et al.*, 1951; Bovet, 1958).

The data set out in Table 7 also show that if one considers those com-pounds with an interonium chain consisting of ten carbon atoms, then the potency of the esters is of the same order of magnitude as that of decamethonium (Table 7l) and considerably greater than that of the ethers (Table 7h), the amides (Table 7i, j), and the carbamates (Table 7k). We will return to this point later.

(b) *Inter-onium distance.* Because of the ease of hydrolysis of the mole-cule by cholinesterases the interpretation of the data in the case of the aliphatic esters of bis(triethyl-ammonium) is rather complex.

TABLE 7. DERIVATIVES OF SUCCINYLCHOLINE
(The chain joining the two trimethylammonium groups containing ten atoms—
for (g) twelve atoms)
(After Fusco *et al.*, 1951)
HDD = head-drop dose (rabbit, i.v.)

		HDD
(a)	$ME_3N^+CH_2CH_2O\ CO\ CH_2CH_2\ CO\ O\ CH_2\ CH_2N^+Me_3$	0.2 mg/kg
	(succinylcholine)	
(b)	$Me_3N\ CH_2CH_2O\ CO\ CH_2CH_2CH_2CH_2CH_2CH_2N^+Me_3$	0.2
(c)	$Me_3N^+CH_2CH_2CO\ O\ CH_2CH_2O\ CO\ CH_2CH_2N^+Me_3$	0.1
(d)	$Me_3N\ CH_2O\ CO\ CH_2CH_2CH_2CH_2CO\ O\ CH_2N^+Me_3$	5.0
(e)	$Me_3N\ CH_2CO\ O\ CH_2CH_2CH_2CH_2O\ CO\ CH\ N^+Me_3$	100.0
(f)	$Me_3N\ CH_2CO\ O\ CH_2CH_2O\ CO\ CH_2NMe_3$	100.0
(g)	$Me_3N\ CH_2CH_2CH_2O\ CO\ CH_2CH_2CO\ O\ CH_2CH_2CH_2N^+Me$	2.0
(h)	$Me_3N\ CH_2CH_2O\ CH_2CH_2CH_2CH_2O\ CH_2CH_2N^+Me$	1.5
(i)	$Me_3N\ CH_2CH_2CO\ NH\ CH_2CH_2NH\ CO\ CH_2CH_2N^+Me_3$	100.0
(j)	$Me_7N\ CH_2CH_2NH\ CO\ CH_2CH_2CO\ NH\ CH_2CH_2N^+Me_3$	25.0
(k)	$Me_3N\ CH_2CH_2O\ CO\ NH\ NH\ CO\ O\ CH_2CH_2N^+Me_3$	100.0
(l)	$Me_3N\ CH_2CH_2CH_2CH_2CH_2CH_2CH_2CH_2CH_2CH_2N^+Me_3$	1.5
	(decamethonium)	

TABLE 8. EFFECT OF AN ANTI-CHOLINESTERASE[†] ON THE
NEUROMUSCULAR BLOCKING ACTIVITY OF SUCCINYLCHOLINE
AND ITS HIGHER HOMOLOGS (After Danilov, 1966)
$$Me_3N^+(CH_2)_2OCO\ (CH_2)_nCOO\ (CH_2)_2N^+Me_3$$

		Neuromuscular blocking activity Cat, sciatic–gastrocnemius preparation ED_{50} mol/kg	
n		Normal	After anticholin-esterase[†]
(a) 2 (Succinylcholine)		0.08	0.02
(b) 6		1.0	0.005
(c) 8		1.2	0.02
	Carbolonium	0.005	0.005

[†] *p*-Nitrobenzyl ester of *O*-ethyl-ethylphosphinic acid.

In the normal animal, maximal activity resides in succinylcholine in which the chain comprises ten carbon atoms, as in the case of decamethonium (Bovet *et al.*, 1948; Bovet, 1958) (Tables 8 and 9).

By contrast, in animals pretreated with a cholinesterase inhibitor (*p*-nitrophenyl ester of *O*-ethyl-ethylphosphinic acid) the maximum activity resides in suberyldicholine (Table 8b) in which the chain contains fourteen carbon atoms (Danilov, 1966).

TABLE 9 (After Fusco *et al.*, 1951)

$$(CH_2)n\ \diagup\overset{\textstyle COOCH_2CH_2—R}{}\ \diagdown\underset{\textstyle COOCH_2CH_2—R}{}$$

n	R= —N$^+$(CH$_3$)$_3$.I	—N$^+$(CH$_3$)$_2$ | C$_2$H$_5$.I	—N$^+$(CH$_3$)$_2$ | C$_2$H$_5$.I	—N$^+$(C$_2$H$_5$)$_3$.I
1	HDD: 2 mg/kg			15
2	0.2	0.8	15	12
3	0.5			20
4	0.5	0.5	10	10

HDD = head-drop dose (rabbit).

TABLE 10. NEUROMUSCULAR BLOCKING ACTIVITY OF SUCCINYL-BIS-METHYLCHOLINES
(After Bovet, 1959)
HDD = head-drop dose (rabbit)

(a) $CH_2COOCH_2CH_2N^+(CH_3)_3$ $CH_2COOCH_2CH_2N^+(CH_3)_3$	HDD	0.2 mg/kg	Depolarizing
(b) $CH_2COOCH(CH_3)CH_2N^+(CH_3)_3$ $CH_2COOCH(CH_3)CH_2N^+(CH_3)_3$		30 mg/kg	Depolarizing
(c) $CH_3COOCH_2CH(CH_3)N^+(CH_3)_3$ $CH_2COOCH_2CH(CH_3)N^+(CH_3)_3$		0.8 mg/kg	Competitive

(c) *Nature of the substituents on the quaternary ammonium center.* In the case of a linear interonium chain, the replacement of a methyl group by an acidic radical always leads to reduction of the depolarizing activity (Table 9).

The activity of the bis-pyrrolidinum homologue is identical with that of succinylcholine, whereas the bis-piperidine derivative is less potent (Kimensis, 1960).

TABLE 11. MODE OF NEUROMUSCULAR BLOCKADE PRODUCED BY PHENYLSUCCINYL-CHOLINES (After Bovet, 1959)
ED = effective neuromuscular blocking dose (dog i.v.)
HDD = head-drop dose (rabbit i.v.)
CD = dose producing muscular contraction in bird and frog (s.c.)

		Dog (ED mg/kg)	Rabbit (HDD mg/kg)	Bird (CD mg/kg)	Frog (CD cont. mg/kg)
(i) $CH_2COOCH_2\ CH_2\ N^+Me_3$ | $CH_2\ COOCH_2\ CH_2\ N^+Me_3$	L	0.1	0.3	0.01	0.05 1.0

(ii) C_6H_5—CH—$COOCH_2\ CH_2\ N^+Me_3$
   |
  $CH_2.COOCH_2CH_2\ N^+Me_3$
	L	5.0	10.0	0.02	0.05 1.0

(iii) $C_6\ H_5$—CH—$COOCH_2\ CH_2N^+\ Me_3$ | $C_6\ H_5$—CH—$COOCH_2\ CH_2\ N^+\ Me_3$	P	2.0	5.0	—	0.5 —

(iv) $(C_6\ H_5)_2$—C—$COOCH_2\ CH_2\ N^+\ Me_3$
    |
  CH_2—$COOCH_2\ CH_2\ N^+\ Me_3$
	P	5.0	5.0	—	2.0 —

L = leptocurare, P = pachycurare

(d) *Branching of the chain.* Branching of the interonium chain modifies both the potency and the mechanism of neuromuscular blockade.

In the succinic ester series, the derivatives of α-methylcholine (Table 10c) have properties similar both qualitatively and quantitatively to those of succinylcholine. By contrast, the succinic esters of β-methylcholine (Table 10b) are relatively more potent and have properties resembling those of the competitive neuromuscular blocking agents (Rosnati, 1950; Vander-haeghe, 1951).

A subsequent study showed that the $(+)(+)$, $(-)(-)$ and $(+)(-)$ isomers of α-methylcholine esters have a depolarizing mechanism of action; the same is true for the $(+)(-)$ isomer in the case of β-methyl-choline esters, whereas the $(+)(+)$ and $(-)(-)$ isomers have a competitive mechanism of action (Lesser, 1961). A number of aromatic derivatives of succinic acid (Rosnati, 1957; Rosnati *et al.*, 1958) and of glutaric acid (Smith and Ryan, 1961) have been prepared.

The introduction of an aromatic ring into the structure generally results in a reduction in the potency of the compound and may cause a change in its mode of action (Table 11).

11.2.6. ALIPHATIC DERIVATIVES WITH AN ETHER OR CARBAMIC ESTER FUNCTION: HEXACARBACHOLINE— STRUCTURE WITH C-16

Two aliphatic series containing a linear chain homologous with deca-methonium constitute glaring exceptions to the "rule of 10 carbon atoms".

In the case of the ether oxides, the maximal activity resides in chains of eleven (Levis *et al.*, 1953) (15a) to sixteen (Girod and Häfliger, 1952) (15b) carbon atoms.

TABLE 12. POTENCIES OF HEXACARBACHOLINE HOMOLOGS
(After Cheymol, 1953; Cheymol *et al.*, 1954)

	n	Units in chain	Rabbit HDD (mg/kg)
(a) $Me_3.N^+.(CH_2)_2.O.CO.NH.(CH_2)_n.NH.CO.O(CH_2)_2$ N^+Me_3 $2 \times {}^-$	0	10	33
(b)	1	11	0.8
(c)	2	12	1
(d)	4	14	0.3
(e)	5	15	0.1
(f) (hexacarbacholine)	6	16	0.03
(g)	10	20	0.09

$$Me_3N^+(CH_2)_5 \cdot O \cdot (CH_2)_5N^+Me_3 \qquad (15a)$$

Oxydipentonium (Brevatonal)
Rabbit head-drop dose = 0.7 mg/kg

$$Me_3N^+CH_2CH_2O\,(CH_2)_{10} \cdot O \cdot CH_2CH_2N^+Me_3 \qquad (15b)$$

Rabbit head-drop dose = 0.8 mg

In the case of carbamic esters, the maximum activity resides in compounds with a chain length of fifteen to twenty carbon atoms (Table 12).

In both these series the member with ten atoms in the chain has a considerably lower potency than that of decamethonium or of succinylcholine (Table 7).

The prototype of drugs in this class was hexamethylene-biscarbanylcholine iodide, otherwise known as hexacarbacholine (Imbretil) (Table 12f).

Hexacarbacholine bromide acts by a depolarizing mechanism at doses comparable to those of decamethonium. Its effects are only partially antagonized by neostigmine. The drug is used in surgical anesthesia.

The hypothesis according to which those compounds with a linear chain consisting of sixteen atoms produce a distinct type of neuromuscular paralysis was put forward by Khromov *et al.* (1966).

It takes into consideration the existence of two distinct peaks at C-10 and C_{16} in the polymethylene-bis-methonium series, and to the common pharmacological properties of hexadecamethonium (Fig. 1), suberylcholine (Table 8b) and KB 72 (Danilov, 1966) (16).

According to Michelson *et al.* (1965) the "C-16 structure" is from the phylogenetic standpoint a more primitive configuration than that of the C-10 structure.

$$Me_3N^+(CH_2)_2NH.SO_2 \underset{}{\overset{}{\bigcirc}}\!\!\!\!\bigcirc\!\!\!\!\underset{}{\overset{}{\bigcirc}} SO_2NH.(CH_2)_2N^+Me_3 \qquad 2I^- \qquad (16)$$

KB 72

In addition to a specific criterion for the mechanism of action, the limits to assess to this group of neuromuscular blocking agents presents a problem which has not yet been resolved.

It appears that optimal neuromuscular blocking activity requires the presence of an active (carbamic, sulfamic ether) center in the interonium chain to facilitate the binding of the antagonist with the receptor.

271

11.2.7. AROMATIC COMPOUNDS: GALLAMINE AND BENZOQUINONIUM

In the course of the discussion of structure/activity relationships with the relatively simple compounds considered previously, the effect of the introduction of an aromatic nucleus has been mentioned.

The presence of an aromatic ring usually is accompanied by a competitive (pachycurare) mechanism of action of neuromuscular blockade.

Three curaromimetic drugs which have been introduced into clinical practice are, like *d*-tubocurare, phenolic ethers.

These are gallamine triethiodide (Bovet, Depierre and De Lestrange, 1947) (17), diplacine bromide (Kuzovskov *et al.*, 1952) (18), and mediatonal iodide (Levis, Préat and Dauby, 1952, 1953) (19).

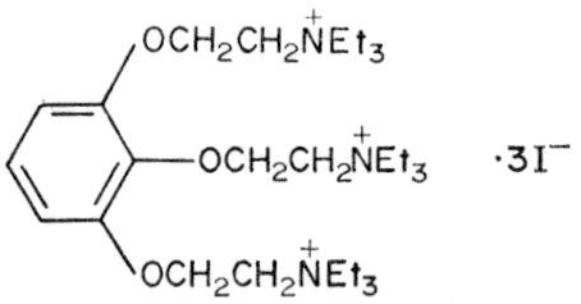

$$(17)$$

Gallamine triethiodide HDD = 0·4 mg/kg

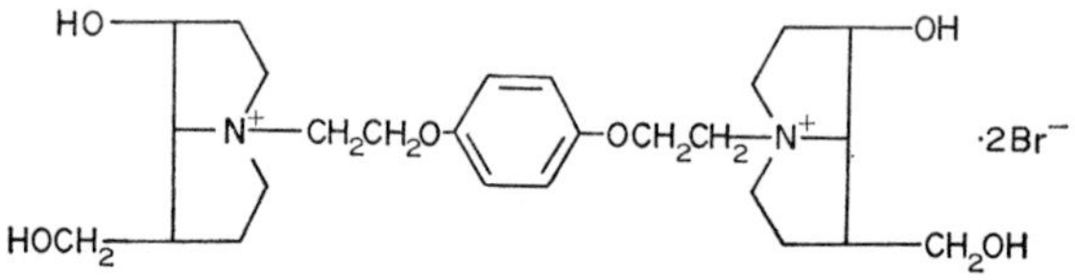

$$(18)$$

Diplacine bromide

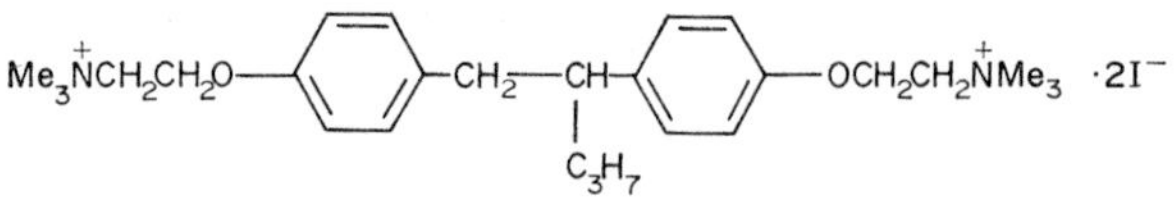

$$(19)$$

Mediatonal iodide HDD = 0·25 mg/kg

Although gallamine triethiodide; 1,2,3-tris (2-diethylamino ethoxy) benzene tris (ethyliodide); flaxedil (17) was the first synthetic muscle relaxant to be introduced into clinical practice, it remains to this day one of the most widely used, and together with succinylcholine has a place in the *International Pharmacopoeia*.

The activity of gallamine is related to that observed many years previously in the ethers of choline (Simonart, 1934) and also to the potentiating effect of a second quaternary group in the molecule.

The effect of gallamine is of the competitive type and is antagonized by neostigmine.

Studies carried out with *N*-alkyl derivatives indicate that progressive replacement of the ethyl groups attached to the quaternary nitrogen atom leads to a decrease in activity (Riker and Wescoe, 1951). In addition, the neuromuscular blocking properties of the molecule are largely due to the introduction of a third onium center into the molecule (Table 2).

2,6-bis(2-diethylaminoethoxy) benzophenone bis(ethyliodide) (20) possess neuromuscular blocking activity comparable with that of gallamine and considerably greater than that of 1,3-bis(2-diethylaminoethoxy) benzene bis(ethyliodide) (21)

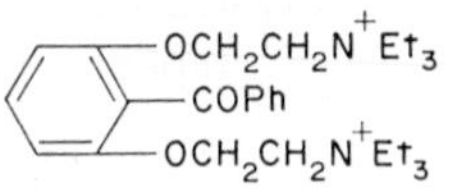

$$-OCH_2CH_2\overset{+}{N}Et_3$$
$$-COPh \qquad (20)$$
$$-OCH_2CH_2\overset{+}{N}Et_3$$

SKF 2015.　　　Head-drop dose = 0·3 mg/kg

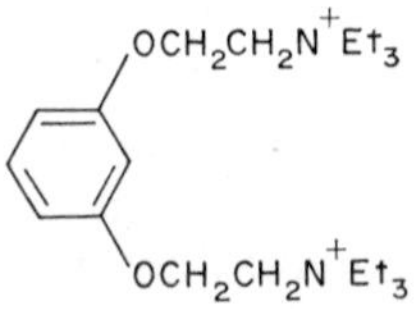

$$OCH_2CH_2\overset{+}{N}Et_3 \qquad (21)$$
$$OCH_2CH_2\overset{+}{N}Et_3$$

Head-drop dose = 1·0 mg/kg

This has led to the suggestion that the onium group in the 2-position stabilizes the orientation of the onium groups in the 1- and 3-positions to give optional activity.

The most probable configuration resulting from the electrostatic repulsion of the charges would be that in which the three onium groups occupy the corners of an equilateral triangle the sides of which are approximately 9 to 10 Å.

Benzoquinonium chloride (2,S-*p*-benzoquinonylenebis) (1 aminotrimethylene) bis-(benzyldiethylammonium chloride), Mytolon (22), which

273

is also clinically useful, is a derivative of 2,5-amino-benzoquinone. It has a structure typical of neuromuscular blocking agents in that there are two quaternary ammonium centers joined by a bridge of twelve atoms.

Although its action is of the competitive (curaromimetic) type, it is only partially reversed by prostigmine. The study of chemically related compounds has led to the finding of neuromuscular blocking activity not only in mono-quaternary derivatives but also in some tertiary amines of this series (Hoppe, 1951).

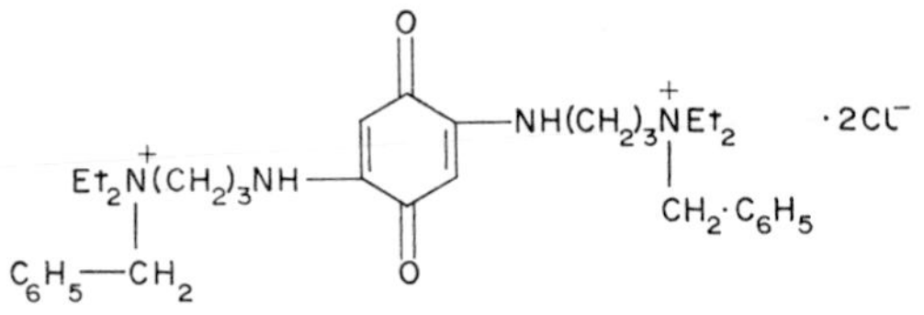

Benzoquinonium chloride (mytolon)

$$(22)$$

It has already been stated that in the polymethylene-bis-trialkyl ammonium series and in the series of esters of aliphatic acids the following generalizations could be made:

(a) In the compounds with short chains (C_6) whose structure resembled that of pachycurares, the ethonium compounds were more active than the corresponding methonium derivatives. Furthermore, both types possessed a competitive mechanism of action.

(b) In the compounds with long chains (C_{10}) whose structure resembled that of the leptocurares, the methonium compounds were more potent than the ethonium derivatives, and the compounds had a depolarizing (acetylcholinomimetic) action.

The data obtained from the study of arylaliphatic compounds previously discussed showed that the introduction of an aromatic ring tends to give the molecule a competitive mechanism of action.

In general, in those compounds whose chemical structure corresponds to a competitive mechanism of action, the triethylammonium compounds are more potent than the trimethylammonium compounds (Table 13a). That is Et_3N^+R compounds $>$ Me_3N^+R compounds so that the index

$$\frac{\text{active dose of triethylammonium compound}}{\text{active dose of trimethylammonium compound}}$$

is less than unity.

TABLE 13. ACTIVITY OF VARIOUS COMPOUNDS ON NEUROMUSCULAR
TRANSMISSION
Comparison between the trimethylammonium and the corresponding
triethylammonium compound. Index of activity Me_3/Et_3
(After Bovet, 1959)

	Curarizing dose		Index Me_3/Et_3	
	Me_3N^+-R	Et_3N^+-R		
$Et_2N^+R > Me_3N^+R$				
$\equiv N^+(CH_2)_6\ N^+\equiv$	26.0	1.0	0.04/1	HDD Rabbit mg/kg
$\equiv N^+CH_2CH(CH_3)OCOCH_2CH_2COOCH(CH_3)CH_2N^+\equiv$	1800.0	4.00	0.22/1	ED (rat diaphragm) mg/l
$\equiv N^+CH_2CH_2$⟨ring⟩$CH_2CH_2\ N^+\equiv$	7.0	3.0	0.15/1	HDD Rabbit
$\equiv N^+CH_2CH_2N$⟨CH_2CH_2/CH_2CH_2⟩$NCH_2CH_2\ N^+\equiv$	93.0	11.0	0.12/1	HDD Rabbit
$\equiv N^+(CH_2)_3\ NH$⟨O=quinone=O⟩$NH(CH_2)_3\ N^+\equiv$	0.4	0.09	0.02/1	HDD Rabbit
$Me_3N^+R > Et_3N^+R$				
$\equiv N^+(CH_2)\ ION^+\equiv$	0.01	0.94	94/1	ED Bird
$\equiv N^+CH_2CH_2OCOCH_2CH_2COOCHCHN^+\equiv$	0.2	12.0	60/1	HDD Rabbit
$\equiv N^+(CH_2CH_3OCO$⟨ring⟩$COO(CH_2)_3\ N^+\equiv$	0.02	1.0	50/1	ED Dog
$\equiv N^+CH_2CH_2OCOCH_2$⟨ring⟩$CH_2COOCH_2CH_2N^+\equiv$	0.5	10.0	20/1	ED Dog
$\equiv N^+CH_2CH_2O$⟨ring⟩$C=C$⟨ring⟩$OCH_2CH_2\ N^+\equiv$ (Et, Et)	0.08	0.08	3.3/1	HDD Rabbit

In the series of depolarizing leptocurares (Table 13b) in which the methonium compounds are always depolarizing, the same index is greater than unity.

Table 14 sets out the data obtained from a homologous series of hydroquinone ethers. There is a sharp change in the value of the index when the number of atoms on the chain attached to each side of the aromatic ring changes from n=4 to n=5.

TABLE 14. NEUROMUSCULAR BLOCKING ACTION OF HYDROQUINONE ETHERS

Comparison between the activity of trimethylammonium compounds and the corresponding triethylammonium derivative. Index of activity Me_3/Et_3.

$$O \cdot (CH_{2n})N^+ \equiv$$

$$2X^-$$

$$O \cdot (CH_2)_n N^+ \equiv$$

(After Bovet, 1959)

n	Rabbit head-drop dose (mg/kg i.v.)			Dog, neuromuscular prep. (mg/kg i.v.)			Mechanism	
	Effective dose		Index	Effective dose		Index		
	Me_3N^+R	Et_3N^+R	Me_3/Et_3	Me_3N^+R	Et_3N^+R	Me_3/Et_3	Me_3 N^+R	Et_3 N^+R
2	2.0	1.5	0.75/1	10.0	2.0	0.2/1	C	C
3	1.5	0.5	0.33/1	1.0	0.5	0.5/1	C	C
4	0.25	0.4	1.6/1	0.005	0.5	80/1	D	C
5	0.25	0.3	1.2/1	0.5	5.0	10/1	D	C

C = competitive.   D = depolarizing.

11.2.8.   SHORT-ACTING NEUROMUSCULAR BLOCKING AGENTS

Interest in short-acting muscle relaxants has previously been mentioned with reference to succinylcholine.

Because of the inconveniences associated with the depolarizing mechanism of action of succinylcholine, many attempts have been made to develop a short-acting neuromuscular blocking agent with a competitive action.

The first solution to this problem was provided by the synthesis of Prodeconium bromide [Decamethylenebis (oxyethylene)] bis[(carboxymethyl) dimethylammonium bromide] dipropyl ester; dioxahexadeconium bromide: Prestonal (Frey, 1955) (23)

$$Me_2N^{\pm}(CH_2)_2O(CH_{12})_{10}O(CH_2)_2N^+Me_2 \quad 2Br^- \quad (23)$$
$$CH_2COOPr \qquad\qquad\qquad CH_2COOPr$$

Prodeconium bromide (Prestonal). Head-drop dose = 0·075 mg/kg.

Subsequently a series of compounds combining the properties of succinylcholine with those of bisquinoleinium derivatives (Collier *et al.*, 1958) (24) or with those of bis-tropeinium (Haining *et al.*, 1960) (25) was studied.

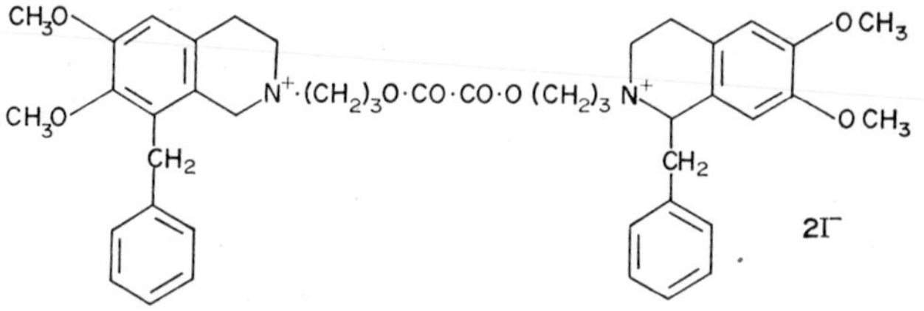

(24)

γ-oxalolaudonium. Head-drop dose = 1·0–2·0 mg/kg

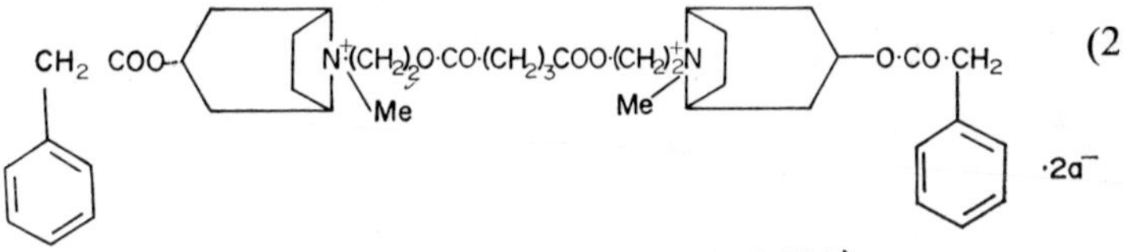

(25)

Bis-tropeinium derivative (epimer of DF 596)

On the other hand, α-truxillic acid has been the starting point of numerous esters some of which have a short duration of action, notably, truxillonium (26a), cyclobutonium (26b) and anatrixonium (26c) (Mharkevich, 1965, 1966).

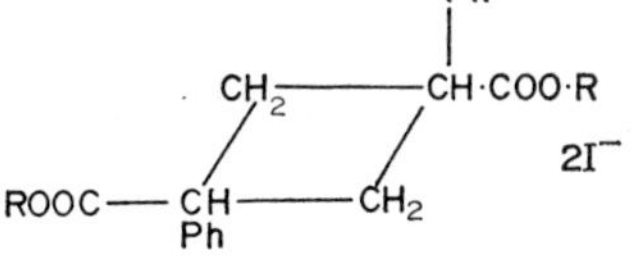

(26)

		Head drop dose (mg/kg)
a) Truxillonium	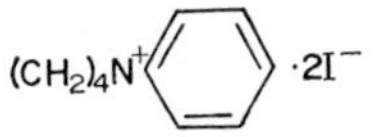 $(CH_2)_4N^+$⟨⟩ ·2I⁻	0·03
b) Cyclobutonium	$(CH_2)_3N^+Et_2Me$ ·2I⁻	0·037
c) Anatrixonium	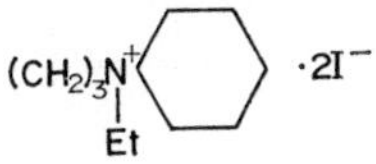 $(CH_2)_3N^+$⟨⟩ ·2I⁻ Et	

277

Piprocurarium (Brevicurare) (27) is also a competitive muscle relaxant with a short duration of action (Cheymol *et al.*, 1960):

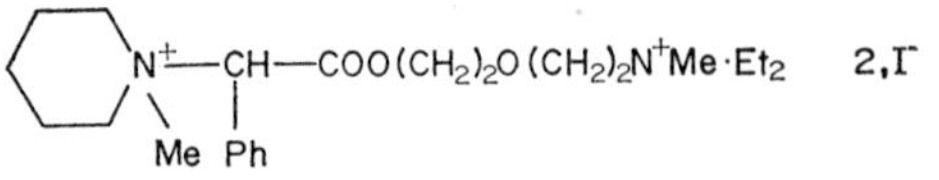

$$\text{\Large\bigcirc}N^{\pm}-CH-COO(CH_2)_2O(CH_2)_2N^+Me\cdot Et_2 \quad 2,I^- \qquad (27)$$
$$Me\ Ph$$

Piprocurarium (Brevicurare)

In the aromatic series, the esters of terephthalic acid and of phenyl-diacetic acid (28) with choline and its homologues have been synthesized. In general, these compounds have a short duration of action due to their hydrolysis by serum cholinesterase (Rosnati, 1957).

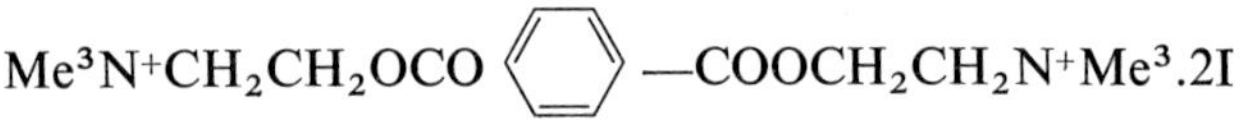

$$Me_3N^+CH_2CH_2OCO \text{\Large\bigcirc} -COOCH_2CH_2N^+Me_3 \cdot 2I \qquad (28)$$

phenyldiacetylcholine

11.2.9. AMINO-AMMONIUM DERIVATIVES. ISOCURINE AND NOBUTANE

Aliphatic polyonium compounds with a branched (29) (Kensler *et al.*, 1954) or straight (30) (Edwards *et al.*, 1961; Stenlake, 1963) chain have a relatively weak activity which is often accompanied by central side effects.

$$[R_3N^+(CH_2)_n]_3CH \qquad\qquad R_3N^+(CH_2)_nN^+(CH_2)_nNR_3$$
$$R_2$$

$$(29) \qquad\qquad\qquad\qquad (30)$$

R = Et, n = 4   R = Et, N = 8

Head-drop dose = 1.25 mg/kg   Head-drop dose = 0.14 mg/kg

According to Stenlake (1963) (who has written an exhaustive revue of work in this field) the neuromuscular block produced by these compounds depends on the interonium distance, the whole length of the chain being relatively unimportant.

Whilst the introduction of an additional quaternary ammonium group profoundly alters the activity of compounds in the polymethylene-bis-onium series, the introduction of a tertiary amino group is relatively unimportant.

It is interesting to compare the activity of members of the three series of amino-ammonium compounds with that of decamethonium.

The presence of one (Hazard *et al.*, 1950) (31) or two (Boissier *et al.*, 1960) (32) piperazine rings, or of the bicyclic structure of bicyclononane (Rubstov and Maschkovskiy, 1961) (33) confers depolarizing activity on the molecule.

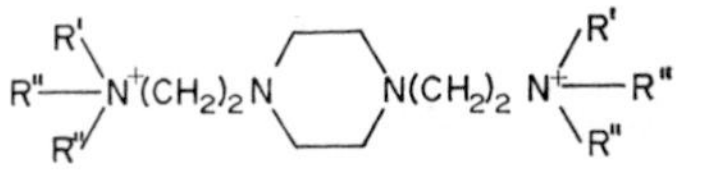

$$R^{''}\!\!-\!\!\underset{R^{'''}}{\overset{R^{'}}{\underset{|}{\overset{|}{N^+}}}}\!(CH_2)_2\,N\!\!\diagdown\!\!N(CH_2)_2\,N^+\!\!-\!\!R^{''} \qquad\qquad (31)$$

R' =R" = Et   292 HO   Head drop dose =10 mg/kg
R' =Et; R" = $CH_2C_6H_5$ Insocurine   Head drop dose = 1·6 mg/kg
Neuromuscular blocking dose in the cat 1/10th *d*–tubocurarine

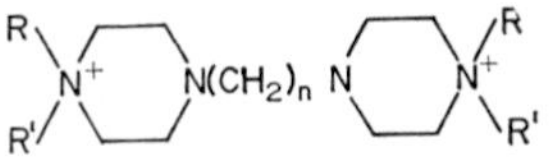

$$(32)$$

R=Me   R'=Et   S.D   211.10
Head drop dose = 0·2 & 0·4 mg/kg

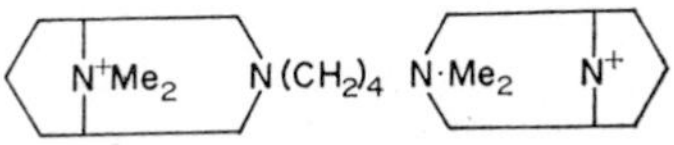

$$(33)$$

No butane   DNB   n.1478
Head drop dose =0·25 mg/kg

11.2.10. ACTIVITY OF "RIGID MOLECULES"

Although the compounds of the various bis-ammonium series mentioned thus far are, in general, flexible molecules, it appears that this is not an essential requirement for activity.

The various hypotheses concerning the relationship between activity and interonium distance makes the study of rigid structures of particular interest.

1. The curare alkaloids possess semi-rigid (*d*-tubocurarine) or rigid c-toxiferine I.

In the case of *d*-tubocurarine chloride none of the four isomers is an entirely rigid structure. The number of atoms between the nitrogen atoms is ten, whilst the maximum distance is from 11 to 14 Å.

In the case of toxiferine, the number of intermediary atoms is nine whilst the distance is 7 Å.

2. Amongst synthetic compounds one of the derivatives of 3-fluorene 9(p-methoxyphenyl) fluorene-2-7-bis-trimethylammonium, iodide (34) has seven interonium carbon atoms, and the structure is completely rigid. Its activity is greater than that of *d*-tubocurarine (Medesan and Stoica, 1960) (34).

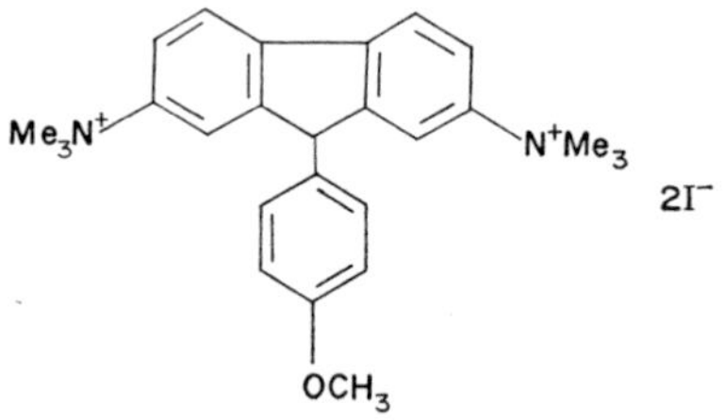

(34)

3. There are three compounds in which the quaternary ammonium centers are separated by nine carbon atoms and which possess very hgh neuromuscular blocking activity.

One is a diaromatic compound with high activity (Torf *et al.*, 1952)

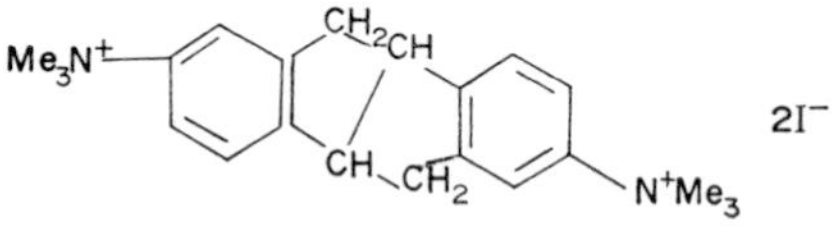

(35)

(35); two others are androstane derivatives (Biggs *et al.*, 1964 (36); Allaudin *et al.*, 1965).

M and B 9105, 3 17-bispyrrolidine-1'yl-5-androstane bis (methyliodide) possesses an entirely rigid structure. The two N^+ atoms are approximately 11 Å apart. It is active in the rabbit at a dose of 0.33 mg/kg.

4. In the case of Malouetine 3β-20α-bis(dimethylamino)-5-pregnane bis (methochloride) (37) the two quaternary ammonium centers are

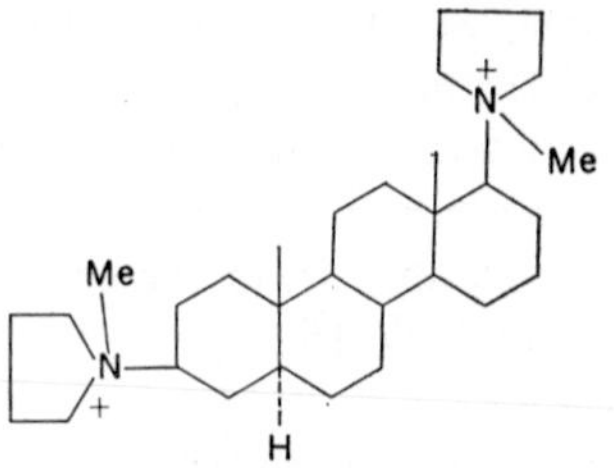

(36)

M and B 9105. Head–drop dose
= 0·033 mg/kg

separated by ten carbon atoms. Although the center of the molecule is rigid, the rotation of the side chain enables the distance between the two quaternary nitrogen atoms to vary from 11 to 12.5 Å. Its activity is comparable with that of *d*-tubocurarine (Janot *et al.*, 1962; Quevauvillier, 1960; Khuong-Huu *et al.*, 1964).

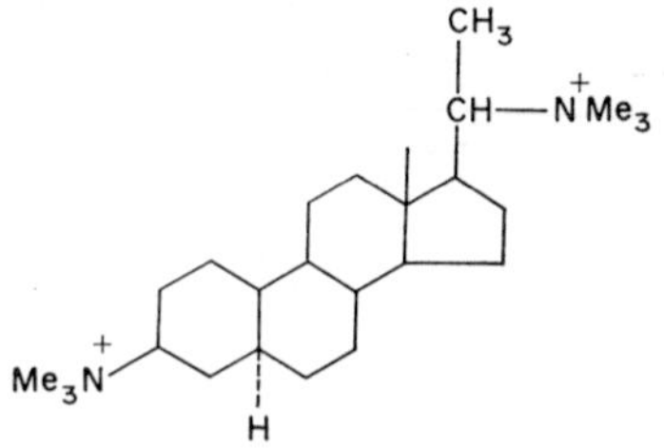

(37)

Malouetine

Comparison between derivatives of Malonetine and of androstane suggests that stereoisomerism of steroid bis-quaternary salts has some effect on activity.

The cost suggestive data on the effect of steric configuration on activity are those obtained from the study of the stereoisomers of succinyl methylcholine and of *d*-tubocurarine.

11.3. CONCLUSIONS

11.3.1. TYPES OF NEUROMUSCULAR BLOCKING AGENTS

The structure–activity relationships of synthetic inhibitors of neuromuscular transmission have been extensively studied because of the value

281

of these compounds as muscle relaxants in anesthesia (McIntyre, 1947). These drugs are based upon either the aliphatic (e.g. decamethonium, suxamethonium), aromatic (e.g. gallamine) or heterocyclic (e.g. *d*-tubocurarine, toxiferine) series, and the molecules may contain ester, ether or (more rarely) carbamide or amine groups, or, in the case of heterocyclic compounds, another nitrogen atom (Table 15).

TABLE 15. MAIN TYPES OF INHIBITORS OF NEUROMUSCULAR TRANSMISSION USED CLINICALLY (CURARIZING AGENTS)

Aliphatic derivatives	Aromatic derivatives	Heterocyclic derivatives
(a) Decamethonium iodide (Table 1a; HDD = 0.1)	Paramion iodide (14; HDD = 0.07)	Hexafluorenium bromide mylaxene (11d; HDD = 0.08)
(b) Ethers Oxydipentonium chloride (15; HDD = 0.7)	Gallamine triethiodide Gallium iodide (Table 2c; HDD = 0.4)	*d*-Tubocurine chloride (DHD = 0.15)
Prodeconium bromide or dioxadecadenium, Prestonal (23; DHD = 0.075)	Anetocurare iodide methdiatonal (19; HDD = 0.25)	Methyltubocurarine iodide methyltubocurarine (9b; HDD = 0.02) Laudenium metho-sulfate laudolissine (Table 5n; HDD 0.03)
(c) Esters Succinylcholine suxamethonium (6; HDD = 0.2)	Pipocurarium brevicurarine (27)	
(d) Nitrogenous compounds Hexacarbacholine bromide (Table 12g; HDD = 0.03)	Benzoquinonium chloride, Mytolon (22; HDD = 0.03)	Toxiferine (DHD = 0.003) Allyltoxiferine (DHD = 0.013)

HDD = Head-drop dose
(rabbit, i.v. mg/kg.)

It seems surprising at first sight that such diverse molecules possess similar properties. The reasons for this are that in all cases (a) they are bases forming strongly-ionized salts, which hence are water-soluble, (b) they possess two onium (quaternary nitrogen) groups—or in the case of *d*-tubocurarine one tertiary amino and one quaternary ammonium—separated by a distance of between 7 and 20 Å. It is generally agreed that the latter are the functional groups of the molecules; they could also be responsible for the binding of the molecules to the cholinergic receptors of the neuromuscular junction, because acetylcholine also has an onium group.

It is probable, at least in the case of compounds whose actions are rapidly and completely reversible, that these curarizing agents exert their main effect postsynaptically, although some workers (Riker *et al.*, 1959; Bowman *et al.*, 1962) disagree. However, the possibility of a presynaptic action must be taken into account when considering derivatives in the hemicholinium group (Schueler, 1960).

11.3.2. STRUCTURAL CHARACTERISTICS OF NEUROMUSCULAR BLOCKING AGENTS

Two factors need to be considered when assessing the relationship between the structure of neuromuscular blocking agents: (a) ionic charge and (b) steric effects (Cavallito, 1959, 1962).

11.3.2.1. *IONIC CHARGE*

There are several lines of evidence to support the view that the electrostatic charge on the onium groups is involved in the blocking action:

(a) Replacement of the quaternary amines with tertiary amine groups leads to a marked reduction in activity, as shown for *d*-tubocurarine (Wintersteiner, 1959) and gallamine (Roberts *et al.*, 1953).

(b) Replacement of the quaternary nitrogen atom with sulfonium, phosphonium and arsonium ions

$$Me_4N^+, Me_4P, Me_4As^+$$

leads to a change in potency that is directly proportional to the charge density on the central atom (Holmes *et al.*, 1947). Similarly, replacement of a piperidine with a morpholine nucleus leads to a reduction in the blocking potency, correlated with diminution in charge density on the onium group (Hazard, 1953; Cavallito *et al.*, 1950).

(c) No curaromimetic compound contains a strongly anionic group; this is well known, for example, for the betaines.

(d) When the onium groups are sufficiently close, their mutual interaction leads to both a decrease in charge density and to loss of pharmacological activity. The best known examples are the short-chain (n = 2–4) polymethylene compounds (Stenlake, 1963).

11.3.2.2. *STERIC EFFECTS*

The second factor to be considered is the steric arrangement of the molecule. It is believed that the inhibitor binds to the receptor by a reciprocal fitting, the distance between the functional groups and the degree of mobility of the molecule would govern the type and intensity of pharmacological action at the cholinergic receptor. As long ago as 1949 Ing suggested that steric hindrance at the cationic groups was important in determining the binding of these groups to the surface of the receptor. Many examples of such effects have already been given:

(a) The effect of introducing aromatic or other large radicals into the inter-onium structure of penta- or hexa-methonium is shown in Tables 12 and 13.

(b) When radicals of different dimensions are introduced into the neighborhood of the onium groups in the decamethonium series, there is a large increase or decrease in neuromuscular blocking potency that can be correlated with steric effects.

(c) There is extensive literature showing the significance of the aromatic nuclei in the gallamine, diplacine and anetocurare series. This shows that the structure of the chain connecting the two onium groups, as well as the nature of the radicals attached to the onium groups, is important. This is also shown by a comparison of the succinic esters of α- and β-methylcholine.

(d) Experiments with the derivatives of androstane and malouetine have confirmed the results obtained in studies with the natural alkaloids related to *d*-tubocurarine, establishing the role of steric hindrance in curarizing activity.

11.3.3. OVERALL MOLECULAR STRUCTURE OF THE LEPTOCURARES AND PACHYCURARES

Analysis of the structure-action relationships of neuromuscular blocking agents cannot usefully be pursued without differentiating between depolarizing (leptocurares) and competitive (pachycurares) modes of action. The concept that these drugs can be classified into one or other group is upheld by observations on the methonium/ethonium index, which expresses the ratio of activities of the trimethyl- and triethylammonium compounds. It has frequently been observed that, in the case of depolarizing agents, the trimethylammonium compounds have a greater activity than the corresponding triethylammonium derivatives (index is greater than unity), whereas the converse is true for competitive blockers (index is less than unity) (Bovet, 1959; Stenlake, 1963; Triggle, 1965).

However, the hypothesis that a distinction between lepto- and pachycurares ca.1 be made on a purely stereochemical basis is not substantiated in the case of tridecamethonium (C_{13}) (Zaimis, 1953) and certain poly-onium derivatives (Edwards *et al.*, 1961) which have no depolarizing action in spite of their chain length. These anomalies can be explained by an additional hypothesis namely that in molecules with an inter-onium chain length greater than the optimum, the ends twist in towards each other to give a more compact structure assuming a configuration more similar to that of the branched pachycurares.

Several workers have postulated that instead of making a distinction between two groups, acetylcholine-mimetic and acetylcholine-competitive, the curarizing agents of the bis-onium series comprise a unique group, other such agents being competitive neuromuscular blockers. However, (a) the existence of molecules possessing both types of action, (b) the fact that many substances exert a depolarizing or a competitive action depending upon the type of nerve-muscle preparation being investigated and (c) the transition between lepto- and pachycurares that exists in several homologous series, all argue in favor of the concept already discussed.

11.3.4. THE STRUCTURE OF CHOLINERGIC RECEPTORS

Important contributions and reviews have recently been published in the field of structure of cholinergic receptors.

It has frequently been suggested that the study of agonists and antagonists to the action of acetylcholine could assist in the formulation of hypotheses on the nature of cholinergic receptors. Such hypotheses must take into consideration the existence of anionic and cationic centers, and of steric effects in the drug molecules, and van der Waals forces between drug and receptor. In particular, the receptor should contain:

(a) An *aromatic center* that corresponds to the cationic group in the drugs, i.e. an area of ionic bonding.

(b) An area of *van der Waals bonding* situated in the immediate vicinity of each anionic center. One such hypothesis by Barlow (1964) takes into consideration the results of previous workers on compounds with a muscarinic (Ing, 1949) and a nicotinic (Gill and Ing, 1958) action. The model proposed for cholinergic receptors of autonomic ganglia and smooth muscle show two concentric areas, the central zone being an area of ionic bonding, surrounded by an annular area in which van der Waals forces operated.

(c) The model of Wilson and Bergman (1950) includes a third characteristic of cholinergic receptors. They propose that, in the case of acetylcholinesterase, the anionic center (to which the substrate is anchored) is separated by about 5 Å from an *"esterasic"* center (at which the substrate is hydrolyzed).

(d) In addition, observations on the stereospecificity of parasympathomimetric (muscarinic) drugs, parasympatholytic (atropinic) drugs, and drugs which stimulate or depress the autonomic ganglia, have suggested the existence of *accessory centers* which, according to the concept formulated by Hunt (1926), give the cholinergic receptors a mosaic structure.

In the special case of cholinergic receptors of smooth muscle, studies of stereochemical factors involved in the activity of muscarinic derivatives suggest that six different points of attachment exist between drug and receptor (Waser, 1961, 1962; Barlow, 1964); of particular importance are the areas of van der Waals bonding, each situated about 6 Å from the area of primary anionic bonding, and at least one of these projects from the receptor surface: in addition there is a center of attraction between partial charges on drug and receptor. The structure of the cholinergic receptor at autonomic ganglia would be less complex (Gill and Ing, 1958; Gill, 1959).

(e) A fifth factor to be taken into consideration is the *interrelationship between receptor molecules* on the carrier protein. Since acetylcholine possesses only one cationic center, the receptor presumably contains only one complementary anionic center. The tense blocking action of the bis-quaternary compounds has frequently been attributed to attachment to two such anionic centers, suggesting that the receptors are regularly arranged with respect to each other (Barlow, 1960; Stenlake, 1963; Khromov-Borisov and Michelson, 1966).

It is a general agreement that the different types of cholinergic receptor (at autonomic ganglia, smooth muscle and skeletal muscle) may possess very different structures.

11.3.5. FACTORS DETERMINING THE SPECIFICITY OF ACTION ON NEUROMUSCULAR TRANSMISSION

Within the framework of the previous discussion we can now consider the special case of curarizing compounds. Of the five factors mentioned previously, the three that appear to be most significant are (a) anionic centers, (b) areas of van der Waals bonding in the vicinity of these and (c) the interrelationship between receptor molecules. By way of contrast it seems that the specificity of these inhibitors for the neuromuscular junction is due to the absence in the receptors of (c) esterasic centers and

(d) accessory centers, which appear to be essential for cholinergic receptors at the other sites (sympathetic ganglia, adrenal medulla and smooth muscle) and even for the presynaptic effects of hemicholinium. Thus postulated differences between cholinergic receptors at these different sites would be of particular importance in determining the specificity of different groups of agonist and antagonist drugs (e.g. atropinic, ganglion-blocking, and neuromuscular-blocking drugs). However, the structure-action relationships cannot be considered solely on the basis of bond-formation between drug and receptor molecules.

It has already been mentioned that neuromuscular blocking agents are specific for their site of action, not having secondary, and therefore possibly toxic, effects at other cholinergic sites. This is, of course, of great importance to the clinician.

In order to assess the specificity of these drugs most accurately, large doses are administered to an animal whose respiration is controlled. Thus a normally lethal dose in a rabbit can be exceeded nearly always by ten times, and occasionally by a hundred times, if the animal's respiration is maintained artificially. Drugs classified as "minor curarizing agents", however, have such a variety of pharmacological properties (Bovet, 1959) that with such procedure the protection would be ineffectual.

Among the drugs used in anesthesia, the dose required to affect ganglionic transmission (e.g. at the cerebral ganglion of the cat) represent 80 times, in the case of C-toxiferine I, and 100 times, in the case of decamethonium, the effective neuromuscular blocking dose. The specificity of drugs that block transmission at smooth muscles (i.e. with an atropinic action) is even greater.

A final point that should be considered is the existence of the so-called "non-specific" or "silent" receptors. Neuromuscular blocking agents lend themselves particularly well to study of this aspect because in most cases they are poorly metabolized in the organism.

It is known that, in the rabbit, the "head-drop" dose of intravenous C-toxiferine I is 3.4 μg/kg. This is equivalent to about 5 nmole/kg. In order to produce a comparable effect, doses of other blocking agents required are some 20 (d-tubocurarine), 70 (decamethonium) and 140 (gallamine) times greater. These figures are enough to establish that only a minute proportion of the molecules used in a normal clinical dose reach, and bind to, the cholinergic receptors of the motor end-plate. The great majority are fixed in an inactive form to foreign proteins which act as "silent receptors", and thus are prevented from reaching their pharmacological site of action.

This is yet another factor, apart from the variables represented by the distribution of the different types of cholinergic receptor and by the variety of mechanisms by which these interact with the active molecules, that makes analysis of the relationship between structure and action appear particularly complex.

11.3.6. THE STUDY OF CARRIER PROTEINS

Even granting that acetylcholinesterase can be considered as a good model for cholinergic receptors, our ignorance of the exact way in which acetylcholine mediates its effects at the molecular level means that there are major obstacles to defining the mechanism of curarization. It is essential not to overlook the fact that even the terms "depolarizing" and "competitive" for the blocking agents constitute only very simple images; they do not explain their mechanism of action. This is a fundamental problem that faces both the pharmacologist and the physiologist.

Various attempts have been made to isolate the carrier protein of the receptor. They are mainly based on the isolation of membrane fractions from the electric organ of *Electrophorus electricus* that bound to molecules with quaternary ammonium groups. Chagas (1962) has described the isolation of an acidic mucopoly-saccharide which formed complexes with dimethyl-*d*-tubocurarine, gallamine and other quaternary bases. Ehrenpreis (1960) has isolated on electrophoretically-homogeneous protein that bound *d*-tubocurarine and other neurotropic amines, displacing acetylcholine and decamethonium.

Although the interpretation of these results is still not clear, many promising lines of enquiry have opened up. The isolation and characterization of proteins which selectively bind mono- or bis-quaternary ammonium compounds, including those with curarizing properties, is leading to further progress in the analysis of problems encountered in interpreting the exact relationship between chemical structure and pharmacological action with such drugs. It is in this field, the meeting-place of biophysics and pharmacodynamics, that the relationship between acetylcholine and its inhibitors at the neuromuscular junction can be clearly established.

REFERENCES

(*a*) *General Reviews*

Ariens, E. J., Simonis, A. M. and de Groot, W. M. (1955) Affinity and intrinsic activity in the theory of competitive and non-competitive inhibition. *Arch. int. Pharmacodyn.* **100**; 298–322.

BARLOW, R. B. (1955) A series of polymethylene-bis-acetoxyethylammonium salts. *Brit. J. Pharmacol.* **10**: 168–72.

BARLOW, R. B. (1960) Steric aspects of the chemistry and biochemistry of natural products. *Biochem. Soc. Symp. No. 19*, p. 46. Cambridge University Press.

BARLOW, R. B. (1964) Introduction to chemical pharmacology. Methuen, London (1st ed., 1955).

BARLOW, R. B. and ZOLLER, A. (1964) Some effects of long chain polymethylene-bis-onium salts on junctional transmission in the peripheral nervous system. *Brit. J. Pharmacol.* **23**: 131–150.

BATTERSBY, A. R. and HODSON, H. F. (1965) Alkaloid of calabash curare and *Strychnos* species, in: R. H. F. MANSKE (ed.), *The Alkaloid*, p. 515. Academic Press, New York.

BOEHM, R. (1923) Curare and curare alkaloide, in: A. HEFFTER (ed.), *Handbuch der experimentellen Pharmakologie*, 1/2: 179–248. Springer, Berlin.

BOURILLET, F. and CHEYMOL, J. (1966) Pharmacologie des substances curarisantes. *Bull. Schw. Akad. mediz. Wissensch.* **22**: 463–82.

BOVET, D. (1951) Some aspects of the relationship between chemical constitution and curare-like activity. *N.Y. Acad. Sci.* **54**: 407–37.

BOVET, D. and BOVET-NITTI, F. (1948) *Structure et activité pharmacodynamique des médicaments du système nerveux végétatiff*. Karger, Bâle.

BOVET, D. and BOVET-NITTI, F. (1955) Succinylcholine chloride, curarizing agent of short duration of action. *Scientia Medica Italica* **3**: 484–513.

BOVET, D., BOVET-NITTI, F., GUARINO, S., LONGO, V. G. and FUSCO, R. (1951) Recherches sur les poisons curarisants de synthèse. III: Succinylcholine et dérivés aliphatiques. *Arch. int. Pharmacodyn.* **88**: 1–50.

BOVET, D., BOVET-NITTI, F. and MARINI-BETTÓLO, G. B. (1959) *Curare and Curare-like Agents*. Elsevier, Amsterdam.

BOVET, D., DEPIERRE, F., COURVOISIER, S. and DE LESTRANGE, Y. (1949) Recherches sur les poisons curarisants de synthèse. II: Ethers phénoliques à fonction ammonium quaternaire. Action du tri-iodoéthylate de tri(diéthylaminoethoxy)benzène (2559 F.). *Arch. int. Pharmacodyn.* **80**: 172–88.

BOVET, D. and VIAUD, P. (1951) Curares de synthèse: chimie et pharmacologie. *Anesthésie et analgésie* **8**: 328–84.

BOVET-NITTI, F. (1959) Les curares à brève durée d'action, in: BOVET, D., BOVET-NITTI, F. and MARINI-BETTÓLO, G. B. (eds.), *Curare and Curare-like Agents*, pp. 230–43. Elsevier, Amsterdam.

BOWMAN, W. C. (1962) Mechanisms of neuromuscular blockade, in: ELLIS, G. and WEST, G. B. (eds.), *Progress in Medicinal Chemistry* **2**: 88–131. Butterworth, London.

BRÜCKE, F. (1956) Dicholinesters of ω-dicarboxylic acids and related substances. *Pharmacol. Rev.* **8**: 265–335.

BURGER, A. (1960) Curare and curareform drugs, in: *Medicinal Chemistry* (2nd ed.). Interscience, New York.

CAVALLINI, G. (1955) Farmacosintesi di stilbene e difeniletano. *Il Farmaco ed. scient.* **10**: 644–69.

CAVALLITO, C. J. (1959) Some interrelationship of chemical structure, physical properties and curaromimetic action, in: D. BOVET, F. BOVET-NITTI and G. B. MARINI-BETTÓLO (eds.), *Curare and Curare-like Agents*, pp. 288–303. Elsevier, Amsterdam.

CAVALLITO, C. J. (1968) Some relationship between chemical structure and pharmacological activities. *Ann. Rev. Pharmacol.* **8**: 39–66.

CAVALLITO, C. J. and GRAY, A. P. (1960) Chemical nature and pharmacological actions of quaternary ammonium salts, in: JUCKER, F. (ed.), *Fortschritte Arzneimittelforschung* **2**: 135–226. Birkhäusen, Basel.

CHAGAS, C. (1962) The fate of curare during curarization, in: DEREUCK, A. V. S. (ed.), *Curare and Curare-like Agents*, Churchill, London.

CHEYMOL, J. (1954) Curares et anticurares de synthèse. Méchanisme d'action. *Actualités pharmacologiques*, **7**: 35–71. Masson, Paris.

CHEYMOL, J. and BOURILLET, F. (1960) Pharmacologie des substances curarisantes, in: *Actualités pharmacologiques* **13**: 63–107. Masson, Paris.

COLLIER, H. O. J. (1952) The effect of chain-length on curarizing potency in three homologous series. *Brit. J. Pharmacol.* **7**: 392–7.

COLLIER, H. O. J. (1953) Descendants of decamethonium. *Brit. J. Anaesth.* **25**: 100–16.

CRAIG, L. E. (1948) Curariform activity and chemical structure. *Chemical Review* **42**: 285–410.

D'ARCY, F. P. and TAYLOR, E. P. (1962) Quaternary ammonium compounds in medicinal chemistry, I–II. *J. Pharm. Pharmacol.* (*London*) **14**: 129–46, 193–216.

DE BEER, E. J., CASTILLO, J. C., PHILLIPS, A. P., FANELLI, R. V., WNUCK, A. L. and NORTON, S. (1951) Synthetic drugs influencing neuromuscular activity. *Ann. New York Acad. Sc.* **54**: 362–72.

DE REUCK, A. V. S. (ed.) (1962) *Curare and Curare-like Agents.* Ciba Foundation Study Group No. 12. Churchill, London.

FOLDES, F. F. (1954) The mode of action of quaternary ammonium type neuro-muscular blocking agents. *Brit. J. Anaesth.* **26**: 394.

FUSCO, R., ROSNATI, V., BOVET-NITTI, F. and BOVET, D. (1951) Qualche considerazione sul tema: struttura chimica e attività dei curari di sintesi. *Rend. Ist. Sup. Sanità* **14**: 690–716.

GROB, D. (1961) Neuromuscular pharmacology. *Ann. Rev. Pharmacol. U.S.A.* **1**: 237–60.

GYERMEK, L. and NÁDOR, K. (1957) The pharmacology of propane compounds in relation to their steric structure. *J. Pharm. Pharmacol.* **9**: 209–29.

HAINING, C. G., JOHNSTON, R. G. and SMITH, J. M. (1960) The neuromuscular blocking properties of a series of bis-quaternary tropeines. *Brit. J. Pharmacol. Chemotherapy* **15**: 71–81.

HAZARD, R., CHEYMOL, J., CHABRIER, P. and BOURILLET, F. (1959) Synthèse et étude de quelques curares et anticurares, in: D. BOVET, *Curare and Curare-like Agents*, pp. 318–26. Elsevier, Amsterdam.

HOPPE, J. O. (1951) A new series of synthetic curare-like compounds. *Ann. New York Acad. Sc.* **54**: 395–406.

HUNT, C. C. and KUFFLER, S. W. (1950) Pharmacology of the neuromuscular junction. *J. Pharmacol.* Part II, **93**: 96–120.

ING, H. R. (1936) The curariform action of onium salts. *Physiol. Rev.* **16**: 527–44.

ING, H. R. (1949) Structure–action relationship of the choline group. *Science* **109**: 264–6.

JACOB, J. and TAZIEFF-DEPIERRE, F. (1959) Actions neuromusculaires des composés anticholinestérosiques, in: D. BOVET, F. BOVET-NITTI and G. B. MARINI-BETTÓLO (eds.), *Curare and Curare-like Agents*, pp. 304–18, Elsevier, Amsterdam.

KARCZMAR, A. G. (1957) Neuromuscular pharmacology. *Ann. Rev. Pharmacol.* **7**: 241–76.

KARRER, P., SCHMID, H. and WASER, P. (1960) Kurzer Überblick über die Chemie und Pharmakologie der Calebassen-curare-Alkaloide. *Il Farmaco* **15**: 126.

KHROMOV-BORISOV, N. V. and MICHELSON, M. J. (1966) The mutual disposition of cholinoreceptors of locomotor muscles, and the changes in their disposition in the course of evolution. *Pharmacol. Rev.* **18**: 1051–90.

LEWIS, J. J. and MUIR, T. C. (1959) The laboratory estimation of curare-like activity in natural and synthetic products. *Laboratory Practice* (*London*) **8**: 333–8, 364–8, 404–7.

LÜLLMANN, H., MONDON, A. and SEIDEL, P. R. (1967) Über das Curare-artig Wirkprinzip des Erytrine Alkaloide. *Arch. Pharmak. exp. Path.* **258**: 91–107.

Synthetic Inhibitors of Neuromuscular Transmission

McINTYRE, L. (1947) *Curare, its Natural History and Clinical Use.* Univ. of Chicago Press, Chicago.

MICHELSON, M. J. and KHROMOV-BORISOV, N. V. (1965) On the "secondary structure" of cholinoreceptive membrane of the cell. (Russian.) *Pharmacology and Chemistry*, pp. 213–14. All. Union Pharmacol. Soc.

MNJOYAN, A. L. and MNJOYAN, O. L. (1958) The synthesis of ditilin and some of its analogues. Report at the All. Union Conference devoted to Ditilin and its clinical application. Academy of Science of the Armenian SSR Institute of Fine Organic Chemistry, Erevan.

MOLITOR, H. and GRAESSLE, O. E. (1950) Pharmacology and toxicology of antibiotics. *Pharmacol. Rev.* **2**: 1–60.

NACHMANSOHN, D. (1952) Chemical mechanism of nerve activity, in: *Modern Trends in Physiology and Biochemistry*, pp. 229–76. Academic Press, New York.

NACHMANSOHN, D. (1963) The chemical basis of Claude Bernard's observations on curare. *Biochem. Zeitschrift* **338**: 454–73.

ORGANISATION MONDIALE DE LA SANTÉ (1967) Spécifications pour le contrôle de la qualité des préparations pharmaceutiques. Deuxième édition de la Pharmacopée internationale. Pharmacopoea internationalis. Editio secunda. OMS, Gèneve. Gallemini trieshidum. Suxemethonii chloridum. Tubocurarini chloridum.

OSWALD, K. (1924) *Chemische Konstitution und physiologische Wirkung.* Berlin.

PATON, W. D. M. (1949) The pharmacology of curare and curarizing substances. *J. Pharm. Pharmacol.* **1**: 273–86.

PATON, W. D. M. and ZAIMIS, E. (1949) The pharmacological actions of polymethylene-bis-trimethyl-ammonium salts. *Brit. J. Pharmacol.* **4**: 381–409.

PATON, W. D. M. and ZAIMIS, E. (1952) The methonium compounds. *Pharmacol. Rev.* **4**: 219–52.

PFANKUCH, E. (1930) in: J. HOUBEN (ed.), *Fortschr Heilstoffchemie*, II, Abt. 1, 1042. Berlin.

PRADHAM, S. N., VARADAN, K. S., RAY, C. and DE, N. N. (1954) Studies in synthetic neuromuscular blocking agents, II. *J. Scient. Ind. Research* **13B**: 118–21.

RANDALL, L. O. (1951) Synthetic curare-like agents and their antagonists. *Ann. New York Acad. Sc.* **54**: 460–79.

RANDALL, L. O. and JAMPOLSKY, L. M. (1953) Pharmacology of drugs affecting skeletal muscle. *Am. J. Physical Medicine* **32**: 102–25.

RAVENTOS, J. (1937) Pharmacological actions of quaternary ammonium salts. *Quart. J. exper. Physiol.* **26**: 361–74.

RIKER, JR., W. F. and WESCOE, W. C. (1951) The pharmacology of Flexedil with observations on certain analogs. *Ann. New York Acad. Sc.* **54**: 373–94.

ROBSON, J. M. and KEELE, C. A. (1956) *Recent Advances in Pharmacology*, 2nd ed. Churchill, London.

SCHMID, H. (1966) Chemie des Calebassencurare. *Bull. Schw. Akad. mediz. Wissensch.* **22**: 415–28.

SCHUELLER, F. W. (1960) The mechanism of action of the hemicholinisms. *Int. Rev. Neurobiol.* **2**: 77–97.

SCHWEIZERISCHE AKADEMIE DER MEDIZINISCHEN WISSENSCHAFTEN (ed.) (1966–7) Curare. *Bull. Schw. Akad. med. Wissensch.* **22**: 391–527 (1966); **23**: 5–138 (1967). Schwabe & Co., Basel (1967).

STENLAKE, J. B. (1963) Some chemical aspects of neuromuscular block, in: G. P. ELLIS and G. B. WEST (eds.), *Progress in Medicinal Chemistry* **3**: 1–51. Butterworth, London.

TAYLOR, D. B. (1951) Some basic aspects of the pharmacology of synthetic curariform drugs. *Pharmacol. Rev.* **3**: 412–44.

TAYLOR, D. B. and NEDERGAARD, O. V. (1965) Relation between structure and action of quaternary ammonium neuromuscular blocking agents. *Physiol. Rev. U.S.A.* **45**: 523–54.

THESLEFF, S. and QUASTEL, D. M. (1965) Neuromuscular pharmacology. *Ann. Rev. Pharmacol.* **5**: 263–84.

TRENDELENBURG, P. (1923) Quartäre Ammonium Verbindungen, in: A HEFFTER (ed.), *Handbuch der experimentellen Pharmakologie* I/1: 539–64. Springer, Berlin.

TRIGGLE, D. J. (1965) Chemical aspects of the autonomic nervous system. Academic Press, London.

VAN ROSSUM, J. M. and ARIENS, E. J. (1959) Pharmacodynamics of drugs affecting skeletal muscle. Structure–action relationship in homologous series of quaternary ammonium salts. *Arch. int. Pharmacodyn.* **118**: 393–417.

WASER, P. (1965) in: G. B. KOELLE, W. W. DOUGLAS and A. CARLSSON (eds.), *Pharmacology of Cholinergic and Andrenergic Transmission*. Pergamon Press, Oxford.

WASER, P. G. (1960) The cholinergic receptor. *J. Pharm. Pharmacol. (London)* **12**: 577–97.

(b) Other references

ALEXANDROVA, E. and FILATOV, B. N. (1965) *Pharmacol. and Chemistry (Moscow)* 10.

ALLAUDDIN, M., CADDY, B., LEWIS, J. J., MARTIN-SMITH, M. and SUGRUE, M. F. (1965) *J. Pharm. Pharmacol.* **17**: 55.

BARLOW, R. B., BLASCHKO, H., HIMMS, J. M. and TRENDELENBURG, U. (1955) *Brit. J. Pharmacol.* **10**: 116.

BARLOW, R. D. and ING, H. R. (1948) *Nature* **161**: 718; *Brit. J. Pharmacol.* **3**: 298.

BARLOW, R. B. and ZOLLER, A. (1962) *Brit. J. Pharmacol.* **19**: 485.

BARLOW, R. B. and ZOLLER, A. (1964) *Brit. J. Pharmacol.* **23**: 131.

BARZAGHI, F., MANTEGAZZA, P. and RIVA, M. (1965) *Brit. J. Pharmacol. Chem.* **24**: 282.

BENNETT, A. E. (1941) *Am. J. Med. Sc.* **202**: 102.

BIGGS, R. S., DAVIS, M. and WEIN, R. (1964) *Experientia* **20**: 119.

BOEHM, R. (1897) *Arch. Pharm.* **235**: 660.

BOVET, D., BOVET-NITTI, F., GUARINO, S., LONGO, V. G. and MAROTTA, M. (1949) *Rend. Ist. Super. Samità (Roma)* **12**: 106.

BOVET, D., COURVOISIER, S., DUCROT, R. and HORCLOIS, R. (1946) *Compt. rend. Acad. Sc. (Paris)* **223**: 597.

BOVET, D., DEPIERRE, F. and DE LESTRANGE, Y. (1947) *C.R. Acad. Sc. (Paris)* **225**: 74.

BOWMAN, W. C., HEMSWORTH, B. A. and RAND, M. J. (1960) *Brit. J. Pharmacol.* **19**: 198.

BUCHNER, E. (1861) *Jahresber.* **1861**: 767.

BURMAN, M. S. (1939) *Arch. Neurol. Psychiat.* **41**: 307.

BUTAEV, V. M. (1953) in: S. V. ANITCHKOV (ed.), *Pharmacology of New Drugs.* (In Russian.) p. 82, Leningrad.

CAVALLITO, C. J. SCHLIEPER, D. C. and O'DELL, T. B. (1954) *J. Org. Chem.* **19**: 826.

CAVALLITO, C. G., SORIA, A. E., HOPPE, J. O. (1950) *J. Am. Chem. Soc*, **72**: 2661.

CHASE, H. F. and LEHMAN, A. J. (1942) *J. Pharmacol. exp. Ther.* **75**: 265.

CHASE, H. F., LEHMAN, A. J. and RICHARD, E. E. (1944) *J. Pharmacol. exp. Ther.* **82**: 266.

CHEYMOL, J. (1953) *Bull. Acad. Med. (Paris)* **137**: 83.

CHEYMOL, J., DELABY, R., CHABRIER, P., NAJER, H. and BOURILLET, F. (1954) *Arch. intern. Pharmacodyn.* **98**: 161.

COLLIER, H. O. J. and MACAULEY, B. (1952) *Brit. J. Pharmacol.* **7**: 398

COLLIER, H. O. J. and TAYLOR, E. P. (1949) *Nature* **164**: 491.

CRUM-BROWN, A. and FRASER, T. (1868–9) *Trans. Roy. Soc. Edinburgh* **25**: 151, 693.

DALLEMAGNE, M. J. and PHILIPPOT, E. (1950) *Arch. intern. Pharmacodyn.* **84**: 189.

DALLEMAGNE, M. J. and PHILIPPOT, E. (1951) *Arch. intern. Pharmacodyn.* **87**: 127.

DANILOV, A. F. (1966) *Farmakol. Toksikol. (Moscow)* **29**: 308.
EDWARDS, D., LEWIS, J. J. and MARREN, G. (1966) *J. Pharm. Pharmacol.* **18**: 670.
EDWARDS, D., STENLAKE, J. B., LEWIS, J. J. and STATHERS (1961) *J. Med. Pharm. Chem.* **3**: 369.
EHRENPREIS, S. (1959) *Science* **129**: 1613.
EVERETT, A. J., LOWE, L. A. and WILKINSON, S. (1970) *Chemical Communications 1970*, 1020.
FREY, R. (1955) *Proc. World Congress of Anesthesia, Scheveningen*, p. 252.
FUSCO, R., CHIAVARELLI, S., PALAZZO, G. and BOVET, D. (1949) *Gazz. Chim. Ital.* **79**: 129.
GILL, E. W. (1959) *Proc. Roy. Soc.* **B 150**: 181.
GILL, E. W. and ING, H. R. (1958) *Il Farmcao* **13**: 244.
GIROD, E. and HÄFLIGER, F. (1952) *Experientia* **8**: 233.
GRIFFITH, H. R. and JOHNSON, G. E. (1942) *Anesthesiology* **3**: 418.
HAINING, C. G., JOHNSTON, R. G. and SMITH, J. M. (1960) *Brit. J. Pharmacol. Chemotherapy* **15**: 71.
HAZARD, R., CHEYMOL, J., CHABRIER, P., CORTEGGIANI, E. and NICOLAS, F. (1959) *Arch. intern. Pharmacodyn.* **84**: 237; *Therapie* **5**: 129.
HOLMES, P. E. B., JENDEN, D. J. and TAYLOR, D. B. (1947) *Nature* **159**: 86.
HUGUENARD, P. and MARTIN, C. (1950) *Anesthésie et analgésie* **7**: 336.
HUNT, R. (1926) *J. Pharmacol.* **28**: 367.
HUNT, R. and TAVEAU, R. DE M. (1911) *Hyg. Lab. Bull. Nr.* 73—Publ. Health Marine Hosp. Serv. U.S.A.
JACOB, J. and DEPIERRE, F. (1950) *Arch. intern. Pharmacodyn.* **83**: 1.
JANOT, M. M., LAINE, F., KHUONG-HUU, Q. and GOUTAREL, R. (1962) *Bull. Soc. Chem. France* **1962**: 111.
KHARKEVICH, D. A. and KRAVCHUK, L. A. (1961) *Farmakol. e Tocsicol.* **3**: 318.
KHUONG-HUU-LAINE, F. and PINTO-SCOGNAMIGLIO, W. (1964) *Arch. intern. Pharmacodyn.* **147**: 209.
KIMURA, K. K., UNNA, K. R. and PFEIFFER, C. C. (1949) *J. Pharmacol.* **95**: 149.
KING, G. H. (1935) *J. Chem. Soc.* **1935**: 1381.
KULZ, F. (1928) *Arch. exp. Pathol.* **98**: 339.
KUZOVKOV, A. D., MASHKOVSKIU, D. D., DANILOVA, A. V. and MEN'SHIKOV, G. P. (1952) *Doklady. Akad. Nauk. SSR.* **103**: 251.
LEHMAN, A. J., CHASE, H. F. and YONKMAN, F. F. (1942) *J. Pharmacol. exp. Ther.* **75**: 270.
LESSER, E. (1961) *J. Pharm. Pharmacol.* **13**: 703.
LEVIS, S., PRÉAT, S. and DAUBY, J. (1953) *Arch. intern. Pharmacodyn.* **93**: 46.
LÜLLMAN, H., MONDON, A. and SEIDEL, P. R. (1967) *Arch. exp. Path.* **258**: 91.
LUTTRINGHAUS, A., KERP, L. and PREUGSHAS (1957) *Arzneimittel Forsch.* **7**: 222.
MACRI, F. (1954) *Proc. Soc. exp. Biol. Med.* **85**: 603.
MNDJOYAN, A. L. and MNDJOYAN and BABIYAN (1954) *Doklady. Akad. Nauk. Armyan SSR* **18**: 45; **19**: 93.
O'DELL, T. B. and NAPOLI, M. D. (1957) *J. Pharmacol.* **120**: 438.
PATON, W. D. M. and ZAIMIS, E. J. (1948) *Nature* **161**: 718.
PHILIPPOT, E. and DALLEMAGNE, M. J. (1952) *Experientia* 273.
PREYER, R. (1865) *Compt. rend. Acad. Sc. (Paris)* **60**: 1346.
QUEVAUVILLIER, A. and LAINE, F. (1960) *Ann. Pharm. Fr.* **18**: 678.
RABUTEAU (1873) Goulstonian Lecture. *Brit. M.J.* **1**.
RIKER, W. K. and SZRENIAWSKI, Z. (1959) *J. Pharmacol. exp. Ther.* **126**: 233.
ROBERTS, J., RIKER JR., W. J. and ROY, B. B. (1953) *Feder. Proc.* **12**: 361.
ROSNATI, V. (1950) *Gazz. Chim. Ital.* **80**: 663.
ROSNATI, V. (1957) *Gazz. Chim. Ital.* **87**: 215, 228, 386.
ROSNATI, V. and ANGELINI-KOTHNY, H. (1958) *Gazz. Chim. Ital.* **88**: 1284.

ROSNATI, V., ANGELINI-KOTHNY, H. and BOVET, D. (1958) *Gazz. Chim. Ital.* **88**: 1293.
ROSNATI, V. and BOVET, D. (1951) *Rend. Ist. Sup. Sanità (Roma)* **14**: 473.
ROSNATI, V. and PUSCHNER, H. (1957) *Gazz. Chim. Ital.* **87**: 1240.
ROULIN, J. and BOUSSINGAULT, J. (1829) *Ann. Chim.* **39**: 24.
RUBSTOV, M. V., MASCHKOVSKIY, M. D., NIKITSKAYA, E. C., MEDVEDEV, B. A. and
    USOVSKAYA, V. S. (1961) *Journ. Medic. Pharmac. Chem.* **3**: 441.
SACHS, T. (1878) *Ann. Chem.* **191**: 354.
SANTESSON, C. G. and KORAEN, G. (1900) *Skand. Arch. Physiol.* **10**: 201.
SIMONART, A. (1934) *Arch. Int. Pharmacodyn.* **48**: 328.
STENLAKE, J. B. (1963) in: ELLIS, G. P. and WEST, G. B. (eds.), *Progress in Medical
    Chemistry.* Butterworth, London.
TAYLOR, E. P. (1952) *J. Chem. Soc.* **1950**: 142, 1309.
TAYLOR, E. P. and COLLIER, H. O. J. (1950) *Nature* **165**: 602.
TAYLOR, E. P. and COLLIER, H. O. J. (1951) *Nature* **167**: 602.
THESLEFF, S. and UNNA, K. R. (1954) *J. Pharmacol. exp. Ther.* **111**: 99.
TORF, S. F., KHROMOV, N. V., BUTAEV, B. M. and GREBENKIN, M. A. (1952) *Pharmacol.
    i Toxicol.* **15**: 12.
UNNA, K. R. and GRESLIN, J. G. (1944) *J. Pharmacol. exp. Ther.* **80**: 53.
UNNA, K. R., KNIASUK, M. and GRESLIN, J. G. (1944) *J. Pharmacol. exp. Ther.* **80**: 39.
VANDERHAEGHE, H. (1951) *Nature* **167**: 527.
WEST, R. (1935) *Proc. Roy. Soc.* **28**: 565.
WEST, R. (1935) *Lancet* **1**: 242.
WILLSTAETTER, R. and HEUBNER, W. (1907) *Ber. deut. Chem. Ges.* **40**: 3869.
WILSON, I. B. and BERGMANN, F. (1950) *J. Biol. Chem.* **185**: 479; **196**: 683.
WINTERSTEINER, O. (1959) in: D. BOVET, F. BOVET-NITTI and G. B. MARINI BETTÓLO (eds.),
    Curare and Curare-like Agents. Elsevier, Amsterdam.
ZAIMIS, E. (1953) *J. Physiol. (London)* **122**: 238.

C. PHARMACODYNAMICS OF
NEUROMUSCULAR BLOCKING AGENTS

CHAPTER 12

INHIBITORS OF POST-SYNAPTIC RECEPTORS

J. Cheymol and F. Bourillet

Paris

ABBREVIATIONS

NM	neuromuscular
ACh	acetylcholine
ChE	cholinesterase
d-Tc	*d*-tubocurarine
C10	decamethonium
SCh	succinylcholine

12.1. INTRODUCTION

The standardization and the analysis of the mode of action of different neuromuscular blocking agents has been at the origin of their increasingly systematic utilization in anesthesiology and the great progress in our knowledge of the detailed functioning of this synapse.

Indeed more than a century ago the work of Claude Bernard led to the utilization of curare to reduce certain states of contracture. The inconsistency of the results obtained linked to the variation in the activity of the samples led to the abandoning for a long time this clinical indication. It was not until 1941 that the preparations of well-defined activity were obtained with the use of the rabbit head-drop test. Extracts of a Menispermacea, the *Chondrodendron tomentosum* and subsequently *d*-tubocurarine which was isolated from it, made possible the general utilization of curarization in surgical procedures.

Subsequently a very large number of molecules, the most part bisquaternary ammonium salts, were synthesized, some of these are widely used at the present time. The study of their mode of action and of their metabolism has made possible their more precise administration in man

297

and the utilization of appropriate antagonists. Furthermore, it has made it possible to elucidate the successive steps in neuromuscular transmission. The various disciplines, chemical, physiological, biological, histological, anesthesiological and pharmacological, which are intimately related at the myoneural junction has made possible one of the best constructed chapters in pharmacology.

Some drugs producing paralysis act on the central nervous system at the cerebral or spinal level; these are muscle relaxants* which are not discussed in this chapter. Drugs producing peripheral paralysis are almost entirely constituted by substances inhibiting the neuromuscular (NM) junction. This junction may be considered in its widest sense, that is from the motor nerve terminals to the muscle membrane, or be limited to the receptors of the postsynaptic membrane. Since it is possible for the same substance to simultaneously act before and after the synapse,† it seems difficult not to consider the junction in its widest sense. Nevertheless, presynaptic inhibitors have been studied in detail in a separate chapter.‡ We voluntarily limit the scope of this chapter to substances whose main action is on the motor end-plate. These postsynaptic inhibitors may be divided into two main classes, which are antagonists one of the other; the curarizing or competitive blockers (*d*-tubocurarine) and the depolarizing (decamethonium) agents.

After analysis of the possible modes of study in animals, we will describe the various types of paralysis which these drugs can produce. After that we will discuss the cholinergic receptor and their interaction with paralysing substances, finally we will attempt to classify these postsynaptic inhibitors.

12.2. ANIMAL EXPERIMENTATION

The effects produced by a paralysing agent may vary considerably according to the animal species used and the experimental conditions under which the effect is produced. Thus in the study of a new molecule, the choice of the experimental procedures, and the interpretation of the results obtained, must take into consideration certain fundamental principles if one wishes to predict, without too large a risk of error, what is likely to happen in man.

The majority of inhibitory substances of the neuromuscular junction

---

* This term is sometimes used in the clinic, it should in no case be utilized to define inhibitors of the neuromuscular junction.

† See p. 140.

‡ See Chapters 8 and 13.

which are known at the present time are highly ionized molecules, water-soluble but which pass with difficulty barriers in the body and particularly the alimentary canal and the blood–brain barrier. The compounds should thus be administered directly into the circulating venous or arterial blood or possibly by the rectal route.

The animal species which has a sensitivity and reactivity resembling man to the greatest extent is the cat. It is thus this animal which would normally be chosen for preclinical studies of a new neuromuscular blocking agent, for the actual experimentation, or to confirm the results obtained in other animal species.

On the same animal, the various skeletal muscles may react in a very different manner; for example, those muscles causing movement as compared to those holding posture. The particular case of respiratory muscles takes considerable importance in the use of neuromuscular block agents in man. Indeed these muscles perform a vital function, their low sensitivity to a given blocking agent gives it a large margin of safety.

Once the activity of a new neuromuscular blocking agent has been found, it is important to determine the mode of action before comparing its potency with that of a known substance. Some substances act by antagonizing the depolarizing effects of acetylcholine, others, on the other hand, act by producing a prolonged depolarization of the acetylcholine receptors. Subsequently a more careful study of the mode of action will enable the new drug to be classified, at least approximately, according to known molecules.

Some of the most widely used tests will be reviewed without a detailed description being given whilst nevertheless emphasizing essential or possibly peculiar points in each and outlining the conclusions that may be drawn from their use.

12.2.1. DETECTION OF NEUROMUSCULAR BLOCKING ACTIVITY*

12.2.1.1. *IN NON-ANESTHETIZED MAMMALS*

This is a rapid method of verifying neuromuscular blocking effects, for example during the determination of intravenous LD_{50} in, for example, the mouse, the rat, the rabbit. Successive stages include: a progressive flaccidity of the posterior, then anterior, legs, the neck, which may or may not be preceded by fasciculations, tremors, respiratory embarrassment,

---

* See Cheymol, 1957.

an asphyxic reaction and finally death by respiratory arrest. Artificial respiration enables the animals to survive. Opening the thorax makes it possible to determine whether the heart is still beating.* Since death is directly linked to the neuromuscular blocking effects the value of the LD_{50} gives an indication of the active dose in the particular species.

12.2.1.2. *IN AMPHIBIA*

The injection of a neuromuscular blocking agent into the dorsal lymphatic sac of the frog, for example, leads to a suppression of the righting-reflex but the animal survives by its cutaneous respiration. It is on such animals that the "witch-doctors" of the Amazon tribes verified the activity of their preparations of curare.

12.2.2. RAPID DIFFERENTIATION OF THE MODE OF ACTION

Determination of whether or not the new substance is depolarizing.

12.2.2.1. *ON AVIAN MUSCLE* (Buttle and Zaimis, 1949; Cheymol, 1957).

The intravenous administration of a depolarizing substance into the axillary vein of the pigeon or in the jugular vein of an 8-day chick produces an instantaneous contracture of the muscles of the neck and the legs. If the dose is carefully chosen the wings and the respiratory muscles are not affected.

A non-depolarizing substance produces a generalized flaccidity comparable to that observed in mammals.

12.2.2.2. *ON THE BATRACIAN ISOLATED* RECTUS ABDOMINIS MUSCLE (Garcia de Jalòn, 1947; Cheymol, 1957).

The addition of a depolarizing substance to the organ bath produces a contracture of the preparation whilst an antidepolarizing substance on the contrary inhibits such a contracture produced by a depolarizing substance, for example acetylcholine. Whilst this test guarantees the peripheral action of the drug, it is not absolutely specific for neuromuscular blocking agents since some ganglion blocking agents also inhibit the contracture produced by acetylcholine.

---

* In an animal who has just died it is possible to detect the reactivity of certain muscles (diaphragm, tibialis anterior, etc.) by indirect (phrenic, sciatic nerve) or direct electrical stimulation.

12.2.3. EVALUATION OF THE NEUROMUSCULAR BLOCKING ACTIVITY

12.2.3.1. *RABBIT HEAD-DROP TEST* (Varney *et al.*, 1949; Cheymol, 1957).

This is the method of choice to compare the muscle relaxant activity of a neuromuscular blocking agent in comparison with a reference molecule. It possesses a number of advantages:

The relaxation produced is similar to that sort in anesthesiology.

This atonia corresponds to an early action of the blocking agent, the method is thus very sensitive.

The response of a given rabbit is very constant with time.

Each animal receives the substance under test and the reference drug; this makes it possible to obtain a very satisfactory precision for a biological assay (5% with six rabbits for a trained technician).

It is possible by using a slow perfusion of the neuromuscular blocking agent to determine, in addition to the head-drop dose (HDD), the dose producing respiratory arrest (RAD), and cardiac arrest (CAD) the ratio HDD/RAD constitutes an indication of the margin of safety. A CAD which is very near to the RAD may be an indication that the compound possess cardiotoxicity.

Finally this technique allows analysis of the kinetics of the neuromuscular blocking action. Either by noting the latency between the onset of head-drop following injection and the duration of action, or by slow discontinuous infusion, note being taken of the number of times the infusion is arrested and recommenced in order to maintain the head-drop during a given time (1 hour for example).

The disadvantages of this technique are minor:

It is not absolutely specific for neuromuscular blocking agents but the specificity can be confirmed on other species.

It is carried out on the rabbit whose reactions are not necessarily quantitatively or qualitatively similar to those of man.

12.2.3.2. *RAT ISOLATED PHRENIC NERVE-DIAPHRAGM PREPARATION* (Bülbring, 1946; Burn, 1950).

This method is useful to determine the activity with a high degree of precision. It has, however, the disadvantage of being an *in vitro* test, that is to say, very different to conditions of use in man. It also has the disadvantage of using a muscle which theoretically should be only slightly sensitive to a good neuromuscular blocking agent. It is indispensable to know in advance the mechanism of action of the substance under study in order to compare it with the reference substance which it resembles most closely.

12.2.3.3. *FROG ISOLATED* RECTUS ABDOMINIS *MUSCLE PREPARATION* (Garcia de Jalòn, 1947; Cheymol, 1957).

This test may be used to evaluate neuromuscular blocking activity, but with the supplementary disadvantage in comparison with the techniques described above that it applies to an amphibian which is less sensitive than a mammal to neuromuscular blocking agents.

12.2.4. ANALYSIS OF THE MECHANISM OF ACTION

All neuromuscular preparations *in situ* or isolated can constitute a technique for the study of neuromuscular blocking agents. A large number of preparations have been suggested to analyze more and more closely the site of action. Without enumerating all of these, we will discuss first the classical *in vivo* or *in vitro* nerve–muscle techniques; and secondly the more or less specific techniques to study a given mechanism of action at the neuromuscular junction.

12.2.4.1. *CLASSICAL* IN VIVO *TECHNIQUES*

The technique which is the most widely utilized and the richest in teaching is without doubt the sciatic nerve–anterior tibialis muscle preparation of the cat. As previously mentioned the reactivity and the sensitivity of the cat resembles closely that of man. In addition the anterior tibialis—a rapid muscle—is very reproducible in the quality of its reaction with neuromuscular blocking agents, this gives the technique a high degree of specificity. It was originally described by Brown (1938);* we shall mention here only a few important practical details.

Anesthesia by an extemporaneous mixture of chloralose (80 mg/kg) and pentobarbitone (10–15 mg/kg) immediately produced by intravenous administration without a phase of excitation. Anesthesia continues for a number of hours without depression of the cardiovascular or respiratory system.

---

* A very careful study of this technique has been carried out by Bowman (1964).

Insertion of a tracheal cannula so that artificial respiration may be applied if necessary.

Stimulation of the nerve by rectangular pulses of 2–4 V, 0.1–0.2 msec at a frequency of 0.1 Hz (cathode nearest muscle). Avoid cooling of the preparation by placing it horizontally and approaching a lamp near to the muscle after having covered the latter with a thin layer of cotton-wool-soaked physiological solution.

This technique which is applied to the whole animal is comparable to conditions used in man. It guarantees the peripheral action of neuro-muscular blockade since the sciatic nerve is ligated. Nevertheless, it is not able to give precise quantitative data. A number of experimental possibilities can usefully complete this technique, for example by varying the conditions of stimulation:

Variations in the frequency of stimulation, tetanic stimulation; an increase in frequency of stimulation increases the blockade by inhibitors of acetylcholine synthesis by more rapidly depleting the stores of the transmitter. Whether a tetanus is maintained or not gives an indication of the type of neuromuscular blocking agent.

Direct stimulation makes it possible to verify that the drug is or is not acting by depressing the muscle fibers directly. Three fine and flexible electrodes are inserted into the mass of the muscle, two at each end are connected to the anode whilst the central electrode becomes the cathode. The stimulating parameters are as follows: pulse width 0.01–0.05 msec, voltage 70–90 V; this high voltage is necessary in order that the stimulus reaches all the fibers in the muscle. Lower voltages can in a non-paralysed preparation produce a maximal response, the stimulation diffuses to the nerve terminals and partially passes by the synapses. When these are inhibited the amplitude of the contractions diminish without there being any depression of the muscle fibers themselves. In order to avoid an erroneous interpretation the voltage must therefore be maximal.

Alternate indirect (nerve) and direct (muscle) stimulation leads to the best recordings if one takes care to place an isolation unit between the stimulator and the muscle electrodes.

It is also possible to record simultaneously the contraction of a number of muscles or of other parameters.

Simultaneous recording of the contractions of soleus, slow, red muscle, less constant in its reactions than anterior tibialis, rapid, white muscle, and the sensitivity of which varies according to the type of neuromuscular blocking agent.

Simultaneous recording of blood pressure to verify the good cardio-vascular condition (in some cases severe hypotension can depress muscular contraction) or the effect of the neuromuscular blocking agent itself.

Simultaneous recording of respiration: respiratory movements may be recorded through the tracheal cannula or by external pneumocardio-graphy in order to define the degree of respiratory involvement in comparison with paralysis of peripheral muscles.

Recording of membrane potential and action potentials in the nerve and muscle by extra- or intracellular electrodes.

This *in vivo* neuromuscular technique makes it possible to modify the neuromuscular blocking action either by the action of an antagonist or by the utilization of intra-arterial route, or by chronic denervation to eliminate the innervation of the muscle under study.

Action of antagonists: neostigmine, edrophonium or potentiating agents enabled an analysis of the mechanism of action.

Intra-arterial administration instead of using the jugular vein: it is possible to inject drugs against the blood flow into the contralateral external iliac artery after having ligated its collaterals and the median sacral artery. At the moment of injection the arterial blood flow is arrested by pulling on a thread surrounding the artery; this enables more rapid effects to be obtained more transient but more localized and at lower doses. Close intra-arterial injections may also be carried out into the tibial artery, the arterial flow to the muscle being clamped at the moment of injection. By administering in this manner acetyl-choline (1 to 10 mcg),* a muscular twitch is produced which is suppressed only by inhibitors acting by blocking the specific receptors of the motor end-plate.

Chronic denervation: by resection under an anesthesia of a fragment of the peroneal nerve 10 to 14 days before the experiment. Direct electrical stimulation of this muscle produces a contraction which is not inhibited by substances acting on the motor end-plate. Neverthe-less, denervation produces important modifications of the sensitivity of muscle fibers. (The chemo-sensitivity, which in a normal fiber is limited to the motor end-plate, extends to the entire muscle fiber.) The data must thus be interpreted with very great care.

---

* Very rapid injection, always at the same speed, care being taken to wash the catheter with slightly heparinized physiological solution.

Similar *in vivo* neuromuscular preparations may be set up with species other than a cat—for example,* monkey, dog, rabbit, guinea pig, rat, chicken. The interpretation of the results thus obtained is difficult in view of the quantitative and qualitative differences in the sensitivity of the species in relationship to that of man. In the particular case of the chicken one finds that some neuromuscular blocking agents (the depolarizing agents) do not produce paralysis but a contracture as it has been previously pointed out in the relation to the test of differentiation with the pigeon and the chick.

12.2.4.2. *CLASSICAL* IN VITRO *TECHNIQUES*

The data obtained with isolated neuromuscular preparations maintained in so-called physiological solution must be interpreted with considerable care even if the preparations originate from the cat. No artificial solution can reproduce the composition of the extracellular media, and the response to neuromuscular blocking agent thus are modified (Zaimis, 1962, 1966). Such techniques are nevertheless valuable in the study of the mechanism of action particularly because of the simplification due to the suppression of some parameters or some regulatory mechanisms. However, the conclusions should ultimately be compared with data obtained in the whole animal.

A large number of techniques may be employed:

Phrenic nerve–diaphragm preparation of the kitten, the rat, the guinea pig, the mouse, the rectus abdominis preparation of the frog, sartorius preparation of the frog, tenuissimus of the cat (Maclagan, 1962), the biventer cervicis preparation of the chick (Ginsborg and Warriner, 1960) semispinalis of the chick (Child and Zaimis, 1960), obturator nerve-gracilis preparation of the rat (Laity, 1967), sciatic nerve-tibialis anticus of the chick (Van Riezen, 1968). These are of necessity flat and very thin muscles to enable the bathing fluid to readily reach all the muscle fibers.

12.2.4.3. *SPECIAL TECHNIQUES*

The numerous possible points of action of drugs affecting neuromuscular transmission have been pointed out above. The majority of neuromuscular blocking agents act at a number of sites, at their overall action, which usually varies according to the dose, is the result of these different effects. The pharmacological study of these substances necessitates a knowledge of

* See, for example, Zaimis (1953).

these different mechanisms; this is why special techniques are necessary to analyze each of these actions without the intervention of the others. In general isolated organ preparations are useful. Three major sites of action will be considered:

Presynaptic actions.
Postsynaptic actions on receptors of the motor end-plate.
On the muscle fiber itself.

(a) *Presynaptic actions*

By recording the action potential of a nerve either isolated or *in vivo*, it is possible to determine whether a particular inhibitor is acting on the nerve membrane by antagonizing its depolarization. For this the following preparations may be used:
Isolated sciatic nerve preparation of the frog.
Isolated phrenic nerve–diaphragm preparation of the rat.
Sciatic nerve preparation of the cat *in vivo*.
Antidromic potentials in the dorsal roots of the cord (Riker *et al.*, 1957).

Nevertheless the neuromuscular inhibition can be produced at the nerve terminal itself which is less protected and which may not be demonstrated by the above methods. This is why a technique described by Hubbard and Schmidt (1963) and Katz and Miledi (1965) makes it possible to record the action potentials in the region of the nerve ending in the sartorius preparation of the frog. Recordings of the action potentials may be carried out at the same time as those of the motor end-plate with extracellular electrodes.

Two other techniques make it possible to demonstrate a presynaptic inhibition without determination of the precise mechanism of this inhibition:

Recordings from the frog sartorius preparation of the miniature end-plate potentials, the frequency of which decrease in the presence of presynaptic inhibition (Fatt and Katz, 1952).
Determination of the quantity of the acetylcholine liberated at the nerve endings on the rat isolated phrenic nerve–diaphragm preparation (Straughan, 1960; Cheymol *et al.*, 1962). The estimation may be carried on rat blood pressure, on the isolated intestine preparation of a sensitized guinea pig, on the dorsal muscle of the leech, or even on the isolated lung of the frog. Presynaptic inhibition produces a

diminution in the quantity of acetylcholine liberated by nerve stimulation. In contrast to the recording of miniature end-plate potentials, this method does not give an instantaneous recording but gives data spread out over successive periods of 20 minutes.

Finally it should be recalled with inhibitors of the synthesis of acetylcholine the effects of increasing the frequency of stimulation on an *in vivo* cat preparation and antagonism by the addition of choline.

(b) *Action on receptors at the motor end-plate*

The antagonism of the action of acetylcholine on the receptors at the motor end-plate represents the mode of action of many neuromuscular blocking agents particularly curare and curare-like agents. Such an action may be demonstrated on the *in vivo* neuromuscular preparation of the cat by studying the antagonistic effect of anticurares (neostigmine, edrophonium) or of carefully chosen doses of depolarizing agents.

Other more precise techniques may be used:

Recording of miniature end-plate potentials (frog sartorius preparation, isolated rat diaphragm preparation—for instance, with transversely cut preparations, Barstad and Lilleheil, 1968): the amplitudes of the miniature end-plate potentials are reduced.

Recording of end-plate potentials: the amplitudes of these are also reduced (Fatt and Katz, 1951). Nevertheless, before concluding that an action is on the motor end-plate one must be sure that there is no action presynaptically.

Investigation of an antagonistic action against acetylcholine on an *in vivo* preparation (sciatic–anterior tibialis preparation of the cat). Close intra-arterial injection of acetylcholine (1–10 mcg into the tibial artery) produces a contraction of the muscle which is reduced or totally abolished by a curarizing agent. This method is undoubtedly the most certain. Antagonism against acetylcholine may also be demonstrated on isolated preparations such as the denervated diaphragm of the rat, the chick biventer cervicis preparation,* the rectus abdominis preparation of the frog.†

* This preparation has the possibility of being stimulated both by its motor nerve and by the addition of acetylcholine to the bath (Ginsborg and Warriner, 1960).

† This second method may be used according to numerous protocols:

Preventative or curative inhibition of a contracture produced by acetylcholine.

Determination of curves relating the amplitude of contraction to the dose of acetylcholine in the presence of increasing concentrations of the curarizing agent in order to demonstrate the presence of competitive inhibition.

Protecting the specific receptors by prior fixation of a reversible curarizing agent;

Some techniques which are much more specialized and involve the iontophoretic application of acetylcholine in the region of the motor end-plate together with intracellular recording of potential (Del Castillo and Katz, 1957a).

(c) *Direct action on muscle fibers*

This effect can result either from an action on the muscle membrane which is no longer able to propagate an action potential, or by an inhibition of the excitation–contraction coupling mechanism, or even by a direct action on the contractile protein (this is generally irreversible).

The overall effect may be observed in an *in vivo* preparation or an isolated preparation with direct stimulation of the muscle. The best technique consists of alternately stimulating directly and indirectly the anterior tibialis preparation of the cat *in vivo*, the rabbit, the rat, or the isolated diaphragm preparation of the rat. Chronically denervated muscles may also be used: *in vivo* preparations may be used in which recordings are simultaneously made of the twitches of a chronically denervated paw (direct stimulation) and of the normally innervated other paw (direct and indirect stimulation). In the latter case it is necessary to use a stimulus isolation unit. Such experiments make it possible to disassociate presynaptic or curarizing effects from a direct action on the muscle which sometimes is found in the same molecule.

The recording of muscular action potentials with an analysis of the character of their modification makes it possible to determine the mechanism of the inhibition.

In concluding these few pages on the interpretation of experimental results three points will be emphasized:

The great variation in the quantitative and qualitative sensitivity of various animal species in respect to neuromuscular blocking agents.

The differences in reactivity according to the experimental conditions, particularly according to whether an *in vitro* or an *in vivo* preparation is used, the ultimate objective being to extrapolate the data to man.

The majority of neuromuscular blocking agents may act at a number of points at the neuromuscular junction; it is thus essential to determine these before reaching a conclusion on their mechanism of action.

---

if the neuromuscular blocking agent has irreversible action (for example, venoms of some snakes) and acts on specific receptors, their saturation by prior treatment with a reversible curarizing agent (*d*-Tc) prevents the complete blockade of the preparation.

If care is not taken to respect these fundamental points in discussing the results there is a danger of reaching invalid conclusions.

12.3. DIFFERENT TYPES OF PARALYSIS

Amongst known paralysing substances some have a presynaptic action and have been the object of special study. However, the great majority act primarily on the receptors of the motor end-plate. There are two principle types of action:

Paralysis by antagonism of the depolarizing action of acetylcholine.
Paralysis by prolonged depolarization of the motor end-plate.

We will describe the various effects observed in animals after the administration of *d*-tubocurarine and of decamethonium which may be considered as reference substances for the two types of paralysis. We will consider later the existence of heretical or "mixed" paralysis.

12.3.1. PHARMACODYNAMICS OF *d*-TUBOCURARINE (*d*-Tc)

With the conclusions which Claude Bernard reached following his experiments on curare, the essential had been said. The nerve is not affected, the muscle is not affected, curare acts at the junction between the nerve and the muscle. Since that time, numerous studies have confirmed and above all extended this observation. *d*-Tc inhibits neuromuscular transmission by blocking the specific receptors of the synapse, thus antagonizing the depolarizing effects which normally would have been produced by the acetylcholine liberated at the motor nerve endings.

12.3.1.1. *CHARACTERISTICS OF CURARIZATION*

The intravenous administration of *d*-Tc produces in all animal species a progressive flaccid paralysis affecting initially the small muscles of the head and the neck, subsequently those of the paws and the abdominal muscles, finally the respiratory muscles.

The sensitivity to *d*-Tc varies from one species to another in the proportion of 1 to 10 (for a 90% inhibition of the anterior tibialis muscle the effective dose is 40–50 mcg/kg for the rat or the mouse, 350 mcg/kg for the cat, and as much as 400 mcg/kg for the rabbit. Man is intermediate with a sensitivity comparable to that of the cat.) Figure 1 (Zaimis, 1953) compares the differences in sensitivity for *d*-Tc and decamethonium according to the species.

309

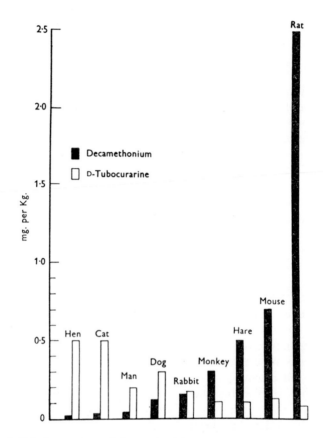

FIG. 1. Relative potency of decamethonium and *d*-tubocurarine in different species. The dose indicated in mg/kg is that required to produce a 90–100% neuromuscular block in all species but mouse where it represents the ED_{50} using the righting reflex test (in Zaimis, 1953).

A lowering of the body temperature reduces the sensitivity to *d*-Tc (Bigland *et al.*, 1958).

The rabbit head-drop requires the infusion of smaller doses (0.15–0.18 mg/kg) in the view of high sensitivity of the test; respiratory arrest is produced with a dose of 0.30 to 0.35 mg/kg.

With repeated administration the preparations become sensitized to *d*-Tc: for example, in an *in vivo* anterior tibialis preparation of the cat, the intravenous doses required to produce successive neuromuscular blockade are: 350 mcg/kg, 250 mcg/kg, 200 mcg/kg, etc.; this sensitization may be explained by the fact that a return of contractions to the maximal amplitude is produced soon as the motor end-plate potential exceeds the threshold for a contractile response (margin of safety). It may also be explained by a progressive saturation of nonspecific sites.

The duration of action varies according to the species; it is short in the case of the rat and the mouse (5 minutes), longer in other species (20 to 45 minutes).

The degree of paralysis varies slightly according to the frequency of stimulation. High rates of frequency produce fatigue of the neuromuscular preparation rendering it more sensitive. In the particular case of tetanic stimulation of a motor nerve, one does not observe a tetanic response of the muscle but simply a contraction followed by paralysis. The tetanus is thus not maintained. This is because at each tetanic stimulus a smaller quantity of acetylcholine is liberated than during low-frequency stimulation. The depolarization of the motor end-plate which is already depressed by d-Tc will thus be subliminal and will not produce a contractile response. After a return to a low frequency of stimulation an antagonist effect is observed (return of the amplitude of contractions) corresponding to the "post-tetanic potentiation". This is due to the stimulation of acetylcholine synthesis during the tetanus, producing an increase in the number of quanta liberated by the influx when the frequency of stimulation is decreased (Fig. 2).

12.3.1.2 *MODIFICATION OF CURARIZATION*

Numerous substances are able to antagonize or to potentiate the effects of d-Tc. These may act at three sites:

On the receptors themselves.

On the amount of acetylcholine liberated at the motor nerve endings (increase, protection, decrease).

On the metabolism of d-Tc (sites of loss).

(a) *Antagonism*

Neostigmine and edrophonium have powerful antagonistic actions on curarization* and these are widely used as in anesthesiology.† Neostigmine has a progressive and prolonged action. In contrast edrophonium has a rapid but transient action. The majority of substances classified as "anticholinesterases" are also capable of antagonizing the actions of d-Tc

---

* See chapter 16.
† See chapter 18.

(eserine organophosphates, oxamides, etc.). The mechanism of this anti-curare action may be explained by the protection they afford to molecules of acetylcholine in the region of the postsynaptic membrane. However, in reality it is much more complex; without going into details, this problem being discussed elsewhere, these compounds are capable, according to the dose, of having a number of effects which can play a role in their anti-curare effect:

Anticholinesterase action both pre- and postsynaptically.

A direct depolarizing effect or by acting through the intermediary of acetylcholine pre- and postsynaptically.

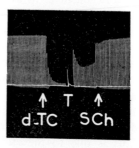

FIG. 2. Effect of a tetanus and succinylcholine on curarization. Maximal twitches of a tibialis anticus muscle of the cat (chloralose + nembutal anesthesia)—stimulation of the sciaticus nerve once every 10 seconds. At *d*-Tc: intravenous injection of *d*-tubocurarine (350 mcg/kg)—at T, tetanus (30 c/sec for 15 seconds); the tetanus was not maintained but induced a post-tetanic potentiation. At SCh: antagonism by succinylcholine (25 mcg in the external iliac artery).

A facilitating action* linked to an increase in the amount of acetylcholine liberated at the nerve endings. This applies not to the content of each quantum but to the number of quanta liberated by the nervous influx.

A direct sensitizing action of the motor end-plate to acetylcholine.

Tetraethylammonium, Ca and K ions, certain phenol derivatives and guanidine have anticurare actions and increase in the region of the nerve ending the number of quanta of acetylcholine liberated by nervous influx.

Depolarizing substances such as C10, succinylcholine (Fig. 2) and acetyl-choline itself (in close arterial injection) antagonize *d*-Tc whilst they are themselves paralyzing agents. The classical representation of neuromuscular transmission situates such an effect in the region of the postsynaptic

* On a normal preparation this "facilitation or potentiation" corresponds to an increase in the amplitude of the contractile response.

receptors. Recent experiments, however, tend to indicate that it is also on the motor nerve terminals that these depolarizing substances exert their anticurare action.

(b) *Potentiation of curarization*

Curarization may be potentiated by numerous drugs. The administration of a first dose of *d*-Tc sensitizes the neuromuscular preparation to a new injection. This "auto-sensitization" which is a property of the myoneural junction may be observed with all other true curarizing agents or curarimimetics (gallamine, toxiferine, erythrina alcaloids, etc.), which when administered at the same time as *d*-Tc, increases the effect of the latter drug by simple addition.

Other substances such as Mg ions, hemicholinium, triethylcholine, botulinus toxin, tetrodotoxine, and saxitoxine, certain antibiotics which by various presynaptic mechanisms reduce the quantity of acetylcholine liberated by each influx, are also able to increase the paralysing action of *d*-Tc.

Finally, other molecules are able to potentiate the effects of *d*-Tc without acting at the neuromuscular junction. This is the case, for example, of SKF 525A, beta-diethylaminoethyldiphenyl, propyl acetate and certain sulphonamides (acetazolamide, chlorothiazide, probenecide), the hypothesis which is usually put forward to explain the action of these substances concern the general metabolism of *d*-Tc. In addition to the specific receptors of the motor end-plate, other, so-called non-specific receptors or sites of loss, fix and thus render inactive a certain number of the molecules of *d*-Tc. These may be liberated or displaced by potentiating agents. The molecules so liberated enter the circulation and are capable of acting at the neuromuscular junction.

12.3.1.3. *ACTION ON POSTSYNAPTIC RECEPTORS*

By its two quaternary ammonium centres which are strongly ionized and by its steric configuration, *d*-Tc is able to combine in a reversible manner with the specific receptors for ACh localized on the postsynaptic membrane. These receptors which are thus blocked can no longer be depolarized by acetylcholine. Nevertheless there appears to be competition between the molecules of *d*-Tc and those of ACh for the occupation of the receptors.

(a) *Fixation on the receptors*

This fixation may be directly or indirectly demonstrated for the majority of species whatever the muscle or whatever the experimental conditions:

Indirectly by demonstrating an antagonistic effect of either endogenous or exogenous acetylcholine.

By recording the end-plate potentials following the administration of *d*-Tc, the amplitudes of the end-plate potentials progressively decrease, in proportion to the number of receptors which are blocked. Under a certain threshold equivalent to 30% to 50% of its amplitude, the end-plate potential can no longer depolarize the muscular membrane; the transmission is thus blocked. It is then possible to record end-plate potentials without the interference due to muscular action potentials.

By recording miniature end-plate potentials intracellularly. Following *d*-Tc there is a diminution not in the frequency but in the amplitude of these spontaneous potentials.

By inhibition of the contractile actions of acetylcholine. *d*-Tc completely inhibits the action of acetylcholine either when it is administered by close arterial injection *in vivo* preparations or when it is added to isolated preparations (rectus, biventer, denervated diaphragm).

Directly by using ^{14}C- or ^{3}H-labeled *d*-Tc. The majority of the radioactivity is localized in the regions identified as the motor end-plate in other sections by histochemical methods. It has been demonstrated that the number of receptors inhibited reaches a maximal limit of 3 to 4 $\times$ 10^6 molecules per end-plate (Waser, 1963) and that these molecules are fixed to the membrane surface. This latter point has been confirmed by the inactivity of *d*-Tc injected into the interior of a cell by iontophoresis.

This fixation on to receptors is the only action of *d*-Tc on the motor end-plate; none of the electrical properties, membrane potential, membrane resistance of the end-plate, are modified.

What is the nature of this reaction with the receptor? Is it an interference with the ability of the transmitter to reach the receptors or is it due to a modification of the properties of the receptors or of the permeability of the postsynaptic membrane. These questions are still without an adequate answer.

(b) *Competitive nature*

This fixation corresponds to an equilibrium and reversible reaction modified by acetylcholine. Indeed curarization is antagonized by ACh itself and by everything which increases its concentration at the end-plate, tetanic stimulation, anticholinesterases, depolarizing facilitating drugs, etc.

This competition may be quantified on the batracian rectus, by the addition of increasing doses of agonist or antagonist (see Fig. 6, p. 336); it occurs in proportion of one molecule of agonist for one molecule of antagonist (Jenkinson, 1960).

This competitive nature has been questioned by Taylor and Nedergaard (1965) basing their findings on the conclusions of Del Castillo and Katz (1957b); the molecules of acetylcholine being present for too short a time to displace those of curare. A better understanding of these complex molecular phenomena which take place at the end-plate, would enable this point to be resolved. One may nevertheless state that at the present time it would appear that there is overall a competitive action.

12.3.1.4 *ACTION ON NERVE TERMINALS*

The presynaptic action of d-Tc has for some time been in question but now appears to be well established (Hubbard *et al.*, 1969). Small doses of d-Tc which are considerably smaller than those required to produce paralysis are able to prevent the effects of stimulation of nerve terminals by ACh, and the hydroxyaniliniums, or that which appear after prolonged tetanic stimulation. The existence of these cholinergic sites at the nerve terminals is now beyond question and it would be surprising if d-Tc was not fixed by them. Standaert (1964) has suggested that d-Tc prevents the postpotentials of the amyelinated terminals and thus antagonizes the generation of a potential or of a repetitive response. A facilitating action on transmission has been shown (Hubbard *et al.*, 1965; Jones and Laity, 1965) with small doses of d-Tc and the presynaptic origin of this action seems very probable.

Autoradiographs obtained with ^3H-d-Tc tend to prove that in addition to a localization of curare on the motor end-plate a preterminal localization of radioactivity is occasionally seen (Cohen *et al.*, 1967).

The important question which must be posed concerns the role of this presynaptic action in the neuromuscular blockade produced by d-Tc. We have shown following the observations of Dale that the quantity of ACh liberated at the nerve terminals was not modified by d-Tc (Cheymol *et al.*, 1962). The experiments of Beani and Bianchi (1961) which tended to show a reduction in the amount ACh liberated have been repeated and formally contradicted by Chang, Cheng, and Chen (1967). The paralyzing action of d-Tc is thus due not to a presynaptic but to a postsynaptic effect. This agrees with the conclusions of Bowen and Merry (1969) and those of Katz and Miledi (1965); d-Tc possesses a powerful postsynaptic paralyzing action whilst its presynaptic effects are comparatively weak or even absent.

12.3.1.5. *ACTION ON MUSCLE FIBERS*

On curarized neuromuscular preparation, direct electrical stimulation produces a normal contractile response. The muscle has preserved the integral electrical characteristics, its excitability, and its contractile properties: only the depression of the motor end-plate prevents the initiation of the muscular action potential.

Nevertheless, chronic denervated muscles sometimes respond by a contracture on injection of *d*-Tc: this paradoxical stimulant effect may be explained by a depolarizing activity which is too weak to act on receptors localized in the motor end-plate in a normal muscle but which is sufficient to stimulate the receptors present on the whole surface of the denervated muscle membrane.

12.3.2. PHARMACODYNAMICS OF DECAMETHONIUM (C10)

Decamethonium (C10), which is little used in anesthesia, has been the subject of numerous pharmacological studies as the main member of a series of substances with a depolarizing mode of action. It is also a bis-quaternary ammonium compound and as *d*-Tc produces a flaccid paralysis in mammals, there being, however, an initial phase of fasciculations. A more thorough analysis of its mechanism action not only differentiates it from *d*-Tc but is different from it in all points. Its mechanism of action is much more complex particularly since there is a fundamental difference according to species and even in the same species according to the muscle. Adding to this the considerable effect of the experimental conditions (*in vivo* or *in vitro*) one understands the difficulty in finding a single mode of action of C10. Should one postulate a distinct action in each type of experiment? In any case C10 cannot be considered as a true curarizing agent or a curarimimetic even if the concept of Claude Bernard is enlarged since both the nerve fiber and the end-plate are affected. The muscle fiber is no longer identical to itself. We will thus speak of a neuromuscular blocking action.

12.3.2.1. *CHARACTERISTICS AND MODIFICATIONS OF THE NEUROMUSCULAR BLOCKING ACTION OF C10*

With the object of avoiding the confusions linked to the diverse experimental results depending on the experimental preparation it seems wiser to describe each separately.

(a) *On neuromuscular preparations of the cat* in vivo

As we have already seen this preparation produces reactions comparable to those observed in man. On the anterior tibialis preparation C10 is first stimulant then neuromuscular blocking.

The *stimulant* phase is only observed after weak doses and is absent during slow infusion. It consists of three distinct phenomena:

(i) Fasciculations appear after a latency in the absence of all stimulus at the lowest dose.

(ii) A contractile response appears without latency at higher doses in the absence of all stimuli.

(iii) A facilitation or potentiation of the maximal twitch obtained after stimulation of the motor nerve.

A *paralyzing* phase progressively develops leading to the disappearance of all traces of stimulant effect. This differs in all respects from curarization, for example:

Tetanic stimulation of the nerve produces a maintained response without antagonizing the paralysis.

d-Tc in contrast antagonizes this action whilst neostigmine, edrophonium increase the paralysis or are without effect.

A lowering of the temperature of the muscle increases the paralysis.

The effects of C10 correspond exactly to those produced by acetylcholine itself when it is protected from hydrolysis by the simultaneous administration of neostigmine.

Red muscles such as soleus which are rich in myoglobine and have slow and tonic contractions and the respiratory muscles are less sensitive than the anterior tibialis. The paralysis produced is not so typical and rapidly changes into curarization, this is also the case for the muscles of the majority of mammals other than the cat.

(b) *On mammals other than the cat*

The first administration of C10 to these animals produces fasciculations and a facilitation but the paralysis which progressively follows has characteristics of curarization: not maintained response to tetanic stimulation, post-tetanic facilitation, antagonism by neostigmine, increase in the paralysis produced by *d*-Tc. This is the "dual block" or paralysis of mixed type described by Zaimis (1953), first a cholinomimetic or depolarizing action followed by competitive block. The importance of the initial depolarizing component in comparison with the "competitive" component varies according to the species or the muscle. This explains the great variation in reactions to C10.

Indeed even on the anterior tibialis preparation of the cat which has a pure depolarizing action, some 7 hours after the slow intravenous infusion the type of paralysis changes and takes on characteristics of curarization since it is increased and not antagonized by *d*-Tc (Dybing, 1960). The diphasic paralyzing action of C10 seems general, the main variation is the time to the onset of the second phase which varies from a few minutes to some hours.

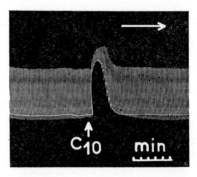

Fig. 3. Substained contracture produced by decamethonium in the hen. Dialbarbitone anesthesia. Maximal twitches of the gastrocnemius muscle elicited by stimulation of the sciaticus nerve once every 10 seconds. At C10, intravenous injection of decamethonium (8 mcg/kg).

A progressive tachyphylaxis to repeated doses of C10 is associated with this mixed action producing a disappearance of the first phase and a considerable variation in the sensitivity from one species to another. The cat, which shows a pure reaction, is the most sensitive (10–20 mcg/kg), the rabbit, the dog, the monkey, and the rat are increasingly less sensitive since paralyzing dose for this latter species is of the order of 1500 mcg/kg (see Fig. 1, p. 310).

The higher C13 homologue (tridecamethonium) of C10 produces in the cat a mixed action comparable to that observed in the rabbit with C10.

(c) *On avian muscle*

The pigeon, the chicken, or the chick, show very characteristic reaction with C10. Immediately following intravenous injection a prolonged contracture of the legs and neck muscles occur—this is made manifest by an extension of the limbs and a retraction of the head while the wings remain flaccid. This contracture ceases without a phase of paralysis. On an *in vivo* sciatic-gastrocnemius preparations a contracture is produced following C10 without the slightest reduction in the amplitude of the contractions (Fig. 3).

SKF-525A (β-diethylaminoethyl,3,3-diphenylpropylacetate) changes this typical reaction into a competitive-like blockade, the mechanism of which is not yet known (Suarez-Kurtz *et al.*, 1969).

(d) *On isolated mammalian preparations*

The results obtained are very different according to the muscle and the experimental conditions; the paralysis may or may not be preceded by contractures and present two successive phases:

The first is a depolarizing type and is rapid and transient, it is insensitive to anticholinesterases, to K ions and to temperature.

The other, which is slower and precedes until complete inhibition or to a level where the amplitudes are small but constant, resembles curarization since it is sensitive to changes in temperature, it is increased by *d*-Tc and it is at least partially antagonized by the anticholinesterases and by K ions. The removal of C10 by washing the preparation leads to a restoration of the maximal amplitude.

In some experiments, only the second phase is observed. Curiously enough the muscles of the cat (for example tenuissimus) which in *in vivo* preparation reacts by pure depolarization, in isolated organ bath shows successively the two types of paralysis (Maclagen, 1962).

The competitive character of the second phase of paralysis is not accepted by all authors. It would appear that in some cases it is really competitive whilst in other cases it is not competitive (very weak reaction to ACh and to anticholinesterases).

(e) *On isolated amphibian preparations*

Certain muscles with multiple innervation, for example the rectus abdominis, react by a prolonged contracture, others show a bi-phasic paralysis as is observed on mammalian muscle.

12.3.2.2. *ACTION ON MOTOR NERVE TERMINALS*

For a few years, attention has been directed to the effects of a number of substances on the motor nerve terminals. It has been shown that C10, as other depolarizing agents, are able to act on the motor nerve terminals at doses below those required to produce paralysis.

The various publications on this subject are still contradictory and the experimental facts will be separated from the interpretations and the consequences attributed to them.

On an *in vivo* neuromuscular preparation of the cat (sciatic tibialis or soleus) simultaneous recordings are made of the action potentials in the ventral roots of motor nerve fibers and the action potentials in the corresponding muscle fiber. After injection of the depolarizing agent it is observed that whilst the motor fiber is orthodromically stimulated, there are repetitive antidromic discharges which precede by a few milliseconds the muscle action potential. With a slightly higher dose of the depolarizing agent, in the absence of all electrical stimulation of the nerve fibers, there is following a slight latency a repetitive antidromic discharge and corresponding muscle action potential.

These repetitive antidromic potentials are only observed during the primary phase of excitation and disappear during inhibition of transmission. They are inhibited by very weak and non-paralyzing doses of d-Tc or other curarimimetic substances.

The purely nervous origin of this repetitive discharge is still under discussion. Indeed some authors consider that this is due to "ephaptic" stimulation of the terminals particularly at high doses. However, there is strong evidence in favor of its nervous origin (Standaert and Riker, 1967).

It is more difficult to explain this phenomena. Is it due to an anticholinesterase effect? Although C10 possesses such properties it has been demonstrated that these are not indispensable. A direct depolarizing action on the terminal membrane may be ruled out since it has been shown that depolarizing substances such as ACh or SCh do not increase the frequency of miniature potentials recorded in the region of the motor endplate. The hypotheses which are accepted at the present time are:

1. An increase and a prolongation in the negative after-potential in the region of the nerve terminal leading to either a repetitive stimulation of the first node of Ranvier, or to an increase in the amount of acetylcholine released by the influx.
2. Or a direct depolarizing of this first node of Ranvier (Hubbard *et al.*, 1965). This depolarization could increase the excitability of the nerve terminals.

Do these presynaptic phenomena explain the first stimulant phase of

320

C10? Some authors accept that the facilitation, fasciculations, contractile response and even inhibition of transmission may be explained by an initial stimulation then an inhibition at high doses of the nerve terminals. In spite of certain contradictory evidence, such as the observations of repetitive muscular responses in the absence of nervous activity and the increase in the discharge of motoneurones due to activation of muscle fibers by depolarizing agents the nervous origin of the facilitation and fasciculations is quite possible.

As regards the contractile response, the hypothesis of a presynaptic origin is more difficult to defend. Indeed as will be shown later, chronically denervated muscle is even more sensitive than normal muscle to the contracture produced by C10.

The inhibition of transmission seems to be the consequence of action of C10 on receptors of the postsynaptic membrane (Bowen and Merry, 1969).

12.3.2.3. *ACTION OF DECAMETHONIUM ON RECEPTORS OF THE POSTSYNAPTIC MEMBRANE*

As *d*-tubocurarine, decamethonium by virtue of its quaternary ammonium functions is able to become fixed to receptors on the motor end-plate. Due to its more slender and flexible molecular structure, it is able to penetrate through the membrane whilst *d*-Tc, a more massive molecule, remains on the surface. The effects which C10 exerts on a motor end-plate are both different and more complex. It produces first of all a depolarization of the membrane producing an inexcitability of this, then a desensitization of the receptors (see a recent analysis by Waud, 1968).

(a) *Fixation on the receptors and penetration through the membrane*

The use of labeled C10 has made it possible to determine the localization and the kinetics of the fixation of C10 at the neuromuscular junction.

Waser (1963) has been able to show by autoradiography of the mouse diaphragm that C10 labeled with ^{14}C on the methyl group becomes fixed in the region of the motor end-plate but also in adjacent regions as far as 1 mm away. This fixation is very different from that of curare since no saturation is observed even after the administration of a number of lethal doses. The quantity fixed increases and can reach a level on the end-plates some 20 times higher than those of curare (7×10^7 molecules per end-plate) and a corresponding amount on adjacent regions.

The proportion and the localization varies according to the time after injection, the concentration of C10 in the region of the end-plate increases rapidly (in a few seconds) and then progressively increases (during the following 20 minutes). Around end-plate the concentration rapidly reaches a plateau then after 10 minutes increases further but more slowly. The size of the radioactive zone reaches a maximum in 30 seconds, decreases and then increases progressively after 10 minutes.

A more recent study on the rat with C10 labeled with tritium on the methyl radical (Creese and MacLagen, 1967; Taylor *et al.*, 1967) has made it possible to confirm the observations of Waser using minimally active doses. C10 is strongly bound in the region of the end-plate and a few hundred mcm around it but it is capable of penetrating into the muscle fibers (observations on transverse sections).

The fixation and the penetration are inhibited by a prior injection of *d*-Tc. The loss in radioactivity is very slow and almost nil after 2 hours. It is hardly 50% after 10 days. It has been shown that the maximal concentration of C10 in the region of the end-plate decreases bit by bit by diffusion of the molecules towards the extremities of the muscle fiber.

(b) *Depolarization and temporary inexcitability of the membrane (Phase I Block)*

C10 depolarizes the postsynaptic membrane as does ACh itself by a local increase in the permeability of the membrane to Na and K ions. This explains the primary manifestations of excitation observed after C10. Nevertheless, cholinesterases which limit in time the effects of acetylcholine are without action on C10. The effects of C10 in the region of the end-plate are similar to those of acetylcholine in the presence of an anticholinesterase. The depolarization is prolonged and its persistence beyond a certain level progressively leads to an inactivation of the transport mechanisms of Na leading to an action potential. The muscle membrane surrounding the end-plate becomes electrically inexcitable. An end-plate potential even if formed is incapable of producing a propagated action potential along the muscle. Transmission is thus blocked. Recordings of end-plate potentials during complete blockade corresponding to a threshold potential shows that this is always higher (up to 3 times) than in the case of curarization. C10 thus increases the threshold of excitability of the end-plate.

d-Tc by becoming fixed to the same receptors without depolarization prevents or antagonizes this blockade. On the contrary the anticholinesterases increase the local concentration of acetylcholine and increase the depolarization.

How may one explain the maintenance of a tetanus during a partial

322

blockade by C10? It is known that each influx of a tetanic stimulus contains fewer quanta of ACh than a stimulation at lower frequencies. Each influx is thus less effective; this lowered efficacy is compensated by a greater sensitivity due to the slight degree of depolarization of the post-synaptic membrane of the still active muscle fibres. When the blockade is total there is no contractile response to tetanic stimulation. This inexcitability of the membrane by persistent depolarization constitutes the mechanism of paralysis produced by C10 on certain muscles of the cat and to the first phase of the complex blockade of transmission in other muscles or animal species.

(c) *Desensitization of the receptors (Phase II Block)*

The second phase of paralysis may appear imperceptibly during blockade of an *in vivo* preparation whilst following experimental conditions, it is generally distinguished from the first phase by a temporary return of the contractions on isolated preparations. Indeed, in spite of the persistence of molecules of C10 in the region of the receptors the end-plate membrane becomes repolarized and thus again becomes electrically excitable. During this repolarization of the membrane the receptors become less and less sensitive to depolarizing agents (explanation of tachyphylaxis) and particularly to acetylcholine which no longer produces an end-plate potential of sufficient amplitude to produce a muscle action potential.

On isolated preparation this phase of desensitization of the receptors is weakly competitive whilst on *in vivo* preparations it has the characteristics of a competitive action. Opinion is still contradictory as to the exact mechanism of this reduced sensitivity of the end-plate. Is it due to true curarization, or does it correspond as has been suggested for isolated preparations to a slow reversible modification of the receptors (Rang and Ritter, 1969) which become incapable of producing or of maintaining an ionic permeability of the postsynaptic membrane under the action of acetylcholine? Theories will be proposed later* on the molecular action of depolarizing substances but decisive experiments are still necessary to prove the mechanism. The prolonged depolarization of the end-plate produces a profound and slowly reversible modification of the ionic equilibrium, particularly that of potassium. This must certainly disturb the normal functioning of the postsynaptic membrane much more on isolated muscles than on *in vivo* muscles.

* See p. 340.

323

12.3.2.4. *ACTION OF C10 ON MUSCLE FIBERS*

We have seen that the electrical inexcitability due to a prolonged depolarization does not remain localized to the motor end-plate but overflows slightly to the adjacent muscle membrane. The inhibition of the muscular conduction around the end-plate may produce a slight reduction in the amplitude of the contraction obtained by direct stimulation of the muscle following injection of high doses of C10.

On chronically denervated muscle, which has chemosensitive receptors on the whole surface of the membrane, the effects of C10 are much more important.

At low doses, the depolarizing effect exerts itself on a limited number of receptors and leads to a contraction with propagated potential.

At moderate doses the entire membrane is depolarized and leads to a contracture which is not propagated.

At high doses, in addition to these preceding phenomena (contraction, contracture), a paralysis of the contractions by direct stimulation, paralysis due to inexcitability of whole muscle membrane by prolonged depolarization.

In concluding this rapid analysis of the paralyzing action of the C10 it may be said at the present state of knowledge the paralysis results from a stimulation followed by blockade of the cholinergic receptors on the presynaptic and postsynaptic membranes. According to the muscle, the animal species, and the experimental conditions one or other of these effects predominates on one or other of the receptors of the membranes leading to very varied paralysis.

Whatever the precise cause it is not due to curarization since the nerve fiber, the motor end-plate, and the muscle fibers are all affected.

12.3.3. OTHER TYPES OF PARALYSIS

Amongst the numerous neuromuscular inhibitors, the main action of which are on the postsynaptic membrane, some may be termed "heretical" and cannot be precisely placed in either the group of *d*-Tc or in that of C10. Two of the most widely studied will be described, these are prodeconium or Prestonal* and benzoquinonium or Mytolon*.

PRODECONIUM (Vallée, 1957; Van Rossum *et al.*, 1958)

$$CH_3—N^+—CH_2 \cdot CH_2 \cdot O \cdot (CH_2)_{10} \cdot O \cdot CH_2CH_2—N^+—CH_3$$

with CH_3 and $C_3H_7O \cdot CO \cdot CH_2$ on the left nitrogen, and CH_3 and $CH_2 \cdot COOC_3H_7$ on the right nitrogen

Prodeconium

Prodeconium produces a very brief and flaccid paralysis both in mammals and in birds, without trace of primary excitatory phenomena. The contractions by direct stimulation of the muscle fibers are not depressed, the muscle itself is not affected. Similarly nervous conduction is not altered by concentrations as much as 100 times the paralyzing concentration. Prodeconium is a weak acetylcholinesterase inhibitor.

Neostigmine is sometimes able to produce a weak return of the contractions but in no case can this be considered as antagonism. More often no effect or a weak synergistic effect is observed. Edrophonium on the contrary increases the paralysis. *d*-Tc and C10,* although mutual antagonists, are in the present case synergistic with prodeconium. This leads to the suggestion that prodeconium does not act directly on specific receptors of the end-plate.

Adrenaline antagonizes the paralysis produced by prodeconium.

This substance behaves as an antagonist of acetylcholine, for example on the rectus abdominis muscle of the frog. It does not produce contracture and antagonizes the effects of depolarizing substances. Nevertheless this antagonism is not competitive. In the presence of highly active concentrations of prodeconium, it is not possible to obtain a maximal contractile response by considerably increasing the concentration of depolarizing substance (see Fig. 7, p. 337).

These overall experimental facts may be summarized by saying that prodeconium, a non-depolarizing substance, antagonizes depolarizing agents by a non-competitive mechanism.

How or where does it act?

It is thought that its short duration of action is linked to the presence of an easily hydrolyzable substituent on the quaternary nitrogen atom.

The mechanism of its action remains for the present unknown. It may be supposed that the molecules of prodeconium become more fixed to

* It should nevertheless be pointed out that the primary excitatory phenomena characteristic of depolarizing substances is prevented by prodeconium.

325

different receptors than the specific receptors and that this fixation produces either a deformation of the specific receptors, which are then no longer able to bind molecules of acetylcholine, or an inhibition of the processes which follow after fixation of acetylcholine molecules onto specific receptors.

The action of prodeconium is probably postsynaptic. Does it have a presynaptic component? At the present time there is no evidence to enable a definite answer to be given to this question.

BENZOQUINONIUM (Hoppe, 1951; Bowman, 1958; Blaber and Bowman, 1962; Christ and Blaber, 1968)

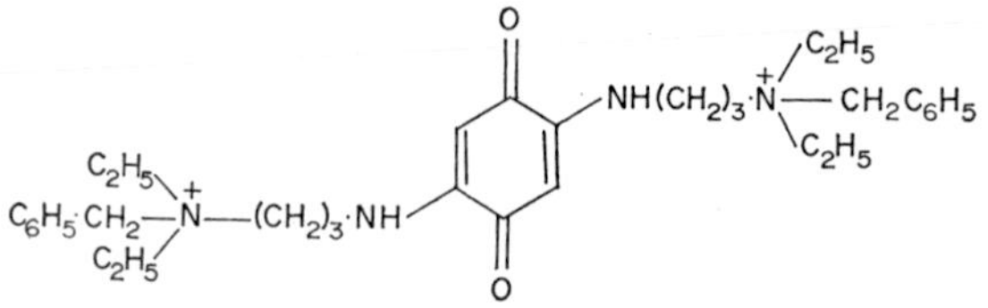

Paralysis produced by benzoquinonium has certain characteristics comparable to those of *d*-Tc:

It is increased by *d*-Tc.
A progressive action with a moderate duration without a primary phase of excitation, nor a depression of direct contraction.
Tetanus is not maintained.
Reciprocal antagonism with depolarizing agents. Endogenous ACh liberated by tetanic stimulation of nerve or exogenously injected ACh antagonize the paralysis. This antagonistic action, which is stronger than in the case for *d*-Tc, is increased by a prior administration of an anticholinesterase. Tetraethylammonium, which is known to increase the liberation of acetylcholine at the nerve terminals, is an antagonist.
On the rectus abdominis muscle of the frog, antagonism with acetylcholine is competitive but with a non-competitive component. No contracture is observed.

In contrast, other properties differentiated clearly from *d*-Tc:

Anticholinesterases and anticurare substances are almost without action on preparations in the cat, and are partial antagonists on chicken preparations.
Benzoquinonium has an anticholinesterase activity *in vitro* which is very marked since it is one-third that of neostigmine. It is thought

that this activity could explain the fact that neostigmine and other anticholinesterases are incapable of antagonizing paralysis produced by benzoquinonium. This hypothesis has now been abandoned.

Benzoquinonium clearly inhibits the facilitation and the anticurare effects of edrophonium, of neostigmine, of eserine, and of TEPP, etc., probably on the nerve terminals.

In the activity of benzoquinonium two effects can be distinguished: a pre-synaptic action, inhibition of the facilitating sites, and a post-synaptic effect, anticholinesterase and antidepolarizing activity.

What is the precise mechanism of paralysis?

Some authors consider the presynaptic inhibition plays an important role. Other authors consider that the postsynaptic antidepolarizing action (possibly only partially competitive) is responsible for the inhibition of transmission. It has to be particularly potent in this respect since it is not antagonized by anticholinesterases.

12.4. THE CHOLINERGIC RECEPTORS OF THE NEUROMUSCULAR JUNCTION—MUTUAL DISPOSITION

Knowledge of the nature and structure of the cholinergic receptors remains a fundamental and difficult problem in the study of neuromuscular transmission. A number of hypotheses have carefully been advanced, these are still incomplete and cannot at the present time constitute a satisfactory reply. Studies nevertheless continue along two different and complementary approaches.

The first approach consists in isolating that fraction of the tissue which is rich in receptors (electric organs of fish, skeletal muscle) and in studying its reactivity with agonists and antagonists. This method has the advantage of eliminating a number of factors which are foreign to the receptors perturbing the reaction of the substances under study. It also has a number of disadvantages:

The purity of the isolated fraction must be very great in order that the results are interpretable, but they are very difficult to obtain.

Does the isolated fraction constitute the specific receptor or secondary points of fixation or of loss?

By supposing that the isolated fraction is truly the specific receptor, are its properties *in vitro* identical to those which it possesses in the living tissue?

These difficulties in interpretation have led a number of workers to use the other approach. That is to study the reactivity of various agonists or antagonists on the receptors *in vivo* as a function of their molecular structure. An important advantage of such a method is that it considers receptors in their "physiological" state. Nevertheless, the interpretation of results obtained is complicated by the interference of numerous factors: tissue diffusion, influence of metabolism, interaction with other receptors, modifying the reactivity of the substances under study with specific receptors.

The various hypotheses concerning cholinergic receptors which are considered to be valid at the present time, and their mutual disposition on the membrane surface of the neuromuscular synapse will be summarized.

12.4.1. THE CHOLINERGIC RECEPTORS

The receptors for acetylcholine or the cholinergic receptors may be considered as a group of atoms which form part of a molecule which is orientated in such a manner that molecules of acetylcholine become preferentially fixed to it. This fixation produces biocellular modifications which constitute the pharmacological response (depolarization with alteration in the permeability to certain ions).

These receptors are functional structures, specific, complementary to ACh and localized in certain special and readily accessible regions of the membrane surface.

There exists various types of cholinergic receptors in proportion to their specificity to certain agonists (muscarine, nicotine, etc.) or antagonists (atropine, hexamethonium, *d*-Tc, etc.). This difference may be related to the structure of cholinergic receptor itself or to the mutual disposition of these receptors in relation one to the other. In all these cases, acetylcholine is the "master key" of all the different "locks".

The fixation of acetylcholine on the cholinergic structure may occur by at least three of its functional atoms or active centers:

The nitrogen atom of the quaternary ammonium function.
The oxygen atom of the ester group.
The oxygen atom of the carboxyl group.

Following the studies of Barlow (1955), it is generally accepted that the cholinergic sites comprise two sites as does cholinesterase (see Fig. 4):

Anionic site, the active center of which could be the carboxyl function of a dicarboxylic amino acid, a function derived from phosphoric acid* or sulfamic or even a thiol function. This site combines with the cationic head provided by the quaternary ammonium function. The presence of "subcenters" are suggested which participate in the fixation of the cationic head.

An esterophilic site, constituted by a dipole system capable of fixing, by dipole–dipole interaction, the strongly polarized ester function.

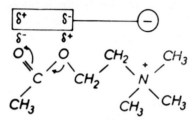

FIG. 4. Scheme of cholinoreceptor (in Khromov-Borisov and Michelson, 1966).

There exists a positive charge on the strongly polarized oxygen atom of the ester, there exists a negative charge on the carbonyl oxygen atom. On the esterophilic site there must correspondingly be two points of fixation respectively positive and negative constituting a dipole moment.

This esterophilic site is considered to be different from the esterase site of cholinesterase. Nevertheless, a number of arguments are currently in favor of assimilating the cholinergic receptors to the anionic site of cholinesterase itself (Ehrenpreis, Beckett, Zupancic, Wurzel and Belleau, in Ehrenpreis, 1967). This hypothesis, which is not accepted by all, of a system of combined cholinesterase and cholinergic receptors forming a functional unity is supported by diverse experimental findings.†

* A number of arguments are in favor of a phosphoric grouping as the anionic site (Cavalitto, 1967):
   It is an essential constituent of a number of biochemical structures (ATP; nucleic acids; coenzyme A, etc.) involved in the ACh synthesis.
   It is readily able to fix certain physiological cations such as Ca.
   It can provide a zone of high electron density favorable for cationic binding.
   It can provide a grid or lattice-type distribution of anionic sites (polyphosphate structures).

† There is a similarity between the equilibrium constant for the fixation of *d*-Tc and of ACh on a preparation of butyryl-ChE and for the fixation of *d*-Tc on cholinergic receptors of living tissue and the anionic centers of ChE of the same tissue. In a number of chemical series of esters of choline, the depolarizing activity varies in parallel with the speed of hydrolysis.

This would explain the fact that ACh is rapidly hydrolyzed without the necessity of becoming disassociated from the cholinergic receptor. In this case is it necessary to postulate that on an anionic site would be dependent an esterase site and an esterophilic site, or should both of these be considered as being identical?

It should be noted that the cationic head plays the major role in the mechanism of approach to the anionic site by the ionic forces proportional to the square of the distance, the dipole–dipole interaction forces of the ester and the esterophilic site are proportional to the 4th power of the distance and only comes into play once the molecules is fixed to the receptor.

12.4.2. MUTUAL DISPOSITION OF TWO NEIGHBORING RECEPTORS

By comparing the activity and the structure of bis-onium neuromuscular blocking agents of different chemical series, one can deduce the distance and the mutual disposition of two neighboring anionic centers (see review by Khromov–Borisov and Michelson, 1966).

12.4.2.1. *DISTANCE BETWEEN TWO ANIONIC CENTERS*

(a) "C-10" *Structures*

The high neuromuscular blocking activity of agents such as *d*-Tc, of succinylcholine, of decamethonium, the distance between the two quaternary nitrogen atoms of which corresponds to a 10-element chain and is approximately 1.4 nm, suggests that two neighboring anionic sites are situated at this same distance.* Such a separation of approximately 1.4 nm has been denoted "C-10 structures".

This structure may be confirmed by "anticurare" activity of a synthetic linear polymer containing sulphonic groups every 1.4 nm and capable of combining with cationic heads of *d*-Tc.

A model has been proposed by Waser (1963–7) which assimilates a receptor with pores of 1.2 and 1.4 nm in diameter.

The activity of succinylcholine, of decamethonium, and of intermediary derivatives containing only a single ester function are almost identical.

---

* Nevertheless there exists some molecules where the separation between the quaternary ammonium groups is a 6-element chain (hexafluorenium) and even a 3-element chain (derivatives of pyridinium propyl (trimethyl) ammonium) (Cavallitto, 1967).

This leads to the supposition that the esterophilic sites do not play a role in "C-10" structures.

(b) "C-16" *Structures*

The hypothesis with structures containing a 10-atom element chain has rightly been accepted by all, but the very high activity of molecules possessing a longer chain makes it necessary to postulate the existence of a second structure, the so-called "C-16 structure", corresponding to a distance of approximately 2 nm between the two neighboring anionic sites.

Amongst the active molecules one can cite anethocurarium, prodeconium, derivatives of diphenyl 3-4 hexane, etc., but particularly hexcarbacholine (606 HC or Imbretil) derived from a series of polymethylene bis-carbamoyl-choline (Cheymol *et al.*, 1954); the study of this series has shown that two maxima of activity appear for an 11-element atom chain and for 16- or 17-element atom chain between the onium functions. The activity is significantly higher in the last, that is where the distance is 2 nm.

In any case the series of initially synthesized decamethonium has been completed by the higher homologues and a second maxima of activity, although weaker than C10, has been observed for the derivatives containing 14 to 18 methylene groupings and having a interonium distance of approximately 2 nm.

A comparison of the more active homologues of these two latter series, bis-carbamoylcholine and methonium, shows the importance of the carbamate groupings in relationship to a simple polymethylene chain. This has led to the suggestion that the carbamates groups participate in the activity by becoming fixed to the esterophilic sites of two adjacent cholinergic receptors the centers of which are already fixed by two cationic heads. "C-16" structures thus play a role both in the anionic sites and the esterophilic sites of two cholinergic receptors.

Other experimental proofs confirm this hypothesis. The removal of one of these cationic centers of hexcarbacholine leads to a derivative which is one-third as active, whilst in the methonium series the activity is considerably reduced when one of the quaternary groups is removed. In a series of quaternary derivatives of diphenyl 4-4-disulphonic acid with the diamide functions strongly polarized, the substitution of an amide function which prevents the approach of the esterophilic sites, leads to a marked decrease of activity.

Nevertheless, the study of the activity of the higher homologs of succinylcholine contradicts this hypothesis of the "C-16 structure", for

331

this derivatives are inactive. In fact, this lack of activity is due to a greater sensitivity to hydrolysis by pseudocholinesterase.*

12.4.2.2. MUTUAL DISPOSITION OF THE CHOLINERGIC RECEPTORS

Is the distribution of receptors on the surface of a motor end-plate uniform? If one accepts the diameter of an end-plate may vary between 8 to 18 mcm and that the number of receptors on a motor end-plate is $3-4 \times 10^6$, the distance between the receptors in the case of uniform distribution would be 3.5–9.0 nm. This distance is incompatible with the existence of "C-10" and "C-16" structures. One must thus accept an heterogeneous distribution with regrouping of a certain number of receptors.

How is this regrouping affected? The existence of "C-10" and "C-16" structures with respectively absence and presence of esterophilic sites suggests different possibilities as to the orientation of the receptors one with respect to the other.

Barlow (1960) has suggested two models:

Anionic sites distributed in a rectangular manner the length of the rectangle corresponding to 2 nm and the width to 1.4 nm.

Anionic sites distributed in a square of 1.4 nm, the diagonal corresponding to a distance of 2 nm.

Nevertheless, to take into account the role played by the esterophilic

---

* Using the high blocking activity of suberyldicholine or sebacyldicholine protected by an anticholinesterase, a new principle of controlled myorelaxation has been recently suggested (Godovikov *et al.*, 1968). It involves the use of three ingredients:

(a) A selective inhibitor of pseudo-cholinesterase, for instance, the compound

$$GT-106 \ (C_2H_5O)_2 \ PO-S-CH_2-CH_2-N-(CH_3)-C_6H_5.$$

(b) A neuromuscular blocking agent which is rapidly and selectively hydrolyzed by pseudocholinesterase, for instance, suberyldicholine

$$(CH_3)_3 \ N^+-CH_2-CH_2-O-CO-(CH_2)_6-CO-O-CH_2-CH_2-N^+(CH_3)_3.$$

(c) A reactivator of cholinesterase, for instance the compound

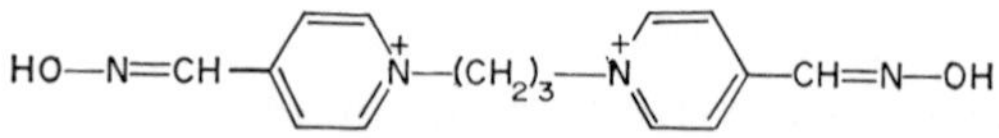

Suberyldicholine is a very weak and very short-acting blocking agent, but after GT-106, its paralyzing potency increases approximately 50-fold and the block lasts many hours. The myoneural transmission can be restored within 5 minutes by injection of TMB 4.

This combination (GT-106–suberyldicholine and TMB 4) does not represent yet a method ready to be immediately used in human surgical practice, but the principle indicates that such a method can be elaborated.

sites, Khromov-Borisov and Michelson (1966) have suggested a tetrameric arrangement of receptor molecules according to the following scheme (Fig. 5):

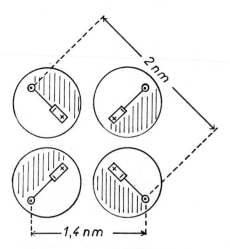

FIG. 5. Suggested tetrameric arrangement of receptor subunits (in **Khromov-Borisov** and Michelson, 1966).

The anionic sites of the four receptor molecules form a square 1.4 nm per side. The esterophilic sites are situated along the diagonals. The sides constitute the "C-10 structures" whilst the diagonals the "C-16 structures".

Such an arrangement of regrouping or clustering by four receptors molecules indicates the nature of the heterogeneous distribution of receptors whilst taking into account the data furnished by the analysis of the pharmacological activity of numerous neuromuscular blocking agents.

12.4.3. EVOLUTION OF "C-10" AND "C-16" STRUCTURES IN THE ANIMAL SERIES

The sensitivity of skeletal muscles of various members of the animal series to various paralyzing or depolarizing mono- or bis-quaternary ammonium compounds gives insight into the evolution of the distribution of cholinergic receptors.

The "C-10" structures are absent in the majority of invertebrate muscles even in the higher invertebrates such as urocordes. Nevertheless, the Annelides such as Hirudines possesses signs of "C-10" structures. The indications of this same structure appear in the muscles of the lower vertebrates such as the cyclostomes fish (lamprey) and is clearer in an amphibia. Finally the "C-10" structures should be considered as characteristic of the higher vertebrates: avia and mammals.

Nevertheless, the muscles of the new-born mammal possesses receptors on all its surface. This chemo-sensitive area is limited bit by bit and in a few days becomes localized to the neural zone. Following chronic denervation the inverse phenomenon is produced since the entire muscular membrane become chemo-sensitive and in the new receptors thus formed "C-10" structures are less important than in the receptors of normal muscle.

"C-16" structures seem to appear earlier in the animal evolution than "C-10" structures. Indeed the signs of "C-16" appear in Echinodermes and in certain cephalopode molluscs with a more highly differentiated musculature. This particular structure is very marked in Hirudines and in the Vertebrates.

In conclusion, it is possible to accept that during evolution the dimer "C-16" structure, which may exist by itself, precedes "C-10" structures which have never been demonstrated in the absence of "C-16" structures.

12.5. INTERACTION BETWEEN RECEPTORS AND PARALYZING AGENTS

The nature of the receptors on the postsynaptic membrane remains, as we have just seen, still unknown in spite of certain partial and fragmentary approaches. The same is the case for the molecular mechanism by which an active molecule becomes fixed to the receptor and produces either an agonistic or antagonistic effect.

Molecules such as acetylcholine, decamethonium, d-Tc, or prodeconium which have an undoubted chemical relationship in view of their quaternary ammonium function act on the same receptors. The great diversity in the effects produced by these substances on the neuromuscular junction have been pointed out: depolarization, depolarization followed by paralysis, competitive neuromuscular blockade, non-competitive neuromuscular blockade.

Are these molecules fixed to the same receptors or to the same elements of the receptors? Do these molecules merely occupy the receptors or do they modify the property of these? What modifications would thus be produced?

In order to answer these questions, which is essential to the understanding of the mechanism of neuromuscular blockade, a number of theories or models have been proposed which attempt to take into account the majority of the experimental data currently available.

12.5.1. THEORY OF THE AFFINITY AND THE INTRINSIC ACTIVITY OR EFFICACY
(Ariens, 1954; Stephenson, 1956)

This very general theory proposes that for each active molecule there are two distinct characteristics: the *affinity* for a given receptor and the *efficacy* or *intrinsic activity* which determines the intensity of the effect produced by the molecule on the receptor.

The reaction between the active molecule and the receptor leads to a dissociation constant K_A;* affinity is defined as the inverse of this constant, thus the logarithm of the affinity is equal to $-\log K_A$.

The occupation of the receptors by active molecules leads to a stimulus S_A which is related to the maximal possible stimulus Sm. This relationship is proportional to the fraction of receptors occupied

$$S_A/Sm = \text{alpha} \times [RA]/r.$$

The coefficient of proportionality alpha is called the *intrinsic activity*.

All molecules depolarizing or not which come into the environmental medium of the receptor (biophase) and possessing sufficient affinity becomes fixed to the receptors. If they possess an intrinsic activity (depolarizing) they produce on the adjacent membrane an increase in permeability to the ions corresponding to the depolarization of that membrane. This is true of acetylcholine, of decamethonium, etc. If on the contrary the intrinsic activity of the molecule is weak or absent, it produces a simple blockade of the receptors. This is true for *d*-Tc. For non-competitive blocking agents the affinity plays a role in relation to different receptors but which are interdependent with those of acetylcholine. The occupation of these will make it impossible for the cholinergic receptors to fix acetylcholine.

The relationship between structure and activity of different molecules

---

* In the bi-molecular reaction between active molecule and receptor there exists the following equilibrium:

$$[R] + [A] \underset{K_2}{\overset{K_1}{\rightleftharpoons}} [RA]$$

in which $[R]$ equals the concentration of free receptors, $[A]$ equals the concentration of active molecules, $[RA]$ is the concentration of occupied receptors. In practice one can calculate the proportion of occupied receptors $[RA]/r = 1/1 + K_A \times [A]$ in which r is the total number of receptors and K_A the dissociation constant.

is made possible by the determination of the affinity constant and the intrinsic activity.

This determination is usually carried out on isolated muscle preparation (rectus abdominis of the frog) in order to reduce the influence of general metabolism on the approach to the receptors and on the modification of the effects produced by the interaction of active substances on the receptors.

Dose/contractile response curves are established with increased doses of the depolarizing substance. The maximal amplitude obtained with the substance in relation to a reference standard corresponds to the intrinsic activity whilst the position on the axis of a dose gives its affinity.*

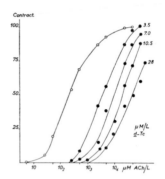

FIG. 6. Cumulative log dose–response curves for *d*-tubocurarine on acetylcholine contracture of the isolated frog's rectus abdominis muscle. The parallel shift of the curves demonstrates a competitive antagonism.

For competitive inhibitors, there is no intrinsic activity but simply affinity. This is determined in relation to a depolarizing substance. A series of curves relating dose of depolarizing substance to contractile response are established in the presence of increasing concentrations of the inhibitor. Each curve corresponds to a given concentration. For a competitive inhibitor these curves remain parallel and the shift for each concentration enables the affinity to be measured (see Fig. 6).†

* The measurement of these two parameters can be made from dose/contractile response curves. The affinity is expressed by $pD2 = -\log [A]$ 50, that is the negative logarithm of the dose producing 50% of the maximal possible effect. The intrinsic activity $a = EAm/ESm$, EAm being the maximal effect produced by the substance and ESm being the maximal effect produced by the standard substance.

† By analogy with pA_2 of Schild, one determines $pA_2 = -\log [B]_x + \log (x - 1)$ in which $[B]_x$ represents the concentration of inhibitor which produces a shift of the curves by a factor x.

In the case of non-competitive antagonism the dose response curves are not parallel one to the other but become parallel to the dose axis at high concentrations. One can determine the non-competitive affinity and a negative intrinsic activity (see Fig. 7).*

This theory has been applied to a very large number of chemical series both of depolarizing substances and/or inhibitors. In these the values of the parameters thus determined varies in a regular manner according to the length of the substituents. The presence of a radical which is long on the onium function reduces the intrinsic activity by lowering the charge

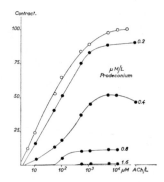

Fig. 7. Cumulative log dose–response for prodeconium on acetylcholine contracture of the isolated frog's rectus abdominis muscle. The decline of the curves and the decrease of the maximal amplitude demonstrate a noncompetitive antagonism.

on the cationic head and by increasing the distance between charge and receptor. The effect produced on the receptor is thus reduced.

Nevertheless, this theory does not explain everything, in particular the precise nature of the reaction between the active molecule and the receptor.

12.5.2. THEORY OF TWO-PHASE INTERACTION
(Del Castillo and Katz, 1957b)

In the first phase, a depolarizing substance S combines rapidly with the receptor R to form an inactive reaction product SR. This reaction product

* For non-competitive affinity $pD'\ 2 = -\log [B]\ 50$, $[B]_{50}$ being the concentration reducing by 50% the maximal depolarizing effect. In this case the intrinsic activity is negative.

transforms in the second phase to a substance SR'—which depolarizes the membrane

$$S + R \leftrightarrows SR \leftrightarrows SR'.$$

This hypothesis of a bi-phasic action is based on the fact that the administration of C10 by iontophoresis to the motor end-plate inhibits the effects of acetylcholine administered almost at the same time by a second micropipette. This supposes that in the action of C10, there is a brief initial phase which is "antiacetylcholine".

This initial phase is the only one observed with true curarizing agents. Thus the reaction constant of the first phase of equilibrium differentiates the curarizing substances from the depolarizing agents.

In addition the prolonged action of a depolarizing substance is able, at least on isolated preparations, to produce a desensitization or inactivation of the receptors (C10 or even acetylcholine in presence of an anticholinesterase). This desensitization corresponds to the disassociation of the reaction product SR' which leaves the receptor R' in a free but inactive form.

The transformation of R' to R (initial form of the receptor) is very slow even if one eliminates the depolarizing substance by washing.

With acetylcholine the reaction sequence may be written as follows:

$$ACh + R \leftrightarrows ACh\,R \leftrightarrows ACh\,R' \rightarrow ACh + R',$$
$$\text{Depolarization} \quad \text{Desensitization}$$

The receptor thus passes through a number of successive states as follows:

Initial free form.

Combination with the active molecule corresponding to a simple blockade of the receptor in the absence of other effect.

Combination with active molecules with depolarizing properties.

A free inactive form which is insensitive and which slowly recovers to its initial state.

These different states are purely hypothetical, since the precise transformation which a molecule undergoes as it passes from one state to the other is not known. This theory constitutes interesting approach but is still very far from giving an accurate picture of the interaction between the molecule of depolarizing substance and the receptor.

338

12.5.3. KINETIC THEORY
(Paton, 1961; Paton and Waud, 1962)

In the combination of a molecule X with a receptor R, the reaction equilibrium may, according to the law of mass action, be written as follows:

$$X + R \underset{K_1}{\overset{K_2}{\rightleftharpoons}} XR.$$

The reaction constant of association and of disassociation are K_1 and K_2 respectively. In general only the equilibrium constant $K = k_2/k_1$ is considered; this may be defined as the proportion of receptors occupied, that is to say the affinity of X for R at equilibrium.

According to the theory of Paton the excitation is proportional, not to the number of receptors occupied but to the velocity of combination of the active molecule with the receptor.

In order to define whether a particular molecule will be stimulant or inhibitor, the reaction velocity constants k_1 and k_2 become important and in particular the dissociation velocity constant k_2.

Indeed, if this constant is increased, that is to say if the dissociation is rapid, the molecules after having combined with the receptor become dissociated and leave the receptor free again for a new association. Thus at all times there is a low occupation of receptors and a large number of associations between active molecules and receptor which produces a stimulation of the receptor. The depolarizing substances have a high dissociation constant (k_2).

In contrast if the dissociation is slow (low value of k_2) the receptors become entirely occupied and do not allow the possibility of new associations. There is no stimulation but on the contrary blockade of the receptor.

For intermediate values of k_2, it is possible to envisage that molecules may be stimulant in a first phase and blocking subsequently.

The differentiation between a depolarizing activity and an inhibitory activity comes from the possibility of the active molecule to dissociate readily or not from the receptor. In other words, the nature of the effect produced depends on the frequency of association with the receptor or on the time during which the molecule remains fixed to the receptor.

This theory provides an explanation for the fact that hindrance of the molecule, increasing its lipophilic character which brings into non-polar interaction forces different from ionic forces, makes the dissociation more difficult. The occupation of the receptors will thus be greater, their activation weaker, the antagonist character of the molecule will thus be enhanced.

Thus in a particular homologous series the more an antagonist is active the slower will be the onset of its action, and the slower its rate of disappearance. Indeed at a constant rate of combination, a reduction in the velocity of dissociation increases both the intensity of the antagonistic effect and the duration of reaction. In contrast, if the more antagonistic molecules are strongly linked, the depolarizing molecules should be only weakly linked. This consequence to this kinetic theory seems *a priori* to be contrary to the observations of Waser (1963) who has shown that depolarizing molecules are fixed some 20 times greater than molecules of curarizing agents. In order to maintain the validity of the kinetic theory, one must suppose that these combinations are occurring at sites other than the receptors themselves.

In spite of certain contradictory arguments and the absence of a direct determination of the dissociation and association constants on which it is based, the kinetic theory agrees in a satisfactory manner with the majority of experimental facts and furnishes a more dynamic conception of the interaction between active molecules and receptors.

12.5.4. THEORY OF THE PENETRATION OF DEPOLARIZING SUBSTANCES

The idea of the penetration of depolarizing substances across the synaptic membrane, which was originally proposed and subsequently abandoned by Paton, has been taken up and to a large extent established by Taylor (1962), Creese *et al.* (1963) and has led Mackay (1963) to propose a theory of the action of drugs and particularly neuromuscular blocking agents. This theory takes into account the blockade by competition produced by certain neuromuscular blocking agents and the blockade in two phases following an initial depolarization produced by other blocking drugs.

Firstly two hypotheses: the fact that drugs penetrate across the postsynaptic membrane and produce a depolarization of this membrane. This penetration is facilitated either by "transporters" or mobile carriers or by fixed sites which are highly specific.

A number of arguments proposed in relation to C10 are in favor of this penetration which takes place in the region of the specific receptor.

There are two possibilities, according to which the active molecule–receptor combination penetrates or does not penetrate across the synaptic membrane.

Firstly, a substance "*A*" capable of penetrating produces an agonist effect that is to say a depolarization. "*A*" forms with the specific site or the carrier a combination related to an affinity constant of the site for "*A*" which may be considered as the partition coefficient between the biophase and surface membrane. "*A*" penetrates from the exterior towards the interior of the membrane according to a penetration coefficient which could correspond to the intrinsic activity of Ariens, and to the thickness of the membrane. The flux of penetration is initially very rapid, reaches a plateau and then decreases with time. It is the initial rapid flux which is supposed to produce the depolarization. Thus when the flux becomes very weak, the membrane repolarizes while the molecules "*A*" are still in the interior of the cell. A second dose of "*A*" produces a weaker effect since the flux of penetration is less extensive. Thus the tachyphylaxis observed with depolarizing agents may be explained.

The second possibility relates to a substance I (inhibitor) which is incapable of penetrating across the postsynaptic membrane. There is no flux of penetration thus no depolarization but I is capable of combining with the site or the carrier on the surface of the membrane. When A and I are both present, there will be competition and the possibility of "*A*" of combining with the sites or with the carrier on the surface of the membrane, will be reduced. The flux of penetration of "*A*" will be reduced, the depolarization will thus be weaker.

If an agonist A_1 has already penetrated into the cell and if the membrane is repolarized when one adds a second agonist A_2, this latter substance will penetrate and depolarize but the flux of penetration of A_2 will be reduced by the presence of A_1. Thus A_1 has secondary competitive properties even when its depolarizing effects have disappeared. By supposing that A_1 is a depolarizing blocking agent and A_2 is acetylcholine, one thus readily explains the two phases of blockade by depolarizing agents.

The analogies between the structures of agonist and antagonist molecules leads to an affinity for the same receptor. Nevertheless, the theory of penetration differentiates one from the other by the weak molecular hindrance for the agonists but the stronger molecular hindrance for the antagonists which thus cannot cross the postsynaptic membrane. There is still missing an explanation of the mechanism by which the penetration produces the depolarization. This explanation would reinforce this interesting theory of the action of neuromuscular blocking agents.

12.5.5. THEORY OF MACROMOLECULAR PERTURBATION

This recent theory suggested by Nachmansohn (1952) has recently been taken up in more general form by Belleau (1964). It supposes that the receptor is a protein macromolecule the structure of which is specific and makes it capable of forming a complex with acetylcholine and chemically related substances.* The configuration of all proteins is adaptable and may be in a number of forms. The fixation of substances on protein leads to a formation of a complex in which one amongst the possible conformations of the protein is favorized and stabilized. This substance leads to a macromolecular perturbation of the protein.

Biophysical studies of the interaction of quaternary ammonium compounds with receptor protein have shown the intervention of hydrophobic molecular forces. There is an elimination of water molecules linked to the transformation of the spatial structure of the protein.

Two types of interaction may be produced:

The first concerns a unique portion of the surface which fixes acetylcholine. This leads to a *specific* perturbation of the protein macromolecular conformation. The form thus stabilized will be an active form. Between the protein P and the stimulant molecule M_s there is an equilibrium as follows:

$$P + M_s \leftrightharpoons P_a \, M_s$$

in which $P_a \, M_s$ constitute the active complex which induces a depolarization on the membrane by altering the permeability to Na and K ions.

The second takes into consideration the interaction with the peripheral hydrophobic portion of the receptor and leads to a *non-specific* perturbation of the protein conformation. The stabilized form will be inactive chaotic form. The reaction of equilibrium may be written by a inhibitor molecule M_i as follows:

$$P + M_i \leftrightharpoons P_c \, M_i$$

in which $P_c \, M_i$ is the inactive complex, that is the complex which does not produce depolarization of the membrane.

A third class of molecule M_{si} leads to the formation of a mixture of

---

* The muscarinic receptor would be comparable although not identical with the anionic site of acetylcholinesterase.

complexes in equilibrium, $P_a\ M_{si}\ P_c\ M_{si}$, this becomes manifest by a partial agonism:

$$P_a\ M_{si} \leftrightarrows P + M_{si} \leftrightarrows P_c\ M_{si}.$$

The variations in free energy do not constitute the biophysical parameter which is sensitive to the specific nature of these different interactions. Indeed there exists a number of possible non-specific interactions. A single mechanism leads to the transformation of the receptor to its active state. All the pure agonists act by this mechanism. The free energy does not vary, it is the entropy and enthalpy which undergo compensatory fluctuations. Thus a comparison of the variation in enthalpy of a homologous chemical series provides evidence of a considerable variation for small changes in chemical structure.

This theory utilizes certain data on the interaction of enzyme–substrate–inhibitor. It is the first to consider a combination of the active molecule and the receptor at the molecular level in the light of biophysical parameters and indicates the specificity of this combination.

CONCLUSION

Each of the theories proposed at the present time emphasizes a particular aspect of the details of the mechanism of action of neuromuscular blocking agents. The difficulties of research in this area are very great and considerable progress is still necessary before one can arrive at an accurate overall view of the phenomena produced by the combination of active molecules and the specific receptor.

12.6. PROVISIONAL CLASSIFICATION

All active molecules at the receptors of the neuromuscular junction possess, as acetylcholine itself, one or two cationic functions which are highly ionized.

Some sulphoniums, arsoniums, phosphoniums, etc., or some tertiary amines are capable of inhibiting transmission but these are mono-derivatives and particularly bis-ammonium quaternary compounds which constitute the great majority of the more active neuromuscular blocking agents. A large number of molecules have been synthesized either with a view of their clinical use, or as models for the study of receptors or the mechanism of action. Each possesses in relation to its nature, the length and importance of its central structure, in relation to its substituents and to its cationic centers, properties which differentiate both qualitatively and quantitatively from other molecules and thus gives its originality.

For clarity and precision, similarities and relationships have been sought in an attempt to group together different substances with comparable actions.

The precise classification of neuromuscular blocking agents presents a number of difficulties:

Insufficient available pharmacological data on certain substances.

An increasing number of exceptions to the various criteria chosen for classification.

A still insufficient knowledge of the molecular events and of the precise mechanism of action which only constitutes a valid criteria.

The diversity of the sites of action on the same molecule along the neuromuscular junction and the difficulty of stating the site of the major effect.

Variations in sensitivity according to the animal species which makes it necessary to choose a species of reference. Should the cat be chosen as the experimental animal since detailed experiments may be carried out, or should preference be given to man since this is the species in which the majority of neuromuscular blocking agents are finally destined?

The progressive change in the mechanism of neuromuscular blockade from one compound to the next derivative in the same homologous chemical series.

Thus all classifications are of necessity imprecise and have their limitations. One must be conscious of these in order to improve the classification as our knowledge of the mechanism action increases. It is nevertheless a valuable tool, which should keep a provisional and evolutionary character if one is to prevent dogmatism.

12.6.1. VARIOUS PROPOSED CLASSIFICATIONS

In addition to the substances whose major site of action is presynaptic (synthesis or release of acetylcholine) and which are not within the scope of the present study* the majority of postsynaptic inhibitors have until the present time been grouped around *d*-tubocurarine or decamethonium. A few other substances, which it is difficult to associate with either of these neuromuscular blocking agents, are now arbitrarily grouped under a heading "heretical".

* See p. 298.

TABLE 1. CLASSIFICATION OF POSTSYNAPTIC NEUROMUSCULAR BLOCKING AGENTS. DIFFERENT TERMINOLOGIES

Type d-tubocurarine	Type Decamethonium	References
Pachycurares	Leptocurares	Bovet et al. (1951)
Competitive	Depolarizing	Paton and Zaimis (1952)
Curaremimetics	Acetylcholino-mimetics	Dallemagne and Philippot (1953)
Anti-depolarizing	Depolarizing	Foldes (1954)
Cholinolytics	Cholinomimetics	van Rossum et al. (1958)
Acetylcholino-competitive	Acetylcholino-mimetics	Cheymol (1963)

The various suggested classifications have been summarized in Table 1 more for the point of view of teaching and clinical use than for research itself. The various terminology employed are a reflection of the evolution in time of the various characteristics chosen as criteria for differentiation.

The first classification established by Bovet *et al.* (1951a and b) emphasized the contrasting molecular forms. The *pachycurares* are substances with large molecules which were hindered by their central structure or their various substituents. Their action is comparable to that of curare. In contrast the *leptocurares* possess narrow, slender molecules where the cationic head is only weakly hindered. These are substances like decamethonium. This classification is retaining interest at the present time, since the hypothesis of mechanism of action depends on the penetration of depolarizing substances across the postsynaptic membrane.*

Paton and Zaimis (1952) have designed for each type of neuromuscular blocking agent the principle characteristic of their effects: *competitive* in one case and *depolarizing* in another. The term competitive may introduce a certain ambiguity if it is accepted that true competition is possible at the molecular level. It is not excluded that some depolarizing agents may themselves act to a certain extent by competition. Intermediary substances produce a mixed or "dual block".

Dallemagne and Philippot (1953) contrast the *curaremimetics* which act like curare to substances which mimic the actions of acetylcholine, the *acetylcholinomimetics*. This classification does not depend on an as yet imprecise molecular phenomenon but on the resemblance to well-known molecules.

The criteria chosen by Foldes (1954) is simple. The molecule is either depolarizing or antidepolarizing. By this simplification, that which is gained by clarity is lost in precision since all molecules which do not have depolarizing action are grouped under the same heading whilst some do not act like curare. It has also been pointed out that depolarizing agents may possess antidepolarizing properties.

The classification suggested by van Rossum *et al.* (1958) of *cholinomimetic* and *cholinolytic* has the same disadvantages but this classification also separates the cholinolytics into competitive and non-competitive. In addition they suggest the existence of intermediary molecules or of transition between each of the proposed groups.

The distinction which we ourselves have put forward in no way refutes the other terminologies which retain their value and their interest.†

* See p. 340.
† The criticisms leveled at the other classifications also apply to our own.

It simply emphasizes the special relationship which exists between a certain group of neuromuscular blocking agents and acetylcholine according to whether there exists competition or in contrast mimetic action. All other molecules which appear to act in a different way are grouped together under the heading "heretical" and await a more extensive study of their mechanism of action.

12.6.2. NEUROMUSCULAR BLOCKING AGENTS OF THE *d*-TUBOCURARINE TYPE

The term "curare" is usually reserved for plant extracts used as arrow poisons and sometimes is extended to include *d*-tubocurarine itself as the main alkaloid. Substances which act like curare are usually termed curarizing agents or curarimimetics (curare-like), pachycurares, competitive agents, acetylcholino competitives, cholinolytics, non-depolarizing or antidepolarizing agents.

This group includes the natural curares as well as synthetic derivatives:

Tube curare (*d*-tubocurarine chloride,* chondrocurines, etc.), calebashe curare (toxiferine, curarines and calebassines),† the Erythrina alkaloids (β-dihydro-erythroidine)‡ which have the unusual characteristic of being a tertiary amine which becomes less active after quaternization.

Dimethyltubocurarine (*d*-Tc-*O*-dimethyl), gallamine tri-ethyiodide (Flaxedil), laudexium methosulfate (Laudolissine), the latter substances are used in anesthesiology; a large number of other synthetic derivatives.

All these molecules possess a highly sterically hindered molecular structure. They are rigid by virtue of their central structure or by the substituents on the nitrogen atom. The distance between the cationic head of the more active molecules is generally of the order of 1.4 nm.

These curarizing agents produce paralysis characterized by the following:

They produce a paralysis which is flaccid for all normally innervated muscles of the majority of the animal species. There is no indication of depolarization.

A tetanus is not maintained.

* See p. 309.
† See chapter 10.
‡ See chapter 10.

Neostigmine, edrophonium, and the anticholinesterases or well-chosen
doses of depolarizing agents antagonize their effects.
The various animal species usually have similar order of sensitivity.

The various hypotheses for the mechanism of action agree that curare
becomes attached in a reversible manner to receptor sites on the postsynaptic membrane and must prevent the fixation on the sites or penetration across it of acetylcholine molecules. This antagonism has competitive
characteristics.

A fixation on cholinoreceptors on the presynaptic nerve membrane is
also produced without there being an inhibition in transmission.

GALLAMINE TRI-ETHYIODIDE (FLAXEDIL)

Gallamine tri-ethyiodide is a neuromuscular blocking agent which is
slightly less active (4 to 6 times) and has a slightly shorter duration of
action than d-Tc.

The mechanism of its action is entirely comparable to that of d-Tc.
Nevertheless, at low doses which do not produce curarization a slight
facilitation of contractions may be observed.

The three side chains do not appear to play identical roles. Only the
cationic centres at the extremities (positions 1 and 3) becomes fixed on the
receptor. The intermediate chain (in position 2) appears to act mainly to
maintain the other two chains at an appropriate separation (1.5 nm).
Indeed the replacement of the side chain in the position 2 by a non-ionized
substituent $—CO—C_6H_5$(SKF2,o15) does not lead to loss of activity.

DIALLYL-NORTOXIFERINE (ALLOFERINE)

Diallyl-nortoxiferine is a neuromuscular blocking agent which is
slightly more active but with a slightly shorter duration of action than
d-Tc. It has recently been introduced into clinical anesthesiology. Its
mechanism of action is entirely comparable to that of d-Tc.

PANCURONIUM BROMIDE

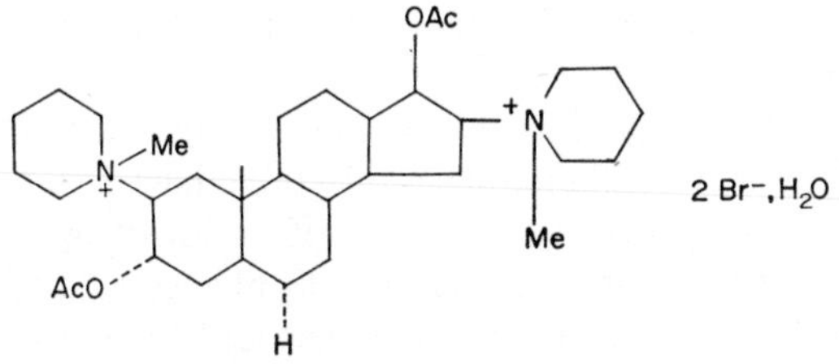

Pancuronium bromide is a bis-ammonium derivative of androstane. It is of competitive type, readily reversed by neostigmine; it possesses 1.5 up to 10 times the potency of *d*-Tc according to the species used for testing while possessing similar duration of action. It has been recently introduced into clinical anesthesiology (Buckett, 1968; Buckett *et al.*, 1968; Bonta and Goorissen, 1968).

TOXINS AND SNAKE VENOMS

The venom of certain Elapides (*Naja, Hemachatus*, etc.) or Hydrophiides (*Enhydrina, Laticauda*, etc.) may produce in man or in animals a paralysis which is slow and not readily reversible (Cheymol *et al.*, 1967 a and b). Toxins responsible for the blockage of neuromuscular transmission have been isolated from these venoms and studied. They are peptides containing 61 or 62 amino acids with a chain maintained in folded form by a number of —S—S— bridges (4 or 5).

Can these peptide molecules be considered as neuromuscular blocking agents? Their massive configuration and the majority of the characteristics of the paralysis they produce argue in favor of this. Nevertheless, the progressive and very prolonged blockade of receptors makes it very difficult to demonstrate a competitive action with acetylcholine or an antagonism by neostigmine or edrophonium.

12.6.3. NEUROMUSCULAR BLOCKING AGENTS OF THE DECAMETHONIUM TYPE

These are all synthetic derivatives which exert their neuromuscular blocking action by a prolonged depolarization of the receptors as would a large excessive dose of acetylcholine, whence their name depolarizing or acetylcholinomimetics. Their molecule is thin, flexible and slender and the cationic centers usually carry methyl radicals which are not sterically hindered (leptocurares).

The complex paralysis which they produce is very variable according to the muscle and the species. These characteristics change more or less rapidly with time.

After a phase of fasciculation and of contracture which is more or less severe, there follows a flaccid paralysis (electrical inexcitability) which has characteristics directly opposite to that of competitive neuromuscular blocking agents. (Tetanus is well maintained, enhancement of the blockade by anticurares, antagonism by curaremimetics.) This is usually followed by a change in the blockade (desensitization of the receptors) resembling a curarization.

Although there are numerous hypotheses, there is at the present time no certainty as to the mechanism of their action at the molecular level* their action extends beyond the motor end-plate to reach the muscle fibers; the nerve terminals are also involved in the action of these depolarizing agents.

SUCCINYLCHOLINE (*Suxamethonium*)

$$Me_3N^+ - CH_2 - CH_2.O.CO.CH_2CH_2.COOCH_2.CH_2N^+Me_3$$

This is a neuromuscular blocking agent which is widely used in anesthesia and is particularly valuable because of its short duration of action. This short duration of action which is linked to its sensitivity to cholinesterase (Hobbiger and Peck, 1969) gives succinylcholine a unique place amongst neuromuscular blocking agents. It is also differentiated from decamethonium by its marked stimulant properties (contracture, fasciculation) which is particularly marked before paralysis. Succinylcholine possesses a presynaptic action which is complex (Standaert and Adams, 1965) and more marked than that of decamethonium: repetitive response to a single stimulus or generation of an action potential independent of all external stimulus.

HEXCARBACHOLINE (606 *HC-Imbretil*)

$$Me_3N^+.CH_2.CH_2.O.CONH - (CH_2)_6 - NH.COO.CH_2CH_2N^+Me_3$$

This is a very active depolarizing molecule similar in many respects to decamethonium. Its peculiarity resides in its interonium distance ("C-16" structure approximately 2 nm); this interonium distance is greater than that in the majority of other neuromuscular blocking agents.

* See pp. 334–343.

TABLE 2.
NEUROMUSCULAR BLOCKING AGENTS WITH MIXED OR "DUAL" ACTION

Group A: Depolarizing and competitives

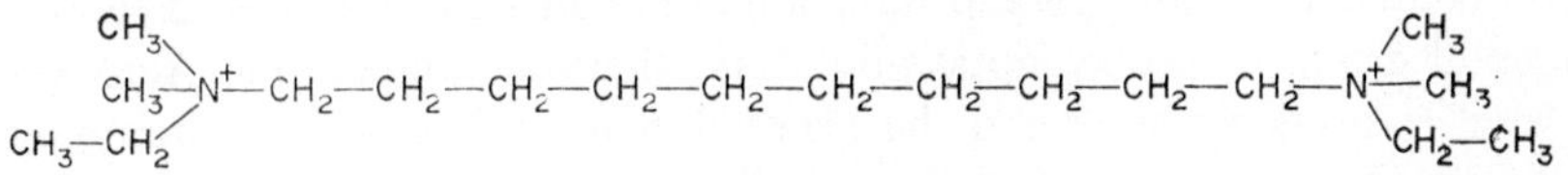

di Me Et–ClO

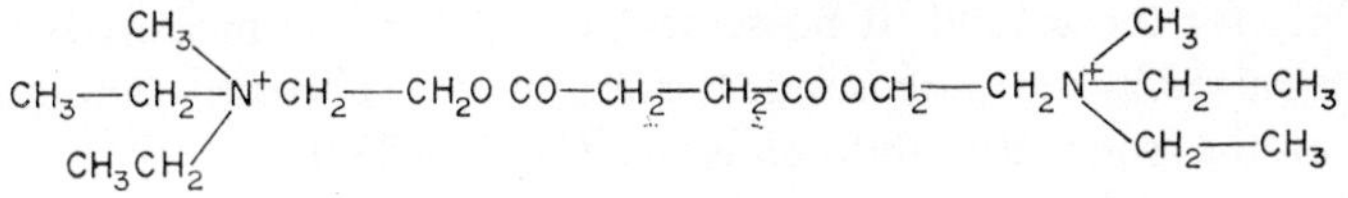

Me di Et Sch

Group B: Competitive and non-competitive

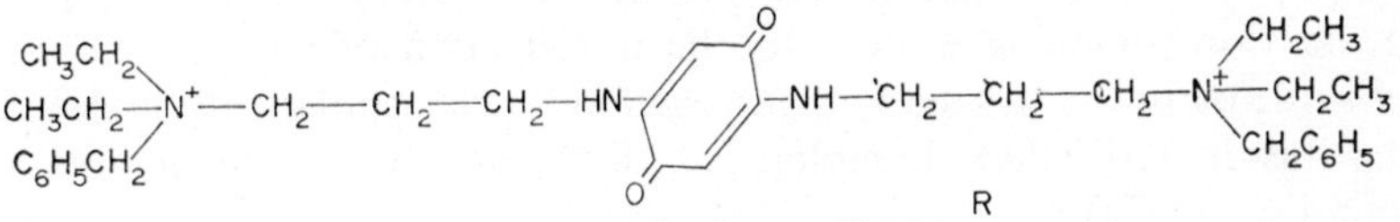

Benzoquinonium or Mytolon

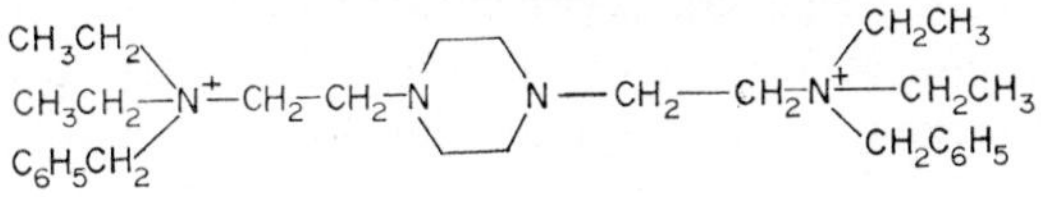

343 H.C.– Isocurine

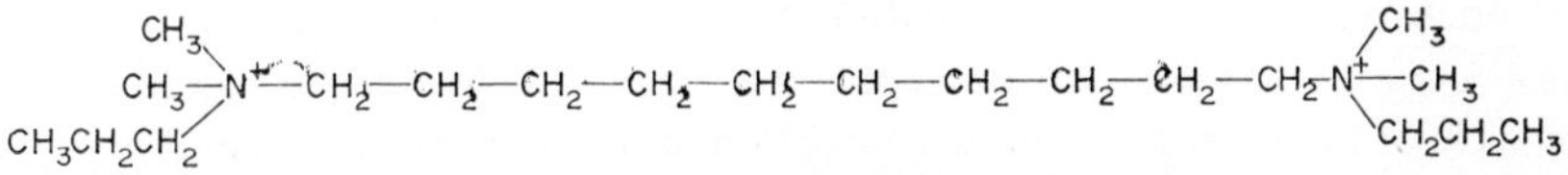

di Me prop ClO

Group C: Depolarizing and non-competitive

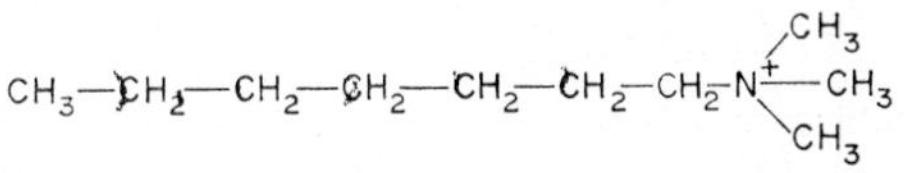

Heptyltrimethylammonium

12.6.4. "HERETICAL" NEUROMUSCULAR BLOCKING AGENTS

This name simply covers without precise definition a certain number of synthetic postsynaptic neuromuscular blocking agents whose mechanism of action are not directly comparable to those of the two main types previously described. A better understanding of their mode of action will

351

probably be obtained in time and will enable these molecules to be separately classified. Such a possible classification has already been suggested by van Rossum and Ariens (1958) who suggested that in addition to the competitive cholinolytics and the cholinomimetics there is a third fundamental group of postsynaptic inhibitors: the non-competitors. Amongst these is prodeconium* and the bis-dimethylheptylammonium homolog of C10. The cationic center of these inhibitors possess a pecularity in having a radical with a long chain CH_2—COO—CH_2—CH_2—CH_3 for the first, and C_7H_{15} for the second. It possesses no depolarizing properties and is not antagonized by the anticurares. It exerts a non-competitive antagonism to ACh on the frog rectus abdominis (see Fig. 7, p.337).

van Rossum and Ariens suggest that in addition there exists intermediary inhibitors between the three main types. These mixed inhibitors may thus be divided into three groups (see Table 2).

Group A. Agents intermediate between depolarizing and competitive agents. Corresponding usually to the introduction of one or two ethyl substituents on the quaternary nitrogen atom of depolarizing molecules (the bis-dimethylethyl homolog of C10 or the bis-methyl-diethyl homolog of SCh).

Group B. Agents intermediate between competitive and non-competitive drugs. Their cationic centers are diethylbenzyl or dimethylpropyl. To this group belong, for example, benzoquinonium, 343HC and the bis-dimethyl-propyl homolog of C10.

Group C. Agents intermediate between the depolarizing and non-competitive agents. This includes heptyltrimethylammonium which produces a non-competitive auto inhibition of the rectus abdominis muscle of the frog. Its cationic center containing both trimethyl and heptyl groups explains its mixed character.

REFERENCES

Many general reviews on the subject have been published, which give an account and a bibliography virtually complete up to 1967. We therefore only mention certain original papers which are among the most important or the most recent.

ACADÉMIE SUISSE DES SCIENCES MÉDICALES (1966) Curare-Symposium. *Bull. Schweiz. Akad. Med. Wiss.* **22**: 391–527; **23**: 5–138.

AESCHLIMANN, J. A. (1951) Curare and anticurare-agents. *Ann. N.Y. Acad. Sci.* **54**: 297–530.

ARIENS, E. J. (1954) Affinity and intrinsic activity in the theory of competitive inhibition. *Arch. Int. Pharmacodyn.* **99**: 32–49.

BARLOW, R. B. (1955) *Introduction to Chemical Pharmacology.* Methuen & Co., Ltd., London; John Wiley & Sons, Inc., New York.

* See p. 325.

BARLOW, R. B. (1960) Steric aspects of drug action. *Biochem. Soc. Symp.* **19**: 46–66.
BARSTAD, J. A. B. and LILLEHEIL, G. (1968) Transversaly cut diaphragm preparation from rat. *Arch. Int. Pharmacodyn.* **175**: 373–90.
BEANI, L. and BIANCHI, C. (1961) L'interferenza della *d*-tubocurarina sulla liberazione di acetilcolina della giunzione neuromusculare: effetto della temperatura e della frequenza di stimulazione. *Boll. Soc. Ital. Biol. Sper.* **37**: 1150–4.
BELLEAU, B. (1964) A molecular theory of drug action based on induced conformational perturbations of receptors. *J. Med. Chem.* **7**: 776–84.
BIGLAND, B., GOETZEE, B., MACLAGAN, J. and ZAIMIS, E. (1958) The effect of lowered muscle temperature on the action of neuromuscular blocking drugs. *J. Physiol. (Lond.)* **141**: 425–34.
BLABER, L. C. and BOWMAN, W. C. (1962) The interaction between benzoquinonium and anticholinesterases in skeletal muscle. *Arch. Int. Pharmacodyn.* **138**: 90–104.
BONTA, I. L. and GOORISSEN, E. M. (1968) Different potency of pancuronium bromide on two types of skeletal muscle. *Europ. J. Pharmacol.* **4**: 303–8.
BOURILLET, F. and CHEYMOL, J. (1966) Pharmacologie des substances curarisantes. *Bull. Schweiz. Akad. Med. Wiss.* **22**: 463–82.
BOVET, D., BOVET-NITTI, F., GUARINO, S., LONGO, V. G. and FUSCO, R. (1951a) Recherches sur les poisons curarisants de synthèse IIIe partie: Succinylcholine et dérivés aliphatiques. *Arch. Int. Pharmacodyn.* **88**: 1–50.
BOVET, D., BOVET-NITTI, F. and MARINI-BETTOLO, G. B. (1959) *Curare and Curare-like Agents.* Elsevier, Amsterdam. 476 pp.
BOVET, D. and VIAUD, P. (1951b) Curares de synthèse: chimie et pharmacologie. *Anesth. Analg.* **8**: 323–78.
BOWEN, J. M. and MERRY, E. H. (1969) Influence of *d*-tubocurarine, decamethonium and succinylcholine on repetitively evoked end-plate potentials. *J. Pharmacol. Exp. Ther.* **167**: 334–43.
BOWMAN, W. C. (1958) The neuromuscular blocking action of benzoquinonium chloride in the cat and in the hen. *Brit. J. Pharmacol.* **13**: 521–30.
BOWMAN, W. C. (1964) Neuromuscular blocking agents. In: *Evaluation of Drug Activities: Pharmacometrics*, pp. 325–51. Academic Press, London and New York.
BROWN, G. L. (1938) The preparation of the tibialis anterior (cat) for close arterial injections. *J. Physiol. (Lond.)* **92**: 22P–3P.
BUCKETT, W. R. (1968) The pharmacology of pancuronium bromide: a new non-depolarising neuromuscular agent. *Irish J. Med. Sci.* (7e) **7**: 565–8.
BUCKETT, W. R., MARJORIBANKS, C. E. B., MARWICK, F. A. and MORTON, M. B. (1968) The pharmacology of pancuronium bromide (ORG. NA 97), a new potent steroidal neuromuscular blocking agent. *Brit. J. Pharmacol.* **32**: 671–82.
BÜLBRING, E. (1946) Observations on the isolated phrenic nerve-diaphragm preparation of the rat. *Brit. J. Pharmacol.* **1**: 38–61.
BURN, J. H. (1950) Curare-like compounds. In: *Biological Standardization*, pp. 345–54. Oxford Medical Publications.
BUTTLE, G. A. H. and ZAIMIS, E. J. (1949) The action of decamethonium iodide in birds. *J. Pharm. Pharmacol.* **1**: 991–2.
CAVALLITO, C. J. (1967) Bonding characteristics of acetylcholine simulants and antagonists and cholinergic receptors. *Ann. N.Y. Acad. Sci.* **144**: 900–12. Some speculations on the chemical nature of post-junctional membrane receptors. *Fed. Proc.* **26**: 1647–54.
CHANG, C. C., CHENG, H. C. and CHEN, T. F. (1967) Does *d*-tubocurarine inhibit the release of acetylcholine from motor nerve endings? *Jap. J. Physiol.* **17**: 505–15.
CHEYMOL, J. (1949) Curares naturels et curares de synthèse. *Actual. Pharmacol.* **1**: 1–52.
CHEYMOL, J. (1954) Curares et anticurares de synthèse—Mécanisme d'action. *Actual. Pharmacol.* **7**: 35–71.

CHEYMOL, J. (1957) Appréciation qualitative et quantitative d'une substance curarisante. *Thérapie* **12**: 321–56.

CHEYMOL, J. (1963) Anticholinergiques inhibiteurs de la jonction neuromusculaire. In: HAZARD, R., CHEYMOL, J., LEVY, J., BOISSIER, J. R. and LECHAT, P. *Manuel de Pharmacologie*, pp. 241–8. Masson, Paris.

CHEYMOL, J. (1969) Acetylcholine, cholinergiques et anticholinergiques. *Prod. Prob. Pharm.* **24**: 6–18.

CHEYMOL, J. and BOURILLET, F. (1960) Etat actuel du problème des substances curarisantes et modificatrices de la curarisation. *Actual. Pharmacol.* **13**: 63–108.

CHEYMOL, J., BOURILLET, F. and OGURA, Y. (1962) Action de quelques paralysants neuromusculaires sur la libération de l'acetylcholine au niveau des terminaisons nerveuses motrices. *Arch. Int. Pharmacodyn.* **139**: 187–97.

CHEYMOL, J., BARME, M., BOURILLET, F. and ROCH-ARVEILLER, M. (1967a) Action neuromusculaire de trois venins d'Hydrophiidés. *Toxicon* **5**: 111–19.

CHEYMOL, J., BOURILLET, F. and ROCH-ARVEILLER, M. (1967b) Actions neuromusculaires comparées des venins de trois Naja. *Arch. Int. Pharmacodyn.* **170**: 193–215.

CHEYMOL, J., DELABY, R., CHABRIER, P., NAJER, H. and BOURILLET, F. (1954) Activité acetylcholinomimétique de quelques dérivés de la carbamoylcholine. *Arch. Int. Pharmacodyn.* **98**: 161–82.

CHILD, K. J. and ZAIMIS, E. (1960) A new biological method for the assay of depolarizing substances using the isolated *semispinalis* muscle of the chick. *Brit. J. Pharmacol.* **15**: 412–16.

CHRIST, D. D. and BLABER, L. C. (1968) The actions of benzoquinonium in the isolated cat tenuissimus muscle. *J. Pharmacol. Exp. Ther.* **160**: 159–65.

COHEN, E. N., RUBINSTEIN, L. J., CORBASCIO, A. N. and HOOD, N. (1967) Localization of *d*-tubocurarine-H3 at the motor end plate. *J. Pharmacol. Exp. Ther.* **157**: 170–4.

CREESE, R., and MACLAGAN, J. (1967) Autoradiography of decamethonium in rat muscle. *Nature (Lond.)* **215**: 988–9.

CREESE, R., TAYLOR, D. B. and TILTON, B. (1963) The influence of curare on the uptake and release of a neuromuscular blocking agent labeled with radioactive iodine. *J. Pharmacol. Exp. Ther.* **139**: 8–17.

DALLEMAGNE, M. J. and PHILIPPOT, E. (1953) La transmission neuromusculaire et son inhibition. Les problèmes qu'elle soulève. *Arch. Ital. Sci. Pharmacol.* **3**: 3.

DEL CASTILLO, J. and KATZ, B. (1957a) A study of curare action with an electrical micromethod. *Proc. Roy. Soc.* B **146**: 339–56.

DEL CASTILLO, J. and KATZ, B. (1957b) Interaction at end-plate receptors between different choline derivatives. *Proc. Roy. Soc.* B **146**: 369–81.

DYBING, F. (1960) The mode of action of decamethonium on neuromuscular transmission in cat. *Acta Pharmacol. Toxicol.* **16**: 291–6.

EHRENPREIS, S. (1967) Cholinergic mechanisms. Introductory remarks. *Ann. N.Y. Acad. Sci.* **144**: 385–6.

EHRENPREIS, S., FLEISH, J. H. and MITTAG, T. W. (1969) Approaches to the molecular nature of pharmacological receptors. *Pharmacol. Rev.* **21**: 131–72.

FATT, P. and KATZ, B. (1951) An analysis of the end-plate potential recorded with an intra-cellular electrode. *J. Physiol. (Lond.)* **115**: 320–70.

FATT, P. and KATZ, B. (1952) Spontaneous subthreshold activity at motor nerve endings. *J. Physiol. (Lond.)* **117**: 109–28.

FOLDES, F. F. (1954) The mode of action of quaternary ammonium type neuromuscular blocking agents. *Brit. J. Anaesth.* **26**: 394–8.

GARCIA DE JALÓN, P. D. (1947) A simple biological assay of curare preparations. *Quart. J. Pharm. Pharmacol.* **20**: 28–30.

GINSBORG, B. L. and WARRINER, J. (1960) The isolated chick biventer cervicis nerve muscle preparation. *Brit. J. Pharmacol.* **15**: 410–11.

GODOVIKOV, N. N., DANILOV, A. F., KABACHNIK, M. I., MICHELSON, M. J. and TEPLOV, N. E. (1968) A new principle of controlled myorelaxation. *Doklady Akademii Nauk SSSR* **183**: 483–5.

HOBBIGER, F. and PECK, A. W. (1969) Hydrolysis of suxamethonium by different types of plasma. *Brit. J. Pharmacol.* **37**: 258–71.

HOPPE, J. O. (1951) A new series of synthetic curare-like compounds. *Ann. N. Y. Acad. Sci.* **54**: 395–406.

HUBBARD, J. I. and SCHMIDT, R. F. (1963) An electrophysiological investigation of mammalian motor nerve terminals. *J. Physiol. (Lond.)* **166**: 145–67.

HUBBARD, J. I., SCHMIDT, R. F. and YOKOTA, T. (1965) The effect of acetylcholine upon mammalian motor nerve terminals. *J. Physiol. (Lond.)* **181**: 810–29.

HUBBARD, J. I., WILSON, D. F. and MIYAMOTO, M. (1969) Reduction of transmitter release by d-tubocurarine. *Nature* **223**: 531–3.

JENKINSON, D. H. (1960) The antagonism between tubocurarine and substances which depolarize the motor end-plate. *J. Physiol. (Lond.)* **152**: 309–24.

JONES, J. J., and LAITY, J. L. H. (1965) A note on an unusual effect of gallamine and tubocurarine. *Brit. J. Pharmacol.* **24**: 360–4.

KARCZMAR, A. G. (1967) Neuromuscular pharmacology. *Annu. Rev. Pharmacol.* **7**: 241–76.

KATZ, B. and MILEDI, R. (1965) Propagation of electric activity in motor nerve terminals. *Proc. Roy. Soc.* B **161**: 453–82.

KATZ, B. (1966) *Nerve, Muscle and Synapse.* McGraw-Hill, Inc., New York.

KHROMOV-BORISOV, N. V. and MICHELSON, M. J. (1966) The mutual disposition of cholinoreceptors of locomotor muscles and the changes in their disposition in the course of evolution. *Pharmacol. Rev.* **18**: 1051–90.

LAITY, J. L. H. (1967) A new nerve muscle preparation: the obturator nerve–anterior gracilis preparation of the rat. *J. Pharm. Pharmacol.* **19**: 265–6.

MACKAY, D. (1963) A flux-carrier hypothesis of drug action. *Nature* **197**: 1171–3.

MACLAGAN, J. (1962) A comparison of the responses of the *tenuissimus* muscle to neuromuscular blocking drugs *in vivo* and *in vitro*. *Brit. J. Pharmacol.* **18**: 204–16.

NACHMANSOHN, D. (1952) *Nerve Impulse*, p. 44. Josiah Macy Jr. Foundation, New York.

NACHMANSOHN, D. (1959) Physiochemical mechanism of nerve activity. Muscular contraction. *Ann. N. Y. Acad. Sci.* **81**: 215–510.

OSSERMAN, K. E. (1966) Myasthenia gravis. *Ann. N. Y. Acad. Sci.* **135**: 1–680.

PATON, W. D. M. (1961) A theory of drug action based on the rate of drug–receptor combination. *Proc. Roy. Soc. London*, B, **154**: 21–69.

PATON, W. D. M. and WAUD, D. R. (1962) Drug receptors interactions at the neuromuscular junction. *Curare and Curare-like Agents*, pp. 34–54. de Reuck, A. S. V. (ed.). Ciba Foundation Study Group no. 12. J. & A. Churchill Ltd., London.

PATON, W. D. M. and ZAIMIS, E. J. (1952) The methonium compounds. *Pharmacol. Rev.* **4**: 219–53.

RANG, H. P. and RITTER, J. M. (1969) Evidence for a molecular change in acetylcholine receptors produced by agonists. *Brit. J. Pharmacol.* **36**: 182 P.

DE REUCK, A. V. S. (1962) *Curare and Curare-like Agents.* Ciba Foundation Study Group no. 12. J. & A. Churchill Ltd., London.

RIKER, W. F., ROBERTS, J., STANDAERT, F. G. and FUJIMORI, H. (1957) The motor nerve terminal as the primary focus for drug-induced facilitation of neuromuscular transmission. *J. Pharmacol. Exp. Ther.* **121**: 286–312.

STANDAERT, F. G. (1964) The action of d-tubocurarine on the motor nerve terminal. *J. Pharmacol. Exp. Ther.* **143**: 181–6.

STANDAERT, F. G. and ADAMS, J. E. (1965) The actions of succinylcholine on the mammalian motor nerve terminal. *J. Pharmacol. Exp. Ther.* **149**, 113–23.

STANDAERT, F. G. and RIKER, W. F. (1967) The consequences of cholinergic drug actions on motor nerve terminals. *Ann. N.Y. Acad. Sci.* **144**: 517–33.

STEPHENSON, R. P. (1956) A modification of receptor theory. *Brit. J. Pharmacol.* **11**: 379–93.

STRAUGHAN, D. W. (1960) The release of acetylcholine from mammalian motor nerve endings. *Brit. J. Pharmacol.* **15**: 417–24.

SUAREZ-KURTZ, G., PAULO, L. G. and FONTELES, M. C. (1969) Further studies on the neuromuscular effects of β-diethylaminoethyl-diphenylpropylacetate hydrochloride (SKF-525-A). *Arch. Int. Pharmacodyn.* **177**: 185–95.

TAYLOR, D. B. (1962) Influence of curare on uptake and release of neuromuscular blocking agent labeled with iodine-131. *Curare and Curare-like Agents*, pp. 21–33. de Reuck, A. S. V. (ed.) Ciba Foundation Study Group no. 12. J. & A. Churchill Ltd., London.

TAYLOR, D. B. and NEDERGAARD, O. A. (1965) Relation between structure and action of quaternary ammonium neuromuscular blocking agents. *Physiol. Rev.* **45**: 523–54.

TAYLOR, D. B., DIXON, W. J., CREESE, R. and CASE, R. (1967) Diffusion of decamethonium in the rat. *Nature (Lond.)* **215**: 989.

THESLEFF, B. and QUASTEL, D. M. J. (1965) Neuromuscular pharmacology. *Annu. Rev. Pharmacol.* **5**: 263–84.

VALLÉE, R. (1957) Le Prestonal, curarisant de synthèse. Etude théorique en fonction d'acquisitions récentes. *Acta Anaesthesiol., Belg.* **1**: 157–74.

VAN RIEZEN, H. (1968) Classification of neuromuscular blocking agents in a new neuromuscular preparation of the chick *in vitro*. *Europ. J. Pharmacol.* **5**: 29–36.

VAN ROSSUM, J. M., ARIENS, E. J. and LINSSEN, G. H. (1958) Basic types of curariform drugs. *Biochem. Pharmacol.* **1**: 193–9.

VARNEY, R. F., LINEGAR, C. R. and HOLADAY, M. A. (1949) The assay of curare by the rabbit "head-drop" method. *J. Pharmacol. Exp. Ther.* **97**: 72–83.

WASER, P. G. (1963) Les récepteurs cholinergiques. *Actual. Pharmacol.* **16**: 169–93.

WASER, P. G. (1967) Receptor localization by autoradiographic techniques. *Ann. N.Y. Acad. Sci.* **144**: 737–55.

WAUD, D. R. (1968) The nature of "depolarization block". *Anesthesiology* **29**: 1014–24.

ZAIMIS, E. J. (1953) Motor end-plate differences as a determining factor in the mode of action of neuromuscular blocking substances. *J. Physiol. (Lond.)* **122**: 238–51.

ZAIMIS, E. (1954) Transmission and block at the motor end-plate and in autonomic ganglia. The interruption of neuromuscular transmission and some of its problems. *Pharmacol. Rev.* **6**: 53–7.

ZAIMIS, E. J. (1962). Experimental hazards and artefact in the study of neuromuscular blocking drugs. *Curare and Curare-like Agents*, pp. 75–86. de Reuck, A. S. V. (ed.). Ciba Foundation Study Group no. 12. J. & A. Churchill Ltd., London.

ZAIMIS, E. J. (1966) Factors which may modify the pharmacological action of curare. *Bull. Schweiz. Akad. Med. Wiss.* **22**: 516–24.

ZAIMIS, E. (1969) General physiology and pharmacology of neuromuscular transmission. In: *Disorders of Voluntary Muscle*, 2nd ed., pp. 57–87. J. & A. Churchill Ltd., London.

CHAPTER 13

INHIBITORS OF ACETYLCHOLINE SYNTHESIS

W. C. Bowman and I. G. Marshall

Glasgow

13.1. ACETYLCHOLINE SYNTHESIS

Acetylcholine (ACh) is synthesized in cholinergic nerve endings from choline and acetyl CoA under the influence of the enzyme, choline acetyltransferase (ChAc) (Korey *et al.*, 1951). ChAc is present in isolated synaptosomes, and density gradient studies on ruptured synaptosomes have shown that most of it is located in the soluble cytoplasm, with some bound to membrane structures (Whittaker *et al.*, 1964; Tuček, 1966; Fonnum, 1966, 1967; Potter, 1968). The degree of solubilization of ChAc depends on the ionic strength of the environment (Fonnum, 1966, 1967) but both the soluble and the bound forms exhibit enzymatic activity (Fonnum, 1968). Subcellular fractionation studies show that ACh itself is located in the microsomal fraction of nerve endings, presumably in the synaptic vesicles (Whittaker *et al.*, 1964; Potter, 1968), and the fact that it is thus separated from its synthesizing enzyme suggests that a mechanism of transporting the synthesized transmitter into its storage particles may be present. Earlier studies by de Robertis and co-workers (1963) had led to the view that both ChAc and ACh were located in the synaptic vesicles. McCaman *et al.* (1965) suggested that species differences in the binding of ChAc to vesicles could account for the discrepancy between the results of de Robertis *et al.* (1963) and those of other workers. However, Tuček (1966) obtained evidence that the fraction studied by de Robertis *et al.* (1963) contained membrane structures other than those of the synaptic vesicles, and that the enzyme was associated with these rather than with the vesicles. The problem of apparent species differences in the localization of ChAc noted by McCaman *et al.* (1965) has been resolved by

357

Fonnum (1970) who found that differences in the surface charge of ChAc from different species leads to different affinities for membranes. The recent report of vesicular synthesis of ACh (Ritchie and Goldberg, 1970) can probably be explained by the fact that the fractions were prepared by the technique of de Robertis *et al.* (1963), and it is hence likely that the vesicle fractions were contaminated with precipitated ChAc.

The identity of the precursor of the acetyl moiety of acetyl CoA for ACh synthesis has also been the subject of some controversy. Pyruvate was suggested by Quastel *et al.* (1936) and acetate and citrate have also been suggested (Lipton and Barron, 1946; Hebb, 1954; Tuček, 1967 a and b). Tuček (1967b) suggested that citrate was the most likely precursor as he found that synthesis of ACh occurred faster in the presence of citrate than in that of acetate, possibly because of the higher extra-mitochondrial localization of ATP citrate lyase. More recent experiments on the synthesis of ACh from radioactively labeled precursors both in brain slices *in vitro* and in the rat brain *in vitro* have shown pyruvate to be the principal precursor (Nakamura *et al.*, 1970; Tuček and Cheng, 1970).

Choline, which is a constituent of diet, is present in extracellular fluids in amounts which differ in different species (Bligh, 1952), and under normal conditions there is enough choline present to support ACh synthesis no matter how heavy the traffic of nerve impulses. However, in experiments with perfused sympathetic ganglia, Birks and MacIntosh (1961) found it necessary to add choline in physiological concentrations (about 10 mcM) to the perfusate, in order to maintain optimal rates of transmitter output in response to nerve stimulation; radioactive choline added to the perfusate is incorporated into ACh, as well as into phosphorylcholine and phospholipid (Friesen *et al.*, 1965; Collier and Lang, 1969; Collier and MacIntosh, 1969).

The fact that choline is a highly ionized quaternary ammonium compound suggested that it would not penetrate lipid membranes from the extracellular fluid to the site of its acetylation within the nerve endings, unless some special transport mechanism were present (MacIntosh, 1963), and more recent evidence indicates that this is in fact so. Radioactive choline is taken up by isolated synaptosomes by a mechanism involving two components, one linear and one saturable (Marchbanks, 1968; Potter, 1968; Bosmann and Hemsworth, 1970). ChAc is present in isolated synaptosomes and a proportion of the choline taken up is converted to ACh (Hebb and Whittaker, 1958; Tuček, 1967a; Marchbanks, 1969). ACh exists within synaptosomes in two compartments, in the cytoplasm and in the vesicles; most of the choline taken up is incorporated into the cytoplasmic ACh (Marchbanks, 1969; Chakrin and Whittaker, 1969). Guth (1969) demonstrated a greater vesicular uptake of ACh at 37°C than did Marchbanks (1969) at 5°C, and he suggests that the low temperature used by Marchbanks may have decreased the kinetic energy of the ACh to a level at which vesicular uptake ceased.

Choline uptake is not a specific property of cholinergic nerve endings. Other cells, including non-cholinergic squid axons (Hodgkin and Martin, 1965), erythrocytes (Askari, 1966; Martin, 1968) and kidney cells (Vander, 1962; Sung and Johnstone, 1965) also possess transport mechanisms for choline. All these transport mechanisms have features in common (Potter, 1968), but some differences may be demonstrated with regard to the specificity of inhibitors. Presumably choline is required in non-cholinergic cells for the synthesis of phospholipid rather than of ACh.

Although glucose and oxygen are necessary for optimal synthesis of ACh (Kahlson and MacIntosh, 1939), there is no convincing evidence that choline uptake into cholinergic synaptosomes is an active, energy-requiring process, since it is not much affected by KCN, DNP or ouabain, and is essentially the same whether the synaptosomes are incubated in a medium containing only tris buffer or in one containing an external energy source (Potter, 1968; Marchbanks, 1968; Diamond and Kennedy, 1969; Bosmann and Hemsworth, 1970; Hemsworth *et al.*, 1971). However, the evidence is consistent with a facilitated uptake mechanism involving a specific carrier molecule in the saturable component of choline transport, since it is temperature dependent, requires a certain ionic milieu, and may be competitively inhibited by drugs (Potter, 1968).

In Potter's (1968) experiments the bulk of the sequestered labeled choline was found in the supernatant fluid after subcellular fractionation, with very little in the microsomal fraction. However, under the conditions of Bosmann and Hemsworth's (1970) experiments the synaptic vesicle fraction contained the highest choline–^{14}C activity; uptake into vesicles was more susceptible to inhibition by ouabain, DNP or KCN than was uptake into whole synaptosomes, but even here the inhibition was unimpressive and required high concentrations. Potter's results appear more compatible with current theories relating to the transmission mechanisms at cholinergic nerve endings, but it is always difficult to correlate *in vitro* results precisely with physiological events *in vivo*. Various factors may influence the results obtained *in vitro*. For example, Burton and Howard (1967) showed that whereas K^+ increases the uptake of choline into nerve-ending fractions, it decreases that into synaptic vesicles. The whole question concerning the role of ions is complex. Synthesis of ACh in intact neurones is dependent on the presence of sodium ions (Wolfgram, 1954; Birks, 1963; Bhatnager and MacIntosh, 1967) and it has been suggested that entry of Na^+ into the axoplasm during the rising phase of the action potential may be the factor that gears synthesis to release. According to Marchbanks (1968, 1969) and Potter (1968), choline uptake by nerve endings is dependent on the presence of Na^+; in Potter's (1968) experiments uptake into isolated synaptosomes was nil when all the sodium was replaced by lithium.

In contrast, Bosmann and Hemsworth (1970) found that omission of Na^+ had little effect on the uptake of choline by whole synaptosomes, but Na^+ lack increased the uptake into the chloroform-soluble (lipid) fraction and into the TCA-insoluble (protein) fraction, as also did lack of K^+ or Mg^{++}. Na^+ was the most powerful inhibitor of uptake into the chloroform-soluble fraction, whereas Mg^{++} was the most powerful in inhibiting uptake into the TCA-insoluble fraction. There is general agreement that absence of K^+ and Mg^{++} has little effect on the incorporation of choline into intact synaptosomes (Marchbanks, 1968; Potter, 1968; Bosmann and Hemsworth, 1970). Bosmann and Hemsworth (1970) speculate that the ionic environment in the immediate vicinity of the subcellular particles may function as a control mechanism determining whether choline is incorporated into lipid, or whether it is made available for acetylation. Thus, a relatively high intracellular Na^+ content associated with a heavy traffic of nerve impulses may inhibit incorporation of choline into lipid and make it available for transmitter synthesis.

In the absence of choline, ACh is taken up into isolated nerve endings by a saturable mechanism, although somewhat less rapidly than is choline (Schuberth and Sundwall, 1968; Potter, 1968; Bosmann and Hemsworth, 1970). Synaptic vesicles also take up ACh to a lesser extent than choline (Burton and Howard, 1967). In the presence of physostigmine, ACh acts as a weak competitive inhibitor of choline transport (Potter, 1968), indicating that both choline and ACh are transported by the same carrier. In Bosmann and Hemsworth's (1970) experiments, the chloroform-soluble fraction of isolated synaptosomes did not take up ACh, indicating that, unlike choline, it is not incorporated into lipid.

Perry (1953) concluded, from experiments on the perfused superior cervical ganglion of the cat, that the choline set free by enzymatic hydrolysis of the transmitter was taken up again by the nerve endings and resynthesized into ACh. More recent studies using radioactive choline have confirmed this conclusion (Collier and MacIntosh, 1969). Since ACh itself may be taken up into isolated nerve endings, re-uptake of intact transmitter must also be considered as an alternative means of inactivation and replenishment (Potter, 1968). It has also been shown that newly synthesized ACh in sympathetic ganglia may be preferentially released by presynaptic nerve impulses, suggesting that it gains rapid access to the readily releasable transmitter pool (Collier, 1969; Collier and MacIntosh, 1969).

Clearly, a lack of any of the factors necessary for the synthesis of ACh will inhibit its formation in cholinergic nerve endings, but the most practical and specific line of attack is by drugs that prevent the action of ChAc, and these may act by direct inhibition or by preventing the access of choline to the site of the enzyme.

13.2. DIRECT INHIBITORS OF CHOLINE ACETYLTRANSFERASE

ChAc was first isolated from cell-free extracts of brain and electric organ by Nachmansohn and Machado (1943) and since that time many chemicals have been examined as potential inhibitors. Amongst the compounds found to have weak inhibitory activity *in vitro* (less than 50% enzyme inhibition at 10^{-3} M) were α-keto acids (Nachmansohn and John, 1944, 1945; Nachmansohn and Weiss, 1948), naphthoquinones (Nachmansohn and Berman, 1946; Nachmansohn and Weiss, 1948), nicotine (Fahmy *et al.*, 1954), barbiturates (Marks, 1956), tetramethylammonium, choline, ACh, neostigmine, decamethonium and succinylcholine (Berman-Reisberg, 1954; Smith *et al.*, 1967). However, it is unlikely that any effects these compounds may exert on cholinergic transmission are mediated by inhibition of ChAc.

Recently Smith *et al.* (1966, 1967) have reported that some members of a series of styryl-pyridine analogs possess potent antiChAc activities. The most potent, which had been previously tested for neuromuscular blocking activity (Cavallito *et al.*, 1964), was hexamethylene-1,4-(1-naphthylvinyl)-pyridinium-6-trimethylammonium, which contains a quaternary pyridinium ring being part of a transconjugated coplanar structure linked by a hexamethylene chain to a trimethylammonium group. This compound produced 50% enzyme inhibition at a concentration of 9×10^{-7} M. However, it was almost equiactive as an inhibitor of acetylcholinesterase. Structural modification of the styryl-pyridine analogs produced more specific inhibitors of ChAc, the most specific being 4-(1-naphthylvinyl) pyridine, although several of these analogs have recently been found to possess an independent action on the hexo-barbitone-metabolizing enzyme system (Goldberg *et al.*, 1971).

4-(1-naphthylvinyl) pyridine

From an analysis of structure–action relationships (Smith *et al.*, 1967; Cavallito *et al.*, 1969, 1970, 1971; Baker and Gibson, 1971) and physico-chemical properties (Allen *et al.*, 1970) within the series it was concluded that for optimal inhibition of ChAc it was necessary to have a π-electron excessive aryl moiety conjugated to a π-electron deficient pyridinium moiety, through a double or triple bond to produce a thin, flat molecule. The trimethylammonium alkane side-chain appeared to be relatively unimportant for antiChAc activity, but it contributed to the anticholin-esterase activity. Studies of the effects of the styryl-pyridine analogs on neuromuscular transmission indicated that *in vivo* the compounds do not exert their primary effect on ChAc, but act directly on the muscle fiber to produce an irreversible block of muscle contractions (Hemsworth and Foldes, 1970). Therefore, as yet, no compounds have been shown to exert their primary effects on cholinergic transmission either *in vivo* or *in vitro*, via direct inhibition of ChAc. Since a prerequisite of any potential inhibitor of ChAc will be an intracellular site of action, it seems likely, in view of the well-known impermeability of biological membranes to quaternary ammonium compounds, that such a substance will be a tertiary or secondary amine.

13.3. INHIBITORS OF CHOLINE TRANSPORT

13.3.1. HEMICHOLINIUMS

During the investigation of the anticholinesterase activity of a number of bisphenacyl derivatives (Long and Schueler, 1954; Schueler, 1955), it was found that the compound α,α'-dimethylethanolamino 4,4'-biaceto-phenone was virtually devoid of anticholinesterase activity, but exhibited an unusual form of delayed toxicity which in some ways resembled that of botulism. This compound contained two choline moieties and in a study of structural analogs of this compound Schueler (1955) found that the original compound was the most potent.

After showing that the compounds underwent hemiacetal formation (Fig. 1), Schueler coined the name "hemicholiniums" for the series. The pharmacology of a,a'-dimethylethanolamino 4,4'-biacetophenone, which is known as hemicholinium-3 or HC-3, has been studied in great detail. Schueler (1960) reviewed much of the earlier work.

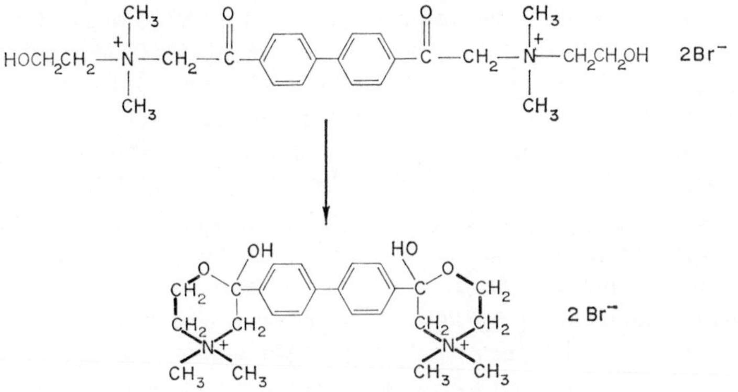

FIG. 1. Hemicholinium No. 3 (HC-3). The thickened lines indicate the two choline moieties.

In all animals studied, death after minimal lethal doses of HC-3 results from a gradually developing respiratory failure. In general, the toxic dose on a body-weight basis is greater, and the time to death longer, in larger animals (Schueler, 1955). This is unusual, since larger animals generally metabolize drugs more slowly, with the result that in most cases the lethal dose for a large animal is lower than that for a small animal. However, smaller animals breathe more rapidly which suggested that respiratory failure after HC-3 is related to breathing rate. The delayed respiratory failure produced by HC-3 is poorly antagonized by anticholinesterase drugs, but pretreatment with choline provides a marked protective effect (Schueler, 1955; Giovinco, 1957).

Kasé and Borison (1958) and Borison (1961) were of the opinion that the respiratory failure produced by HC-3 after systemic administration was mainly due to a depression of the respiratory regulatory mechanism in the brain stem. However, other studies have provided results which appear more consistent with the well-known inability of quaternary ammonium compounds to penetrate the blood–brain barrier (Schueler *et al.*, 1954;

Domer and Schueler, 1960; Dren and Domino, 1968a). Longo (1958, 1959) found little change in phrenic nerve action potentials recorded during full respiratory paralysis produced by HC-3, and subsequent work has provided convincing evidence of a peripheral action which is sufficient to account for its respiratory paralyzing action. Small doses of HC-3, both *in vivo* and *in vitro*, produce a slowly developing failure of neuro-muscular transmission in nerve-skeletal muscle preparations of guinea-pigs, rats, rabbits, cats, dogs and chickens which is dependent upon the frequency of stimulation of the motor nerve (Schueler, 1955; Long and Reitzel, 1958; Reitzel and Long, 1959a; Wilson and Long, 1959; Chang and Rand, 1960; Rand and Chang, 1960; Bowman and Rand, 1961b; Evans and Wilson, 1962, 1964; Bowman *et al.*, 1967; Marshall, 1969; Takagi *et al.*, 1970). Although the necessary pattern of nerve stimulation differs to some extent in different species and under different conditions, in general small doses are ineffective at frequencies of stimulation below 1 Hz and increase in effectiveness as the stimulation frequency is increased. The neuromuscular blocking action of small doses of HC-3 is only weakly and transiently antagonized by anticholinesterase drugs, but is powerfully antagonized by choline, or by reducing the stimulation frequency. Similar effects of HC-3 and choline have been demonstrated at some autonomic cholinergic neuro-effector junctions (Everett, 1966, 1968; Vanov, 1965; Rand & Ridehalgh, 1965; Dhattiwala *et al.*, 1970; Appel and Vincenzi, 1970), and in sympathetic ganglia (Birks and MacIntosh, 1961; Bhatnager *et al.*, 1965). Direct bioassay of the ACh released into the fluid bathing isolated nerve-muscle preparations or into the fluid perfusing a sympa-thetic ganglion shows that HC-3 reduces the output evoked by nerve stimulation (Matthews, 1966; Cheymol *et al.*, 1962; Chang, Cheng and Chen, 1967).

Several analogs of choline have been tested for their ability to reverse the neuromuscular transmission failure produced by small doses of HC-3 (Giovinco, 1957; Reitzel and Long, 1959b). All were found to be ineffective except β-hydroxyethyldimethylethyl ammonium which produced a partial antagonism. Several esters of choline, including ACh, were effective antagonists, but this appeared to be due to the choline set free from them by their rapid hydrolysis, since the antagonism was prevented by treatment with anticholinesterase drugs.

The extracellular fluid in different species contains different levels of free choline (Bligh, 1952) and this is likely to be a factor, in addition to variations in respiratory rate, which contributes to the size of the smallest effective dose of HC-3 in different species. Schueler (1960) observed that even in the same species (mice) there was a wide variation in the smallest effective doses for different batches of animals. This may reflect differences in dietary choline intake, since HC-3 has been shown to be more effective in mice deprived of dietary choline (Angeles *et al.*, 1964). Yet another factor contributing markedly to the size of the minimum effective dose is the activity of the animals (whether restrained, allowed to, or forced to indulge in exercise). In accordance with the dependence of the HC-3 effect on stimulation frequency in nerve–muscle preparations, the drug is more active in paralyzing animals undergoing exercise.

The virtually specific antagonistic action of choline suggested that HC-3 in some way interferes with the choline metabolism of nervous tissue, and thus leads to a decreased synthesis, and hence output, of ACh. HC-3 was found to inhibit the synthesis of ACh by sympathetic ganglia, and by minced brain tissue, but to have no direct effect on ChAc obtained from acetone-dried brain powders (MacIntosh *et al.*, 1956). MacIntosh *et al.* (1956) postulated that HC-3 inhibited ACh synthesis in intact nervous tissue by competing with choline for a specific transport mechanism responsible for carrying extracellular choline to its intracellular sites of acetylation. Gardiner (1961) confirmed this suggestion when he found that HC-3 inhibited ACh synthesis in guinea-pig brain homogenates, but had no effect in homogenates pretreated with ether, a procedure which disrupts membranes surrounding the ChAc (Hebb and Smallman, 1956). HC-3 has also been shown to inhibit active secretion of choline by avian kidney tubules (MacIntosh *et al.*, 1958), and to inhibit choline uptake into erythrocytes (Martin, 1968, 1969) isolated perfused rabbit hearts (Buterbaugh and Spratt, 1968; Buterbaugh *et al.*, 1968), and isolated synaptosomes (Marchbanks, 1968; Potter, 1968; Hemsworth *et al.*, 1971) and synaptic vesicles (Hemsworth *et al.*, 1971). The last-named authors found that, although larger concentration of HC-3 inhibited choline uptake into isolated synaptosomes, smaller concentrations (10^{-5} M) augmented it.

Electron-microscope studies of the effects of HC-3 on synaptic vesicles have shown that, in unstimulated preparations from the rat phrenic nerve (Jones and Kwanbunbumpen, 1968, 1970) and parietal cortex (Csillik and Jóo, 1967), HC-3 reduces the number but not the volume or shape of the vesicles, although Rodriguez de Lores Arnaiz *et al.* (1970) observed no reduction of numbers of vesicles in the rat cerebral cortex. In preparations of the rat phrenic nerve–diaphragm stimulated at 11.3 Hz for 90 minutes in the presence of HC-3, Jones and Kwanbunbumpen (1970) found that mitochondria at the end-plates became swollen with a disordered internal structure, and that vesicle numbers were significantly reduced in comparison not only with control preparations, but also with the unstimulated HC-3 treated preparations. In addition it was shown that HC-3, plus stimulation, produced a significant fall in vesicle volume, although, as in the unstimulated preparations, vesicle shape remained unchanged.

The action of HC-3 is not entirely prejunctional at the neuromuscular junction. In large doses it produces an immediate respiratory paralysis which differs from the delayed effect of small doses in that it may be reversed by anticholinesterase drugs, but not by choline (Schueler, 1955). This suggests that, as might be expected from its chemical structure, large doses exert a postjunctional curare-like block of motor end-plate receptors, and this has been confirmed in experiments on isolated nerve–muscle preparations (Reitzel and Long, 1959a; Bowman and Rand, 1961b; Prasad and MacLeod, 1966; Marshall, 1969; Takagi *et al.*, 1970). The postjunctional blocking action may contribute to a small extent to the paralysis produced by small doses, since even before any transmission failure becomes evident, as judged by the amplitude of the maximal twitch, some depression of responses to ACh and related agonists is observed. Any postjunctional blocking action must become relatively more important as transmitter output fails and normal safety margin in transmitter release (Paton and Waud, 1967) becomes diminished. Transmission failure produced in sympathetic ganglia by HC-3 follows a similar pattern to that at the neuromuscular junction in that it is frequency-dependent and reversible by choline. However, the interonium distance in HC-3 is too great for effective combination with postsynaptic ACh receptors at this site, and here its action is almost exclusively presynaptic (Bhatnager *et al.*, 1965). In smooth muscle HC-3 has been shown to possess some atropine-like action, but this is too weak to contribute much to the transmission failure (Everett, 1966; Bertolini *et al.*, 1967; Györgi *et al.*, 1970).

Intracellular recording techniques at the neuromuscular junction have confirmed that HC-3 possesses both pre- and postjunctional actions. Initial studies showed that HC-3 in large doses blocks neuromuscular transmission and reduces the amplitudes of e.p.p.s and m.e.p.p.s. These effects, which were recorded during low rates of nerve stimulation or in its absence, were associated with a reduced sensitivity to applied ACh, showing that the site of action was postjunctional. They were reversed by physostigmine but not by choline (Martin and Orkand, 1960, 1961; Thies and Brooks, 1961). Elmqvist *et al.* (1963) and Elmqvist and Quastel (1965) performed similar measurements except that preformed transmitter was rapidly released either by nerve stimulation or by KCl.

Under these conditions the amplitudes of the e.p.p.s and m.e.p.p.s were again reduced by HC-3, but by lower concentrations, and in this case the changes occurred in the absence of any decrease in postjunctional chemosensitivity, showing that the effect was located in the nerve endings and was due to a reduction in the size of ACh quanta.

Elmqvist and Quastel (1965) calculated the number of quanta of ACh released in the presence of HC-3, assuming that synthesis was completely blocked, by summing all the e.p.p.s and m.e.p.p.s, and hence they obtained an estimate of the size of the prejunctional store of ACh. In the rat diaphragm this figure was found to be 270,000 ± 70,000 quanta. Similar results were obtained in human intercostal muscles, the mean value being 218,000 quanta (Elmqvist *et al.*, 1964).

The combined results of all these experiments strongly support the postulate of MacIntosh *et al.* (1956) that the main action of HC-3 is to compete with choline for a carrier mechanism in the nerve endings with the result that ChAc is deprived of its substrate for ACh synthesis. Transmission failure becomes evident when the preformed stores of ACh have been partially exhausted by frequent nerve impulses and when synthesis is inhibited to the extent that it cannot keep up with the demand. Excess choline then overcomes the transmission failure by competing more favorably with HC-3 for the carrier mechanism and so restoring substrate to the synthesizing enzyme. Choline, however, possesses additional actions at the neuromuscular junction. It has a weak postjunctional depolarizing action (Hutter, 1952) and it also has some action in increasing the release of preformed ACh (Hutter, 1952). Both of these additional effects could contribute to restoration of transmission failure, and they are probably responsible for the weak, limited and short-lasting anticurare action of choline. It is important to realize therefore that reversal by choline is not by itself a reliable indication of a prejunctional HC-3 type of action, although if the reversal is complete and long lasting it is a strong indication that the transmission failure did arise from such a mechanism. In this connection, the ability of β-hydroxyethyldimethylethyl ammonium, alone among choline analogs tested, partially to restore neuromuscular transmission depressed by HC-3, is of interest (Reitzel and Long, 1959b). The acetyl ester of this compound possesses weak ACh-like activity, and its limited action against HC-3 therefore appears to be an early example of the formation of a "false transmitter".

MacIntosh (1961) has suggested that HC-3, by combining with the choline carrier, may itself be transported to intracellular sites in place of choline, and then compete with ACh for intracellular binding sites, presumably at the level of the synaptic vesicle membrane. Rodriguez de Lores Arnaiz *et al.* (1970) have shown that HC-3 may be acetylated by ChAc, although the efficiency of acetylation is only about 20–25% of that of choline, and they have hence suggested that acetyl-HC-3 may be released as a false transmitter.

Although considerably less effective than at most cholinergic junctions, HC-3 has been shown to block transmission in some sympathetically innervated preparations and this effect is reversed by choline (Rand and Chang, 1960; Chang and Rand, 1960; Brandon and Rand, 1961; Rand and Ridehalgh, 1965). These results have been used in support of the theory of a cholinergic step in adrenergic transmission originally proposed by Burn and Rand (1959), although HC-3 is apparently not effective at all adrenergic junctions (Wilson and Long, 1959; Birks and MacIntosh, 1961; Gardiner and Thompson, 1961; Bevan and Su, 1964; Vincenzi and West, 1965; Leaders, 1965; Everett, 1968; Appel and Vincenzi, 1970). It has been suggested that HC-3 may possess an action on nervous tissue apart from its ability to inhibit the uptake of choline (Frazier, 1968). Frazier *et al.* (1969, 1970) have studied the non-cholinergic effects of HC-3 on squid axons. HC-3 was ineffective when applied externally, but on internal application it reduced the size of the nerve action potential probably by an action on sodium and potassium permeability. It appears unlikely that these effects can account for the actions of externally applied HC-3 on some sympathetic nerves.

Several workers have studied the central actions of HC-3 after intra-ventricular injection of the compound. HC-3 produces a brief period of catatonia on intraventricular injection into conscious animals (Slater, 1968a) followed occasionally by seizures (Shellenberger and Domino, 1967; Slater, 1968a). It also causes a simultaneous reduction of brain ACh (Hebb *et al.*, 1964; Slater, 1968a, b; Dren and Domino, 1968a; Rodriguez de Lores Arnaiz *et al.*, 1970) and this effect is prevented by previous administration of choline (Slater, 1968a). Intraventricular injection of HC-3 reduces the conversion of choline to ACh in the canine caudate nucleus (Gomez *et al.*, 1970). HC-3 antagonizes the tremor produced by tremorine and physostigmine in rats and chicks (Bowman and Osuide, 1968; Slater and Rogers, 1968) and prevents the rise in brain ACh produced by these compounds (Crossland and Slater, 1968). Choline reverses the inhibition of ACh synthesis (Lundgren, 1966; Slater, 1968a) and restores the tremors (Slater and Rogers, 1968). Slater (1968a) was unable to correlate the fall in brain ACh produced by HC-3 with the catatonia and seizures, although Dren and Domino (1968a) associated the fall with various

EEG changes in anesthetized dogs. HC-3 produced high-voltage slow waves in the amygdala and neocortex, and inhibited EEG activation produced by electrical stimulation of the midbrain reticular formation, diffuse thalamic nuclei and posterior hypothalamus. Choline produced a delayed and transient reversal of the HC-3 effects, whereas arecoline, pilocarpine and physostigmine produced EEG activation in the presence of HC-3 (Dren and Domino, 1968b). In a study of the role of ACh in sleep, wakefulness and dreaming in cats, Hazra (1970) found that HC-3 injected intraventricularly facilitated slow wave sleep but virtually abolished paradoxical sleep. He concluded that ACh is involved in maintaining vigilance and the phenomenon of dreaming.

HC-3, applied by iontophoresis, also produces a prejunctional blockade of the collateral endings on Renshaw cells in the cat spinal cord (Quastel and Curtis, 1965), where there is evidence that ACh is the chemical transmitter (Eccles, 1964).

There is evidence that in domestic fowl chicks, the blood–brain barrier is underdeveloped, at least with respect to some drugs (Waelsch, 1955; Zaimis, 1960; Key and Marley, 1962); and some quaternary ammonium compounds which do not penetrate the blood–brain barrier in most mammals or in the adult fowl have been shown to exert central effects in chicks (Bowman and Osuide, 1968). Osuide (1967) found that intravenously injected HC-3 produced a characteristic exercise-dependent paralysis of conscious chicks in doses much smaller than those that depressed spinal reflexes, and that the dose necessary to depress spinal reflexes was in turn much smaller than that necessary to cause peripheral transmission failure in rapidly stimulated nerve-muscle preparations. This suggests that, in the young chick, HC-3 causes failure at cholinergic transmission sites in the brain, the spinal cord and the periphery, and that susceptibility to its action is in that order. All of the effects were reversed by choline, but the paralysis in conscious chicks was also reversed by dimethylaminoethanol (deanol) indicating that this substance is converted to ACh in the brain, as has been suggested by others (Kiplinger *et al.*, 1958; Groth *et al.*, 1958).

Several workers have studied structure-activity relationships in the hemicholinium series, most of the studies involving alterations at the cationic head, or in the biphenyl nucleus. Schueler (1955) showed that HC-15, which is exactly half the molecule of HC-3, exhibited no toxic activity in mice in doses up to 50 mg/kg. Bowman *et al.* (1967) found that the primary action of HC-15 and other monoquaternary analogs of HC-3 on neuromuscular transmission is a postjunctional tubocurarine-like action. However, more recent studies (Hemsworth *et al.*, 1971) on

369

isolated synaptosomes showed that HC-15 is almost as active as HC-3 in inhibiting the uptake of ^{14}C-choline.

Marshall and Long (1959) showed that the introduction of an ether or methylene linkage between the two phenyl rings, produced only a minor decrease in potency, and subsequent studies have shown that the biphenyl moiety may be replaced by a hexamethylene chain (Powers *et al.*, 1962), one phenyl ring (Thampi *et al.*, 1966) or three phenyl rings (Gardiner and Sung, 1969) without appreciable loss of the characteristic HC-3-like activity. The decrease in activity with alteration of the biphenyl nucleus may indicate that in HC-3 the interonium distance is optimal for maximal inhibition of choline transport (Marshall and Long, 1959). In the series of aliphatic hemicholinium derivatives studied by Powers *et al.* (1962), hemicholinium-like activity was retained by one of the compounds, and in this compound the length of the aliphatic chain (hexamethylene) approximated to the length of the biphenyl nucleus.

In this original study of the hemicholiniums, Schueler (1955) found the characteristic activity only in compounds containing an unmasked β-hydroxyl group with respect to the onium centre. This, and spectroscopic evidence led to his suggestion that such compounds underwent hemiacetal formation (Fig. 1). Studies on $\alpha',\alpha',\alpha\alpha$-tetramethyl-HC-3 which can exist in both open-chain and hemiacetal forms, depending upon the experimental conditions, showed that characteristic HC-3-like activity is much more pronounced in the hemiacetal form (Di Augustine and Haarstad, 1967, 1970).

In most studies, the effect of modifying the position of the β-hydroxyl groups and the alkyl substituents on the onium head produced marked changes in pharmacological activity (Schueler, 1955; Marshall and Long, 1959; Long *et al.*, 1967). In a series of close HC-3 analogs, with slightly varying structure at the cationic head, Long *et al.* (1967) were able to demonstrate five different types of pharmacological activity: (1) HC-3 like, (2) tubocurarine-like, (3) ganglion blocking, (4) anticholinesterase, and (5) cocaine-like. On the basis of studies of the α,α-, β,β and α',α'-dimethyl derivatives of HC-3, Di Augustine and Haarstad (1966) have suggested that the α and β parts of the choline moieties rather than the α' part are important in the competition with choline for the choline transport mechanism.

Long *et al.* (1967) also noted that the N-methylpiperidine analog of HC-3 exhibited HC-3-like activity, and subsequent studies (Benz and Long, 1969a, b, 1970) have confirmed that various heterocyclic compounds, lacking a β-hydroxyl substituent are active in this respect, notably the 3-methylpyridinium and 4-methylpiperidinium derivatives. In addition, Benz and Long (1969b) showed that the *N*-allyl derivative of HC-3 possessed high activity. Benz and Long (1969b) have calculated that in the last three named compounds, the terminal methyl groups are separated from the quaternary nitrogen by a distance of 3.7 Å and have concluded that in the bisphenacyl quaternary salt an interonium distance of 14 Å is important for HC-3-like activity, and that this activity can be enhanced if the compound has a non-polar space-filling group 3.7 Å from the onium centre.

Long *et al.* (1967) found that one compound in their series, *a,a'*-bis-(dimethylammonium   acetaldehydediethylacetal)-*p,p'*-diacetyl   biphenyl bromide (DMAE), resembled cocaine in that it potentiated catecholamines and sympathetic nerve stimulation.

α,α'−bis−(dimethyl ammoniumacetaldehyde diethylacetal)−
p,p'−diacetyl biphenyl bromide (DMAE).

Further studies on the mechanism of action of DMAE revealed that it potentiated directly acting catecholamines in normal and reserpinized animals. In these actions DMAE closely paralleled the action of cocaine, and it was suggested that, like cocaine, DMAE inhibited the uptake of noradrenaline into sympathetic nerve terminals (Wong and Long, 1967). However, DMAE differed from cocaine in that it did not antagonize the actions of the indirectly acting sympathomimetic tyramine, and in that it increased the pressor response to angiotensin. Subsequent studies on the interaction between DMAE and angiotensin have led Greenberg and Long (1970) to suggest that DMAE does not inhibit the neuronal reuptake of noradrenaline, but rather that it facilitates the ability of angiotensin to release noradrenaline from sympathetic nerves. DMAE also exerts a profound inhibitory action against the ganglion stimulant substances nicotine, tetramethylammonium and dimethylphenylpiperazinium, while having a much lesser action on transmission through sympathetic ganglia produced by stimulation of the preganglionic nerves (Wong and Long, 1968; Wong *et al.*, 1968; Jaramillo, 1968). This selective effect on ganglion stimulants was much more pronounced than that produced by hexamethonium (Wong and Long, 1968). In the initial study of DMAE (Long *et al.*, 1967),

371

the compound was found to have little effect on neuromuscular transmission. However, recent evidence has shown that DMAE produces a biphasic block of neuromuscular transmission, an initial non-depolarizing block similar to that produced by tubocurarine, and a secondary block of long duration which is reversible by choline (Chiou and Long, 1969). Chiou and Long (1969) have suggested, on the grounds that the ED_{50}s of the two drugs are similar, that DMAE may be converted into HC-3 *in vivo*, with a concomitant inhibition of ACh synthesis.

13.3.2. LINEAR CHOLINE ANALOGS

(a) *Monoquaternary compounds*

Keston and Wortis (1946) demonstrated that the respiratory paralysis and death produced in mice by the triethyl analog of choline [triethyl(2-hydroxyethyl)ammonium; triethylcholine; TEC] could be prevented by the simultaneous administration of choline. They suggested that TEC probably produced neuromuscular block by interfering with the formation of ACh. More recently TEC has been studied in greater detail and shown to be essentially similar to HC-3 in its actions. In conscious animals, it produces muscular weakness which is accentuated by exercise, and in nerve–muscle preparations it produces a slowly developing, frequency-dependent transmission failure. Both of these effects may be reversed by choline but anticholinesterase drugs are only weakly effective (Bowman and Rand, 1961a, b; Bowman *et al.*, 1962a, b; 1967). The mainly prejunctional site of action of the drug is illustrated by the fact that, at the height of the transmission failure, responses of the muscle to ACh are not impaired (Bowman and Rand, 1961b; Bowman *et al.*, 1962a) and direct assay of the released ACh (and the use of radiochemical techniques) showed that the output is reduced, although it may be restored by excess choline (Bowman and Hemsworth, 1965a; Saelens, 1967). A similar effect on ACh output is produced in perfused sympathetic ganglia (Matthews, 1966). Provided that the motor nerve is first stimulated rapidly in the presence of the drug to exhaust the preformed transmitter, TEC produces a choline-reversible decrease in the size of the quantum of transmitter and a reduction in the frequency of the m.e.p.p.s (Elmqvist and Quastel, 1965). Like HC-3, TEC inhibits the synthesis of ACh from choline by homogenates of organized nervous tissue, but has little direct inhibitory activity against ChAc. The inhibition of synthesis is overcome by an increase in the concentration of choline (Bull and Hemsworth, 1963, 1965; Bhatnager *et al.*, 1965; Buterbaugh *et al.*, 1968). TEC inhibits the uptake of labeled choline into isolated synaptosomes (Potter, 1968; Hemsworth *et al.*, 1971), although, as with HC-3, small concentrations have been reported to facilitate choline uptake (Hemsworth *et al.*, 1971). All these results indicate that TEC combines with the choline carrier mechanism in the nerve endings to inhibit the uptake of choline. It is considerably less potent than HC-3, but its postjunctional curare-like action is relatively weaker than that of HC-3, and its effects are more easily reversed by choline. A factor contributing to the easier reversibility by choline may be that TEC is an inhibitor of choline oxidase (Wells, 1954). Injected choline normally disappears rapidly from the circulation (Appleton *et al.*, 1951; Bligh, 1953). As might be expected from its close chemical relationship to tetra-ethylammonium, TEC is relatively more potent than HC-3 in its post-synaptic ganglion blocking action (Bowman and Rand, 1961b; Bhatnager *et al.*, 1965).

Burgen *et al.* (1956) found that TEC was acetylated by ChAc almost as effectively as was choline itself and Bowman and Rand (1961b) suggested that TEC may be transported into the nerve endings in place of choline and there incorporated into a false transmitter. Subsequent authors were unable to demonstrate acetylation of TEC by ChAc (Dauterman and Mehrotra, 1963; Hemsworth and Morris, 1964) but more recently, the original observation of Burgen *et al.* (1956) has been confirmed (Potter, 1968; Hemsworth and Smith, 1970), and TEC has been shown to be transported into isolated synaptosomes and there acetylated to form acetyl-triethylcholine. Acetyltriethylcholine is devoid of either stimulant or blocking activity at the neuromuscular junction (Holton and Ing, 1949; Bowman *et al.*, 1962a) in any concentration that might conceivably be released by nerve endings, so that the direct cause of transmission failure is the absence of ACh, rather than the presence of a false transmitter (Bowman *et al.*, 1962a).

TEC produces an initial increase in ACh release which precedes the transmission failure (Bowman and Hemsworth, 1965a) and this effect is reflected by its anticurare action (Roberts, 1962; Bowman *et al.*, 1962a; Marshall, 1969). In mammals there is only slight repetitive firing and a negligible increase in the amplitude of the maximal twitch of the non-curarized muscle before the onset of transmission failure (Bowman and Rand, 1961b; Bowman *et al.*, 1962a), but these effects are more pronounced in amphibians and avians (Roberts, 1962; Marshall, 1969). In these respects the action of TEC resembles that of the closely related drug, tetraethyl-ammonium (Stovner, 1957, 1958; Koketsu, 1958; Collier and Exley, 1963). Although the transmission failure produced by TEC cannot be attributed

373

to depletion of transmitter resulting from excessive initial release, this effect must contribute to the blocking action by hastening the exhaustion of preformed transmitter. Saelens and Stoll (1965), using a radiochemical technique, found that when synthesis was inhibited by TEC, the diminished output of ACh from the rat phrenic nerve–diaphragm preparation was accompanied by an increased output of choline. Possibly, when TEC is transported into the nerve endings, it initially displaces previously transported choline and preformed ACh from intracellular sites. Then, when the ACh is exhausted, it continues to displace choline from sites inaccessible to the synthesizing enzyme. An initial increase in ACh release does not seem to be an important action of HC-3, although there is a report of it producing this effect in a sympathetic ganglion (Matthews, 1966).

Like HC-3, TEC has proved to be a useful compound for the estimation of prejunctional ACh stores (Elmqvist and Quastel, 1965) and for the pharmacological identification of cholinergic transmission in various preparations (Rand and Ridehalgh, 1965; Bolton, 1967). Locally applied TEC has similar central actions to those of HC-3 (Slater, 1968a, b; Slater and Rogers, 1968).

Bowman and Rand (1962) and Bowman *et al.* (1967) tested a wide range of monoquaternary choline analogs on neuromuscular transmission in the cat, the chick, the isolated phrenic nerve–diaphragm preparation of the rat and the rectus abdominis muscle of the frog. On the basis of mainly indirect evidence, they were able to classify the compounds into three groups according to the characteristics of the primary type of blocking action produced. Generally, analogs with small onium substituents (e.g. trimethyl) possessed postjunctional depolarizing activity, whereas those with large substituents (e.g. propyl or larger) exhibited non-depolarizing postjunctional blocking activity. Compounds with intermediately sized substituents, generally with at least two ethyl groups, produced a blockade with the characteristics of that produced by TEC, in that it was frequency-dependent, slow in onset, reversible by choline and accompanied by an unimpaired response to close-arterially injected ACh. They emphasized, however, that the tests they used did not permit accurate conclusions regarding structure-activity relationships, since they allowed evidence of prejunctional TEC-like activity only when the postjunctional activity of the compound required larger doses, or when it was brief in duration compared to the prejunctional action. Variations in chemical structure, which allowed the demonstration of a prejunctional action in the tests used, may have done so simply by reducing the potency of the postjunctional action relative to that of the prejunctional action.

Bretylium tosylate was one of the compounds studied by Bowman *et al.* (1967). This drug produced a TEC-like transmission failure in the rat diaphragm (Green and Hughes, 1966; Bowman *et al.*, 1967), inhibited the synthesis of ACh by homogenates of organized nervous tissue (Bowman *et al.*, 1967) and reduced ACh output from nerve endings (Chang, Chen and Cheng, 1967). These findings are of interest since they may explain the muscular weakness that was reported sometimes to accompany the antihypertensive action of this drug (Evanson and Sears, 1960; Campbell and Montuschi, 1960).

Bowman *et al.* (1967) found that the compound in which a chlorine group is substituted for the hydroxyl group of TEC was completely inactive at the neuromuscular junction. However, this cannot be taken as evidence that the hydroxyl group is essential, since the tetraethylammonium ion (TEA) itself is active (Bowman *et al.*, 1962a). TEA inhibits the synthesis of ACh by nervous tissue (Bhatnager and MacIntosh, 1967), inhibits the uptake of choline into isolated hearts (Buterbaugh *et al.*, 1968) and erythrocytes (Martin, 1968), and into isolated synaptosomes (Hemsworth *et al.*, 1971), and reduces the output of ACh from the superior cervical ganglion of the cat (Matthews, 1966). Like TEC, it initially increases ACh output from motor nerves (Collier and Exley, 1963) but is more potent than TEC in this respect and it also exhibits weak postjunctional non-depolarizing blocking activity in skeletal muscle (Bowman *et al.*, 1962a; Parsons, 1969) and more powerfully in autonomic ganglia (Burn and Dale, 1915). TEA also affects nerve conduction by blocking potassium channels and thus prolonging the falling phase of the action potential. The falling phase can be prolonged to the extent that re-excitation and repetitive firing result (Hille, 1967). Tetramethylammonium (TMA) is a less potent inhibitor of ACh synthesis than TEA (Bhatnager and MacIntosh, 1967) and is less effective in inhibiting choline uptake into isolated synaptosomes (Hemsworth *et al.*, 1971). However, TMA is much more potent than TEA in inhibiting choline uptake into erythrocytes (Martin, 1969), indicating a basic difference between the transport mechanisms at these sites.

(b) *Bisquaternary compounds*

Bowman and Hemsworth (1965b) studied a series of polymethylene bis-(hydroxyethyl) dimethylammonium salts, which had previously been shown to possess postjunctional blocking activity at the neuromuscular junction (Barlow and Zoller, 1962).

$$HOCH_2CH_2 - \overset{\overset{\displaystyle CH_3}{|}}{\underset{\underset{\displaystyle CH_3}{|}}{\overset{+}{N}}} - (CH_2)_{10} - \overset{\overset{\displaystyle CH_3}{|}}{\underset{\underset{\displaystyle CH_3}{|}}{\overset{+}{N}}} - CH_2CH_2OH \qquad 2\,Br^-$$

Decamethylene bis(hydroxyethyl) dimethylammonium bromide

The penta- and hexamethylene derivatives produced weak prejunctional activity, but the decamethylene compound (C_{10}dichol) was more potent. In slowly stimulated nerve–muscle preparations (0.1 Hz) this compound produced a block with the characteristics of block by depolarization. However, in more rapidly stimulated preparations (1 Hz), a secondary block developed with the characteristics of that due to inhibition of choline transport. The compound was shown to reduce ACh output from the stimulated nerve and to inhibit the synthesis of ACh by nervous tissue (Bowman and Hemsworth, 1965b; Hemsworth, 1971). It also blocks the uptake of choline into isolated synaptosomes (Hemsworth *et al.*, 1971). Both the hexamethylene and decamethylene derivatives are capable of being acetylated by ChAc, at almost the same rate as that of choline, and Hemsworth (1971) has suggested that part of the pharmacological action of these compounds may be due to their incorporation into a false transmitter. Similar biphasic blocks are produced by the α,α-dimethyl and α-ethyl derivatives of succinyldicholine (Bowman *et al.*, 1967), although these compounds have not been studied in detail.

Dowd *et al.* (1968) studied the NN triethyl analog of succinyldicholine and showed that this compound also produced a biphasic block, the second phase of which resembled that produced by TEC. However, in this case, the initial phase was the result of a postjunctional non-depolarizing block. The effects were due to the parent compound rather than to any products of metabolism. A similar type of action was demonstrated for some bicyclic bis-onium esters related to choline in which the onium substituents resembled those of active monoquaternary choline analogs (Marshall, 1968b).

13.3.3. TRIMETHOXYBENZOIC ACID ESTERS

Several trimethoxybenzoic acid esters have been shown to inhibit ACh synthesis in nervous tissue (Bhatnager *et al.*, 1964, 1965; McColl *et al.*, 1964; Chénier *et al.*, 1966). The *in vivo* toxic effects and the *in vitro* inhibition of ACh synthesis are antagonized by choline. The two most potent compounds of the series, troxonium tosylate and troxypyrrolium tosylate, have been studied in the greatest detail. Matthews (1966) showed that troxonium reduced the output of ACh from the superior cervical ganglion of the cat, but, in addition, this compound has marked post-synaptic action at this site (Bhatnager *et al.*, 1965). In the chick biventer cervicis muscle, Marshall (1969) found that troxypyrrolium was the most specific prejunctionally-active drug amongst a series which included HC-3 and TEC.

Bhatnager *et al.* (1964) showed that there was little correlation between the *in vivo* toxicity of the trimethoxybenzoic acid esters and their *in vitro* ability to inhibit ACh synthesis. Further studies have shown that the neuromuscular blocking activity of this series in mammals is more closely related to the toxicity than to inhibition of ACh synthesis (Marshall, 1968c) and it therefore seems that the toxicity and neuromuscular blocking actions of the compounds may reflect a degree of postjunctional non-depolarizing blocking activity.

13.3.4. 2-(4-PHENYLPIPERIDINO) CYCLOHEXANOL (AH 5183)

Potent neuromuscular blocking activity is not usually considered to be a property of tertiary bases such as 2-(4-phenylpiperidino) cyclohexanol (AH 5183), yet Brittain *et al.* (1969a, b) found this compound to be active after both oral and parenteral administration in animals. AH 5183

2-(4-phenylpiperidino) cyclohexanol [AH 5183]

produces a neuromuscular block of slow onset in rapidly stimulated nerve–skeletal muscle preparations of the rat, chicken and cat, which is poorly antagonized by anticholinesterases (Brittain *et al.*, 1969a, b; Marshall, 1970a). The partial antagonism of AH 5183 by choline in the cat led Brittain *et al.* (1969a, b) to suggest that AH 5183 possesses a hemicholinium-like action. These workers also found evidence for an appreciable postjunctional component of action. Marshall (1970a) confirmed that AH 5183 produced a prejunctional block, probably due to reduction of ACh output, but he was unable to demonstrate convincing antagonism by choline, and therefore considered that this drug belongs to a different pharmacological class from the hemicholiniums. The compound does not inhibit ChAc directly (Brittain *et al.*, 1969b). Elimination of other possible sites of action, and consideration of the chemical structure of AH 5183, led Marshall (1970a) to suggest that the compound possesses an intra-cellular action on ACh metabolism, possibly acting by inhibition of ACh uptake into synaptic vesicles. In addition the compound possesses weak local anesthetic activity and a blocking action at α-adrenoreceptors (Marshall, 1970a). Comparison of AH 5183 with its *N*-methyl quaternary analog (AH 5954) revealed that the quaternary compound possessed a different mechanism of neuromuscular blocking action from that possessed by AH 5183 (Marshall, 1970b). AH 5954 was approximately eight times less potent than AH 5183 in blocking neuromuscular transmission, and exhibited the properties of a drug acting extracellularly on the choline transport mechanism.

13.4. CONCLUSION

At the present time, no compound is known with an action entirely confined to the choline transport mechanism. HC-3, TEC, troxonium and troxypyrrolium appear to exert their prime actions at this site, but even these compounds possess postjunctional blocking actions either at the neuromuscular junction or at autonomic ganglia, and, in addition, TEC possesses an initial facilitatory action on cholinergic transmission through which the release of ACh in response to nerve impulses is increased. Another compound which can probably be grouped with these is 3,6-bis(3-diethylamino propoxy) pyridazine bismethiodide. The actions of this compound have not been studied in detail but it produces a frequency-dependent, choline-reversible neuromuscular transmission failure resembling that produced by HC-3 (Gesler and Hoppe, 1956a, b; Gesler *et al.*, 1959; Dhattiwala *et al.*, 1970).

The postjunctional blocking actions of the compounds mentioned above are of the non-depolarizing type. Other compounds, for example, decamethylene bis(hydroxyethyl)dimethylammonium iodide (Bowman and Hemsworth, 1965b), may possess postjunctional depolarizing activity in association with their ability to inhibit choline transport. It thus appears that the latter action may be associated with any of the range of other actions possible at cholinergic transmission sites. Many compounds previously tested under conditions capable of revealing only postjunctional actions might well be found to inhibit choline transport if tested under the appropriate conditions. Some of the dicholine esters and ethers studied by Bovet (1951) and Brücke (1956), particularly those possessing triethyl substitution on the cationic heads, may be examples of this type. When the postjunctional action is powerful, it may completely mask the characteristic signs of choline transport inhibition in experiments on nerve–muscle preparations. Bioassay of released ACh may be complicated by the presence of the drug, and the result of *in vitro* experiments on ACh synthesis, or uptake into isolated synaptosomes, are not always easy to relate to physiological events. Tubocurarine and hexamethonium possess a weak inhibiting action on ACh synthesis (Bhatnager and MacIntosh, 1967) and inhibit choline uptake into isolated synaptosomes (Hemsworth *et al.*, 1971). Hexamethonium also produces a frequency-dependent, choline-reversible transmission failure on the isolated phrenic nerve-diaphragm preparation of the rat (Bowman *et al.*, 1967). Decamethonium is more potent than hexamethonium in inhibiting choline uptake (Hemsworth *et al.*, 1971). Choline uptake into synaptosomes (Hemsworth *et al.*, 1971) or erythrocytes (Martin, 1969) may also be inhibited by physostigmine, neostigmine, ACh, methacholine, carbachol or atropine. However, it is unlikely that an action of this type contributes much, if anything, to the main effects of most of these compounds *in vivo*. Nevertheless, the possibility of inhibited ACh synthesis should be borne in mind when unwanted or unusual effects occur as a result of prolonged drug administration. It has been suggested (Bowman *et al.*, 1967), for example, that such an action of decamethonium and other muscle relaxants of the depolarizing type might contribute to the change in the characteristics of the blockade that often occurs in man after prolonged administration. If such were the case, choline would not be expected to be an effective antagonist, since its postjunctional depolarizing action would summate with that of the muscle relaxant. It is also possible that the metabolites of a drug, rather than the drug itself, might inhibit choline transport. Marshall (1968a) obtained evidence that this was so with members of a series of tris-onium dicholine esters which included a triethyl compound. More recently, Ginsburg *et al.* (1971) have reached similar conclusions with a series of bis-onium dicholine esters. Both series of compounds produced an initial postjunctional block of neuromuscular transmission of the non-depolarizing type. However, in some cases, a secondary phase of block developed with all the characteristics associated with inhibited choline transport. The rate of development of the second phase of block could be correlated with the rate of hydrolysis of the parent drug and the production of the metabolites, which included TEC. Both series of compounds were originally synthesized and tested (Carey *et al.*, 1961; Kitz *et al.*, 1969) in a search for short-acting muscle relaxants to replace succinylcholine. It was hoped that their rapid hydrolysis would give rise to a brief blockade of the non-depolarizing type, and indeed this is the only effect observed under the conventional

379

conditions in which low rates of stimulation of nerve–muscle preparations are used. It thus appears that an action on choline transport is a more important aspect of drug action than has been realized in the past, and it may well be advisable to include tests for it in any programme designed to study the actions of new drugs at cholinergic transmission sites.

The similarities between the symptoms of myasthenia gravis and the effects of HC-3 or TEC, both in conscious animals and in nerve–muscle preparations, have been pointed out (Desmedt, 1958, 1966; Bowman *et al.*, 1962b). The similarities probably simply reflect the fact that a reduced depot of ACh is one of the factors contributing to the subnormal transmission in myasthenia gravis (Elmqvist *et al.*, 1964). There is no convincing evidence for a circulating HC-3-like compound in the disease state, there is no evidence of choline deficiency (Birks and MacIntosh, 1961), administered choline does not increase the size of the acetylcholine quantum in myasthenia, and other differences relating to the m.e.p.p.s and the effects of a tetanus are also demonstrable (Elmqvist *et al.* 1964).

It has been suggested (Bowman and Rand, 1961a) that a drug with a selective inhibitory action on the choline-transport mechanism might be of use in the symptomatic treatment of some types of neurogenic spasticity. In the presence of the drug, the rapid discharge of nerve impulses responsible for maintaining the spasticity would itself lead to transmission failure in the affected muscles, while other muscles whose nerves were firing at a normal rate would be relatively unaffected. TEC was found to relieve the spasticity in the affected muscles of rabbits that had been injected unilaterally with the toxin of *Clostridium tetani*, while other muscles were little affected and the animals continued to breathe adequately (Laurence and Webster, 1961). None of the drugs presently available is sufficiently selective in its action to be of more than experimental interest, but it is possible that a therapeutically useful drug of this type will be found in the future.

REFERENCES

ALLEN, R. C., CARLSON, G. L. and CAVALLITO, C. J. (1970) Choline acetyltransferase inhibitors. Physicochemical properties in relation to inhibitory activity of styrylpyridine analogs. *J. Med. Chem.* **13**: 909–12.

ANGELES, L. T., SCHUELER, F. W., LIM, P. R. T. and SOTTO, A. (1964) Effect of cholinedeficiency on HC-3 action. *Arch. Int. Pharmacodyn.* **152**: 253–66.

APPEL, W. C. and VINCENZI, F. F. (1970) Effects of hemicholinium and bretylium on the release of autonomic transmitters in the isolated sino-atrial node. *Brit. J. Pharmacol.* **40**: 268–74.

APPLETON, H. D., LEVY, B. B., STEELE, J. M. and BRODIE, B. B. (1951) Free choline in plasma. *Fed. Proc.* **10**: 157.

ASKARI, A. (1966) Uptake of quaternary ammonium ions by human erythrocytes. *J. Gen. Physiol.* **49**: 1147–60.

DI AUGUSTINE, R. P. and HAARSTAD, V. B. (1966) The crucial-moiety interference of hemicholinium No. 3. *Pharmacologist* **8**: 191.

DI AUGUSTINE, R. P. and HAARSTAD, V. B. (1967) The active structure of hemicholinium No. 3. *Pharmacologist* **9**: 204.

DI AUGUSTINE, R. P. and HAARSTAD, V. B. (1970) The active structure of hemicholinium inhibiting the biosynthesis of acetylcholine. *Biochem. Pharmacol.* **19**: 559–80.

BAKER, B. R. and GIBSON, R. E. (1971) Irreversible enzyme inhibitors. 181. Inhibition of brain choline acetyltransferase by derivatives of 4-stilbazole. *J. Med. Chem.* **14**: 315–22.

BARLOW, R. B. and ZOLLER, A. (1962) Activity of analogues of decamethonium on the chick biventer cervicis preparation. *Brit. J. Pharmacol.* **19**: 485–91.

BENZ, F. W. and LONG, J. P. (1969a) Investigations on a series of heterocyclic hemicholinium-3 analogs. *J. Pharmacol. Exp. Ther.* **166**: 225–36.

BENZ, F. W. and LONG, J. P. (1969b) Structure-activity relationships of *N*-alkyl and heterocyclic analogs of hemicholinium-3. *J. Pharmacol. Exp. Ther.* **168**: 315–21.

BENZ, F. W. and LONG, J. P. (1970) Further structure-activity relations of heterocyclic analogues of hemicholinium-3. *J. Pharm. Pharmacol.* **22**: 20–5.

BERMAN-REISBERG, R. (1954) Properties and biological significance of choline acetylase. *Yale J. Biol. Med.* **29**: 403–35.

BERTOLINI, A., GREGGIA, A. and FERRARI, W. (1967) Atropine-like properties of hemicholinium-3. *Life Sci.* **6**: 537–43.

BEVAN, J. A. and SU, C. (1964) The sympathetic mechanism of the isolated pulmonary artery of the rabbit. *Brit. J. Pharmacol.* **22**: 176–82.

BHATNAGER, S. P., LAM, A. and McCOLL, J. D. (1964) Inhibition of synthesis of acetylcholine by some esters of trimethoxybenzoic acid. *Nature* **204**: 485–6.

BHATNAGER, S. P., LAM, A and McCOLL, J. D. (1965) Inhibition of acetylcholine synthesis in nervous tissue by some quaternary compounds. *Biochem. Pharmacol.* **14**: 421–34.

BHATNAGER, S. P. and MACINTOSH, F. C. (1967) Effects of quaternary bases and inorganic cations on acetylcholine synthesis in nervous tissue. *Canad. J. Physiol. Pharmacol.* **45**: 249–68.

BIRKS, R. I. (1963) The role of sodium ions in the metabolism of acetylcholine. *Canad. J. Biochem. Physiol.* **41**: 2573–97.

BIRKS, R. and MACINTOSH, F. C. (1961) Acetylcholine metabolism of a sympathetic ganglion. *Canad. J. Biochem. Physiol.* **39**: 787–827.

BLIGH, J. (1952) The level of free choline in plasma. *J. Physiol.* **117**: 234–40.

BLIGH, J. (1953) The role of the liver and the kidneys in the maintenance of the level of free choline in plasma. *J. Physiol.* **120**: 53–62.

BOLTON, T. B. (1967) Intramural nerves in the ventricular myocardium of the domestic fowl and other animals. *Brit. J. Pharmacol.* **31**: 253–68.

BORISON, H. L. (1961) Respiratory depressant effect of HC-3. *Fed. Proc.* **20**: 594–9.

BOSMANN, H. B. and HEMSWORTH, B. A. (1970) Synaptic vesicles: Incorporation of choline by isolated synaptosomes and synaptic vesicles. *Biochem. Pharmacol.* **19**: 133–41.

BOVET, D. (1951) Some aspects of the relationship between chemical constitution and curare-like activity. *Ann. N.Y. Acad. Sci.* **54**: 407–37.

BOWMAN, W. C. and HEMSWORTH, B. A. (1965a) Effects of triethylcholine on the output of acetylcholine from the isolated diaphragm of the rat. *Brit. J. Pharmacol.* **24**: 110–18.

BOWMAN, W. C. and HEMSWORTH, B. A. (1965b) Effects of some polymethylene bis(hydroxyethyl) diethylammonium salts on neuromuscular transmission. *Brit. J. Pharmacol.* **25**: 392–404.

BOWMAN, W. C., HEMSWORTH, B. A. and RAND, M. J. (1962a) Triethylcholine compared with other substances affecting neuromuscular transmission. *Brit. J. Pharmacol.* **19**: 198–218.

BOWMAN, W. C., HEMSWORTH, B. A. and RAND, M. J. (1962b) Myasthenic-like features of the neuromuscular transmission failure produced by triethylcholine. *J. Pharm. Pharmacol.* **14**: 37T–40T.

BOWMAN, W. C., HEMSWORTH, B. A. and RAND, M. J. (1967) Effects of analogues of choline on neuromuscular transmission. *Ann. N.Y. Acad. Sci.* **144**: 471–82.

BOWMAN, W. C. and OSUIDE, G. (1968) Interaction between the effects of tremorine and harmine and of other drugs in chicks. *Europ. J. Pharmacol.* **3**: 106–11.

BOWMAN, W. C. and RAND, M. J. (1961a) The triethyl analogue of choline and neuromuscular transmission. *Lancet.* **i**: 480–1.

BOWMAN, W. C. and RAND, M. J. (1961b) Actions of triethylcholine on neuromuscular transmission. *Brit. J. Pharmacol.* **17**: 176–95.

BOWMAN, W. C. and RAND, M. J. (1962) The neuromuscular blocking action of substances related to choline. *Int. J. Neuropharmacol.* **1**: 129–32.

BRANDON, K. W. and RAND, M. J. (1961) Acetylcholine and the sympathetic innervation of the spleen. *J. Physiol.* **157**: 18–32.

BRITTAIN, R. T., LEVY, G. P. and TYERS, M. B. (1969a) Observations on the neuromuscular blocking action of 2-(4-phenylpiperidino)-cyclohexanol. *Brit. J. Pharmacol.* **36**: 173P–174P.

BRITTAIN, R. T., LEVY, G. P. and TYERS, M. B. (1969b) The neuromuscular blocking action of 2-(4-phenylpiperidino)-cyclohexanol (AH 5183). *Europ. J. Pharmacol.* **8**: 93–9.

BRÜCKE, F. (1956) Dicholinesters of α,ω-dicarboxylic acids and related substances. *Pharmacol. Rev.* **8**: 265–335.

BULL, G. and HEMSWORTH, B. A. (1963) Inhibition of biological synthesis of acetylcholine by triethylcholine. *Nature* **199**: 487–8.

BULL, G. and HEMSWORTH, B. A. (1965) The action of triethylcholine on the biological synthesis of acetylcholine. *Brit. J. Pharmacol.* **25**: 228–33.

BURGEN, A. S. V., BURKE, G. and DESBARATS-SCHONBAUM, M. L. (1956) The specificity of brain choline-acetylase. *Brit. J. Pharmacol.* **11**: 308–12.

BURN, J. H. and DALE, H. H. (1915) The action of certain quaternary ammonium bases. *J. Pharmacol. Exp. Ther.* **6**: 417–38.

BURN, J. H. and RAND, M. J. (1959) Sympathetic postganglionic mechanism. *Nature* **184**: 163–5.

BURTON, R. M. and HOWARD, R. E. (1967) Gangliosides and acetylcholine of the central nervous system. VIII. Role of lipids in the binding and release of neurohormones by synaptic vesicles. *Ann. N.Y. Acad. Sci.* **144**: 411–30.

BUTERBAUGH, G. G., FIGGE, P. K. and SPRATT, J. L. (1968) A comparison of the effects of tetraethylammonium, triethylcholine and hemicholinium on choline uptake by the isolated perfused rabbit heart. *Arch. Int. Pharmacodyn.* **175**: 179–85.

BUTERBAUGH, G. G. and SPRATT, J. L. (1968) Effects of hemicholinium on choline uptake in the isolated rabbit heart. *J. Pharmacol. Exp. Ther.* **159**: 255–63.

CAMPBELL, E. D. R. and MONTUSCHI, E. (1960) Muscle weakness caused by bretylium tosylate. *Lancet* **ii**: 789.

CAREY, F. M., LEWIS, J. J., STENLAKE, J. B. and WILLIAMS, W. D. (1961) Neuromuscular blocking agents. Part IX. Some short-acting linear *NNN*-tris-onium esters. *J. Pharm. Pharmacol.* **13**, 103T–106T.

CAVALLITO, C. J., NAPOLI, M. D. and O'DELL, T. B. (1964) Neuromuscular blocking activities of two short chain linked bis-quaternary ammonium compounds. *Arch. Int. Pharmacodyn.* **149**: 188–94.

CAVALLITO, C. F., YUN, H. S., EDWARDS, M. L. and FOLDES, F. F. (1971) Choline acetyltransferase inhibitors. Styrylpyridine analogs with nitrogen atom modifications. *J. Med. Chem.* **14**: 130–3.

CAVALLITO, C. J., YUN, H. S., KAPLAN, T., SMITH, J. V. and FOLDES, F. F. (1970) Choline acetyltransferase inhibitors. Dimensional and substituent effects among styrylpyridine analogs. *J. Med. Chem.* **13**: 221–4.

CAVALLITO, C. J., YUN, H. J., SMITH, J. C. and FOLDES, F. F. (1969) Choline acetyltransferase inhibitors. Configurational and electronic features of styrylpyridine analogs. *J. Med. Chem.* **12**: 134–8.

CHAKRIN, L. W. and WHITTAKER, V. P. (1969) The subcellular distribution of [N-Me-^{3}H] acetylcholine synthesized by brain *in vivo*. *Biochem. J.* **113**: 97–107.

CHANG, C. C., CHEN, T. F. and CHENG, H. C. (1967) On the mechanism of neuromuscular blocking action of bretylium and guanethidine. *J. Pharmacol. Exp. Ther.* **158**: 89–98.

CHANG, C. C., CHENG, H. C. and CHEN, T. F. (1967) Does *d*-tubocurarine inhibit the release of acetylcholine from motor nerve endings? *Jap. J. Physiol.* **17**: 505–15.

CHANG, V. and RAND, M. J. (1960) Transmission failure in sympathetic nerves produced by hemicholinium. *Brit. J. Pharmacol.* **15**: 588–600.

CHÉNIER, L.-P., LAM, A., CHIZ, J. F. and MCCOLL, J. D. (1966) Structure-activity relationships of some troxypyrrolidinium analogs. *Fed. Proc.* **25**: 228.

CHEYMOL, J., BOURILLET, F. and OGURA, Y. (1962) Action de quelques paralysants neuromusculaires sur la libération de l'acetylcholine au niveau des terminaisons nervenses mortices. *Arch. Int. Pharmacodyn.* **139**: 187–97.

CHIOU, C. Y. and LONG, J. P. (1969) Effects of α,α'-bis-(dimethylammonium-acetaldehyde diethylacetal)-*p,p'*-diacetylbiphenyl bromide (DMAE) on neuromuscular transmission. *J. Pharmacol. Exp. Ther.* **167**: 344–50.

COLLIER, B. (1969) The preferential release of newly synthesized transmitter by a sympathetic ganglion. *J. Physiol.* **205**: 341–52.

COLLIER, B. and EXLEY, K. A. (1963) Mechanism of the antagonism by tetraethylammonium of neuromuscular block due to *d*-tubocurarine, or calcium deficiency. *Nature* **199**: 702–3.

COLLIER, B. and LANG, C. (1969) The metabolism of choline by a sympathetic ganglion. *Canad. J. Physiol. Pharmacol.* **47**: 119–26.

COLLIER, B. and MACINTOSH, F. C. (1969) The source of choline for acetylcholine synthesis in a sympathetic ganglion. *Canad. J. Physiol. Pharmacol.* **47**: 127–35.

CROSSLAND, J. and SLATER, P. (1968) The effect of some drugs on the free and bound acetylcholine content of rat brain. *Brit. J. Pharmacol.* **33**: 42–7.

CSILLIK, B. and JOÓ, F. (1967) Effect of hemicholinium on the number of synaptic vesicles. *Nature* **213**: 508–9.

DAUTERMANN, W. C. and MEHROTRA, K. N. (1963) The *N*-alkyl group specificity of choline acetylase from rat brain. *J. Neurochem.* **10**: 113–17.

DESMEDT, J. E. (1958) Myasthenic-like features of neuromuscular transmission after administration of an inhibitor of acetylcholine synthesis. *Nature* **182**: 1673–4.

DESMEDT, J. E. (1966) Presynaptic mechanisms in myasthenia gravis. *Ann. N.Y. Acad. Sci.* **135**: 209–46.

DHATTIWALA, A. S., JINDAL, M. N. and KELKAR, V. V. (1970) Effects of some drugs on the responses of the rat isolated, innervated urinary bladder to indirect electrical stimulation. *Brit. J. Pharmacol.* **39**: 738–47.

DIAMOND, I. and KENNEDY, E. P. (1969) Carrier-mediated transport of choline into synaptic nerve endings. *J. Biol. Chem.* **244**: 3258–63.

DOMER, F. R. and SCHUELER, F. W. (1960) Synthesis and metabolic studies of C^{14}-labelled hemicholinium number three. *J. Amer. Pharm. Ass. (Sci. Ed.)* **49**: 553–8.

DOWD, H., JENNINGS, S. J., MARSHALL, I. G. and TRACY, B. M. (1968) Effects of the *NN'* triethyl analogue of suxamethonium on neuromuscular transmission. *J. Pharm. Pharmacol.* **20**: 665–72.

DREN, A. T. and DOMINO, E. F. (1968a) Effects of hemicholinium (HC-3) on EEG activation and brain acetylcholine in the dog. *J. Pharmacol. Exp. Ther.* **161**: 141–54.

DREN, A. T. and DOMINO, E. F. (1968b) Cholinergic and adrenergic activating agents as antagonists of the EEG effects of hemicholinium-3. *Arch. Int. Pharmacodyn.* **175**: 63–72.

ECCLES, J. C. (1964) *The Physiology of Synapses.* Springer-Verlag, Berlin.

ELMQVIST, D., HOFMANN, W. W., KUGELBERG, J. and QUASTEL, D. M. J. (1964) An electrophysiological investigation of neuromuscular transmission in myasthenia gravis. *J. Physiol.* **174**: 417–34.

ELMQVIST, D. and QUASTEL, D. M. J. (1965) Presynaptic action of hemicholinium at the neuromuscular junction. *J. Physiol.* **177**: 463–82.

ELMQVIST, D., QUASTEL, D. M. J. and THESLEFF, S. (1963) Prejunctional action of HC-3 on neuromuscular transmission. *J. Physiol.* **167**: 47P–48P.

EVANS, E. R. and WILSON, H. (1962) Some effects of a hemicholinium compound (HC-3) on neuromuscular transmission in the cat. *J. Pharm. Pharmacol.* **14**: 34T–36T.

EVANS, E. R. and WILSON, H. (1964) Actions of hemicholinium (HC-3) on neuromuscular transmission. *Brit. J. Pharmacol.* **22**: 441–52.

EVANSON, J. M. and SEARS, H. T. N. (1960) Comparison of bretylium tosylate with guanethidine in the treatment of severe hypertension. *Lancet* **ii**: 387–9.

EVERETT, S. D. (1966) Pharmacological responses of the isolated oesophagus and crop of the chick. In: *Physiology of the Domestic Fowl*, pp. 261–73. British Egg Marketing Board Symposium No. 1, Horton-Smith, C. and Amoroso, E. C. (eds.). Oliver & Boyd, Edinburgh.

EVERETT, S. D. (1968) Pharmacological responses of the isolated innervated intestine and rectal caecum of the chick. *Brit. J. Pharmacol.* **33**: 342–56.

FAHMY, A. R., RYMAN, B. E. and WALSH, E. O'F. (1954) The inhibition of choline acetylase by nicotine. *J. Pharm. Pharmacol.* **6**: 607–9.

FONNUM, F. (1966) Is choline acetyltransferase present in synaptic vesicles? *Biochem. Pharmacol.* **15**: 1641–3.

FONNUM, F. (1967) The "compartmentation" of choline acetyltransferase within the synaptosome. *Biochem. J.* **103**: 262–70.

FONNUM, F. (1968) Choline acetyltransferase binding to and release from membranes. *Biochem. J.* **109**: 389–98.

FONNUM, F. (1970) Surface charge of choline acetyltransferase from different species. *J. Neurochem.* **17**: 1095–100.

FRAZIER, D. T. (1968) Effect of hemicholinium No. 3 on amphibian nerve. *Expl. Neurol.* **20**: 245–54.

FRAZIER, D. T., NARAHASHI, T. and MOORE, J. W. (1969) Hemicholinium-3: non-cholinergic effects on squid axons. *Science* **163**: 820–1.

FRAZIER, D. T., NARAHASHI, T. and YAMADA, M. (1970) The site of action and active form of local anesthetics. Experiments with quaternary compounds. *J. Pharmacol. Exp. Ther.* **171**: 45–51.

FRIESEN, A. J. D., KEMP, J. W. and WOODBURY, D. W. (1965) The chemical and physical identification of acetylcholine from sympathetic ganglia. *J. Pharmacol. Exp. Ther.* **148**: 312–19.

FRIESEN, A. J. D., LING, G. M. and NAGAI, M. (1967) Choline and phospholipid-choline in a sympathetic ganglion and their relationship to acetylcholine synthesis. *Nature* **214**: 722–4.

GARDINER, J. E. (1961) The inhibition of acetylcholine synthesis in brain by a hemicholinium. *Biochem. J.* **81**: 297–303.

GARDINER, J. E. and SUNG, L. H. (1969) A *p*-terphenyl hemicholinium compound. *Brit. J. Pharmacol.* **36**: 171P–172P.

GARDINER, J. E. and THOMPSON, J. W. (1961) Lack of evidence for a cholinergic mechanism in sympathetic transmission. *Nature* **191**: 86.

GESLER, R. M. and HOPPE, J. O. (1956a) Observations on the neuromuscular blocking activity of a series of bis-quaternary pyridazines, with particular reference to the effects of frequency of stimulation. *J. Pharmacol. Exp. Ther.* **118**: 388–94.

GESLER, R. M. and HOPPE, J. O. (1956b) 3,6-bis (3-diethylaminopropoxy) pyridazine bismethiodide, a long-acting neuromuscular blocking agent. *J. Pharmacol. Exp. Ther.* **118**: 395–406.

GESLER, R. M., LASHER, A. V., HOPPE, J. O. and STECK, E. A. (1959) Further studies on the site of action of the neuromuscular blocking agent 3,6-bis (3-diethylaminopropoxy) pyridazine bismethiodide. *J. Pharmacol. Exp. Ther.* **125**: 323–9.

GINSBURG, S., KITZ, R. J. and SAVARESE, J. J. (1971) The neuromuscular blocking activity of a new series of quaternary N-substituted choline esters. *Brit. J. Pharmacol.* **43**: 107–26.

GIOVINCO, J. F. (1957) Hemicholinium: a new aid in the study of cholinergic mechanisms. *Bull. Tulane Univ. Med. Fac.* **16**: 177–84.

GOLDBERG, M. E., SALAMA, A. I. and BLUM, S. W. (1971) Inhibition of choline acetyltransferase and hexobarbitone-metabolizing enzymes by naphthylvinylpyridine analogues. *J. Pharm. Pharmacol.* **23**: 384–5.

GOMEZ, M. V., DOMINO, E. F. and SELLINGER, O. Z. (1970) Effect of hemicholinium-3 on choline distribution *in vivo* in the canine caudate nucleus. *Biochem. Pharmacol.* **19**: 1753–60.

GREEN, A. F. and HUGHES, R. (1966) Effects of adrenergic neurone blocking agents on voluntary muscle stimulated at different frequencies. *Brit. J. Pharmacol.* **27**: 164–76.

GREENBERG, S. and LONG, J. P. (1970) Potentiation by [4,4′-Biphenylenebis (2-oxoethylene)] bis [(2,2-diethoxyethyl) dimethylammonium bromide] (DMAE) of the sympathetic component of the vasopressor response to angiotensin. *J. Pharmacol. Exp. Ther.* **174**: 35–44.

GROTH, D. P., BAIN, J. A. and PFEIFFER, C. C. (1958) The comparative distribution of C^{14} labelled 2-dimethyl-aminoethanol and choline in the mouse. *J. Pharmacol. Exp. Ther.* **122**: 28A.

GUTH, P. S. (1969) Acetylcholine binding by isolated synaptic vesicles *in vitro*. *Nature* **224**: 384–5.

GYÖRGY, L., PFEIFER, A. K. and KENYERES, J. (1970) The interaction of hemicholinium-3 and oxotremorine in isolated organ preparations. *J. Pharm. Pharmacol.* **22**: 96–100.

HAZRA, J. (1970) Effect of hemicholinium-3 on slow wave and paradoxical sleep of cat. *Europ. J. Pharmacol.* **11**: 395–7.

HEBB, C. O. (1954) Acetylcholine metabolism of nervous tissue. *Pharmacol. Rev.* **6**: 39–43.

HEBB, C. O., LING, G. M., MCGEER, E. G., MCGEER, P. L. and PERKINS, D. (1964) Effect of locally applied hemicholinium on the acetylcholine content of the caudate nucleus. *Nature* **204**: 1309–11.

HEBB, C. O. and SMALLMAN, B. N. (1956) Intracellular distribution of choline acetylase. *J. Physiol.* **134**: 385–92.

HEBB, C. O. and WHITTAKER, V. P. (1958) Intracellular distributions of acetylcholine and choline acetylase. *J. Physiol.* **142**: 187–96.

HEMSWORTH, B. A. (1971) Effects of some polymethylene bis (hydroxyethyl) dimethylammonium compounds on acetylcholine synthesis. *Brit. J. Pharmacol.* **42**: 78–87.

HEMSWORTH, B. A., DARMER, K. I., JR. and BOSMANN, H. B. (1971) The incorporation of choline into isolated synaptosomes and synaptic vesicle fractions in the presence of quaternary ammonium compounds. *Neuropharmacol.* **10**: 109–20.

HEMSWORTH, B. A. and FOLDES, F. F. (1970) Preliminary pharmacological screening of styrylpyridine choline acetyltransferase inhibitors. *Europ. J. Pharmacol.* **11**: 187–94.

HEMSWORTH, B. A. and MORRIS, D. (1964) A comparison of the *N*-alkyl group specificity of choline acetyltransferase from different species. *J. Neurochem.* **11**: 793–803.

HEMSWORTH, B. A. and SMITH, J. C. (1970) The enzymic acetylation of choline analogues. *J. Neurochem.* **17**: 171–7.

HILLE, B. (1967) The selective inhibition of delayed potassium currents in nerve by tetraethylammonium ion. *J. Gen. Physiol.* **50**: 1287–302.

HODGKIN, A. L. and MARTIN, K. (1965) Choline uptake by giant axons of *Loligo*. *J. Physiol.* **179**: 26P–27P.

HOLTON, P. and ING, H. R. (1949) The specificity of the trimethylammonium group in acetylcholine. *Brit. J. Pharmacol.* **4**: 190–6.

HUTTER, O. F. (1952) Effect of choline on neuromuscular transmission in the cat. *J. Physiol.* **117**: 241–50.

JARAMILLO, J. (1968) Ganglionic actions of α,α′-bis-(dimethylammonium acetaldehyde diethylacetal)-*p,p′*-diacetylbiphenyl dibromide (DMAE). *J. Pharmacol. Exp. Ther.* **162**: 30–7.

JONES, S. F. and KWANBUNBUMPEN, S. (1968) On the role of synaptic vesicles in transmitter release. *Life Sci.* **7**: 1251–5.

JONES, S. F. and KWANBUNBUMPEN, S. (1970) The effects of nerve stimulation and hemicholinium on synaptic vesicles at the mammalian neuromuscular junction. *J. Physiol.* **207**: 31–50.

KAHLSON, G. and MACINTOSH, F. C. (1939) Acetylcholine synthesis in a sympathetic ganglion. *J. Physiol.* **96**: 277–92.

KASÉ, Y. and BORISON, H. L. (1958) Central respiratory depressant action of "hemicholinium" in the cat. *J. Pharmacol. Exp. Ther.* **122**: 215–33.

KESTON, A. S. and WORTIS, S. B. (1946) The antagonistic action of choline and its triethyl analogue. *Proc. Soc. Exp. Biol. Med.* **61**: 439–40.

KEY, B. J. and MARLEY, E. (1962) The effect of sympathomimetic amines on behaviour and electrocortical activity of chickens. *Electroen. Neurophysiol.* **14**: 90–105.

KIPLINGER, G. F., SWAIN, H. H. and BRODY, T. M. (1958) The action of dimethylaminoethanol on the isolated heart. *J. Pharmacol. Exp. Ther.* **122**: 37A.

KITZ, R. J., KARIS, J. H. and GINSBURG, S. (1969) A study *in vitro* of new short-acting, non-depolarizing neuromuscular blocking agents. *Biochem. Pharmacol.* **18**: 871–81.

KOKETSU, K. (1958) Action of tetraethylammonium chloride on neuromuscular transmission in the frog. *Amer. J. Physiol.* **193**: 213–18.

KOREY, S. R., DE BRAGANZA, B. and NACHMANSOHN, D. (1951) Choline acetylase V. Esterifications and transacetylations. *J. Biol. Chem.* **189**: 705–15.

LAURENCE, D. R. and WEBSTER, R. A. (1961) The activity of the triethyl analogue of choline in suppressing experimental tetanus. *Lancet* i: 481–2.

LEADERS, F. E. (1965) Separation of adrenergic and cholinergic fibres to the hind limb of the dog by hemicholinium (HC-3). *J. Pharmacol. Exp. Ther.* **148**: 238–46.

LIPTON, M. A. and BARRON, E. S. G. (1946) On the mechanism of the anaerobic synthesis of acetylcholine. *J. Biol. Chem.* **166**: 367–80.

LONG, J. P., EVANS, C. T. and WONG, S. (1967) A pharmacologic evaluation of hemicholinium analogs. *J. Pharmacol. Exp. Ther.* **155**: 223–30.

LONG, J. P. and REITZEL, N. (1958) The neuromuscular blocking properties of a,a′-dimethylethanolamino 4,4′-biacetophenone (hemicholinium). *J. Pharmacol. Exp. Ther.* **122**: 44A.

LONG, J. P. and SCHUELER, F. W. (1954) A new series of cholinesterase inhibitors. *J. Amer. Pharm. Assoc. (Sci. Ed.)* **43**: 79–86.

LONGO, V. G. (1958) Action of hemicholinium No. 3 on phrenic nerve action potentials. *J. Pharmacol. Exp. Ther.* **122**: 45A.

LONGO, V. G. (1959) Actions of hemicholinium No. 3 on phrenic nerve action potentials. *Arch. Int. Pharmacodyn.* **119**: 1–9.

LUNDGREN, G. (1966) Interaction of oxotremorine and hemicholinium on brain acetylcholine formation *in vitro. Life Sci.* **5**: 977–80.

MCCAMAN, R. E., RODRIGUEZ DE LORES ARNAIZ, G. and DE ROBERTIS, E. (1965) Species differences in subcellular distribution of choline acetylase in CNS. *J. Neurochem.* **12**: 927–35.

MCCOLL, J. D., BHATNAGER, S. P. and LAM, A. (1964) Inhibition of acetylcholine synthesis by troxypyrrolium iodide (FWH-399). *Fed. Proc.* **23**: 178.

MACINTOSH, F. C. (1961) Effect of HC-3 on acetylcholine turnover. *Fed. Proc.* **20**: 562–8.

MACINTOSH, F. C. (1963) Synthesis and storage of acetylcholine in nervous tissue. *Canad. J. Biochem. Physiol.* **41**: 2555–70.

MACINTOSH, F. C., BIRKS, R. I. and SASTRY, P. B. (1956) Pharmacological inhibition of acetylcholine synthesis. *Nature* **178**: 1181.

MACINTOSH, F. C., BIRKS, R. I. and SASTRY, P. B. (1958) Mode of action of an inhibitor of acetylcholine synthesis. *Neurology* **8**, Suppl. 1, 90–1.

MARCHBANKS, R. M. (1968) The uptake of [^{14}C] choline into synaptosomes *in vitro. Biochem. J.* **110**: 533–41.

MARCHBANKS, R. M. (1969) The conversion of ^{14}C-choline into ^{14}C-acetylcholine in synaptosomes *in vitro. Biochem. Pharmacol.* **18**: 1763–5.

MARKS, B. H. (1956) Effects of barbiturates on acetylation. *Science* **123**: 332–3.

MARSHALL, F. N. and LONG, J. P. (1959) Pharmacologic studies on some compounds structurally related to the hemicholinium HC-3. *J. Pharmacol. Exp. Ther.* **127**: 236–40.

MARSHALL, I. G. (1968a) The neuromuscular blocking action of some *NNN* and *NN*-bis-onium esters. *Europ. J. Pharmacol.* **2**: 258–64.

MARSHALL, I. G. (1968b) The neuromuscular blocking action of a series of bicyclic bis-onium esters. *Brit. J. Pharmacol.* **34**: 56–69.

MARSHALL, I. G. (1968c) Studies on the neuromuscular blocking activity of some quaternary ammonium compounds. Ph.D. Thesis, University of Strathclyde.

MARSHALL, I. G. (1969) The effects of some hemicholinium-like substances on the chick biventer cervicis muscle preparation. *Europ. J. Pharmacol.* **8**: 204–14.

MARSHALL, I. G. (1970a) Studies on the blocking action of 2-(4-phenylpiperidino) cyclohexanol (AH 5183). *Brit. J. Pharmacol.* **38**: 503–16.

MARSHALL, I. G. (1970b) A comparison between the blocking actions of 2-(4-phenyl-piperidino) cyclohexanol (AH 5183) and its *N*-methyl quaternary analogue (AH 5954). *Brit. J. Pharmacol.* **40**: 68–77.

MARTIN, A. R. and ORKAND, R. K. (1960) Postsynaptic action of HC-3 on neuromuscular transmission. *Fed. Proc.* **20**: 579–82.

MARTIN, A. R. and ORKAND, R. K. (1961) Postsynaptic effect of HC-3 at the neuromuscular junction of the frog. *Canad. J. Biochem. Physiol.* **39**: 343–9.

MARTIN, K. (1968) Concentrative accumulation of choline by human erythrocytes. *J. Gen. Physiol.* **51**: 497–516.

MARTIN, K. (1969) Effects of quaternary ammonium compounds on choline transport in red cells. *Brit. J. Pharmacol.* **36**: 458–69.

MATTHEWS, E. K. (1966) The presynaptic effects of quaternary ammonium compounds on the acetylcholine metabolism of a sympathetic ganglion. *Brit. J. Pharmacol.* **26**: 552–66.

NACHMANSOHN, D. and BERMAN, M. (1946) Studies on choline acetylase III. On the preparation of the coenzyme and its effect on the enzyme. *J. Biol. Chem.* **165**: 551–63.

NACHMANSOHN, D. and JOHN, H. M. (1944) Inhibition of choline acetylase by α-keto acids. *Proc. Soc. Exp. Biol. Med.* **57**: 361–2.

NACHMANSOHN, D. and JOHN, H. M. (1945) Studies on choline acetylase I. Effect of amino acids on the dialyzed enzyme. Inhibition by α-keto acids. *J. Biol. Chem.* **158**: 157–71.

NACHMANSOHN, D. and MACHADO, A. L. (1943) The formation of acetylcholine. A new enzyme "choline acetylase". *J. Neurophysiol.* **6**: 397–444.

NACHMANSOHN, D. and WEISS, M. S. (1948) Studies on choline acetylase IV. Effect of citric acid. *J. Biol. Chem.* **172**: 677–97.

NAKAMURA, R., CHENG, S. C. and NARUSE, H. (1970) A study on the precursors of the acetyl moiety of acetylcholine in brain slices. Observations on the compartmentalization of the acetylcoenzyme A pool. *Biochem. J.* **118**: 443–50.

OSUIDE, G. B. (1967) Personal communication.

PARSONS, R. L. (1969) Mechanism of neuromuscular blockade by tetraethylammonium. *Amer. J. Physiol.* **216**: 925–31.

PATON, W. D. M. and WAUD, D. R. (1967) The margin of safety of neuromuscular transmission. *J. Physiol.* **191**: 59–90.

PERRY, W. L. M. (1953) Acetylcholine release in the cat's superior cervical ganglion. *J. Physiol.* **119**: 439–54.

POTTER, L. T. (1968) Uptake of choline by nerve endings isolated from rat central cortex. In: *The Interaction of Drugs and Subcellular Components in Animal Cells*, pp. 293–304. Campbell, P.N.(ed.). Churchill, London.

POWERS, M. F., KRUGER, S. and SCHUELER, F. W. (1962) Synthesis and pharmacological studies of some aliphatic hemicholinium analogs. *J. Pharm. Sci.* **51**: 27–31.

PRASAD, K. and MACLEOD, D. P. (1966) Effect of hemicholinium-3 on the response of frog rectus abdominis muscle to acetylcholine. *Canad. J. Physiol. Pharmacol.* **44**: 179–87.

QUASTEL, D. M. J. and CURTIS, D. R. (1965) A central action of hemicholinium. *Nature* **208**: 192–4.

QUASTEL, J. H., TENNENBAUM, M. and WHEATLEY, A. H. M. (1936) Choline ester formation in, and choline esterase activities of, tissues *in vitro*. *Biochem. J.* **30**: 1668–81.

RAND, M. J. and CHANG, V. (1960) New evidence for a cholinergic process in sympathetic transmission. *Nature* **188**: 858–9.

RAND, M. J. and RIDEHALGH, A. (1965). Actions of hemicholinium and triethylcholine on responses of guinea-pig colon to stimulation of autonomic nerves. *J. Pharm. Pharmacol.* **17**: 144–56.

REITZEL, N. L. and LONG, J. P. (1959a). The neuromuscular blocking properties of α,α'-dimethylethanolamino 4,4'-biacetophenone (hemicholinium). *Arch. Int. Pharmacodyn.* **119**: 20–30.

REITZEL, N. L. and LONG, J. P. (1959b) Hemicholinium antagonism by choline analogues *J. Pharmacol. Exp. Ther.* **127**: 15–21.

RITCHIE, A. K. and GOLDBERG, A. M. (1970) Vesicular and synaptoplasmic synthesis of acetylcholine. *Science* **169**: 489–90.

DE ROBERTIS, E., RODRIGUEZ DE LORES ARNAIZ, G., SALGANICOFF, L., DE IRALDI, A. P.

and ZIEHER, L. M. (1963) Isolation of synaptic vesicles and structural organization of the acetylcholine systems within brain nerve endings. *J. Neurochem.* **10**: 225–35.

ROBERTS, D. V. (1962) Neuromuscular activity of the triethyl analogue of choline in the frog. *J. Physiol.* **160**: 94–105.

RODRIGUEZ DE LORES ARNAIZ, G., ZIEHER, L. M. and DE ROBERTIS, E. (1970) Neurochemical and structural studies on the mechanism of action of hemicholinium-3 in central cholinergic synapses. *J. Neurochem.* **17**: 221–9.

SAELENS, J. K. (1967) Effects of some quaternary ammonium compounds on choline-C^{14} and acetylcholine-C^{14} efflux from isolated tissue. *Arch. Int. Pharmacodyn.* **166**: 370–3.

SAELENS, J. K. and STOLL, W. R. (1965) The effect of triethylcholine on the efflux of choline and acetylcholine from the rat diaphragm. *Fed. Proc.* **24**: 675.

SCHUBERTH, J. and SUNDWALL, A. (1968) Differences in the subcellular localization of choline, acetylcholine and atropine taken up by mouse brain slices *in vitro. Acta Physiol. Scand.* **72**: 65–71.

SCHUELER, F. W. (1955) A new group of respiratory paralyzants. I. The "hemicholiniums". *J. Pharmacol. Exp. Ther.* **115**: 127–43.

SCHUELER, F. W. (1960) The mechanism of action of the hemicholiniums. *Int. Rev. Neurobiol.* **2**: 77–97.

SCHUELER, F. W., LONGO, V. G. and BOVET, D. (1954) Un nuovo gruppo di parolizzanti centrali. *Arch. Ital. Sci. Farmacol.* **4**: 328–31.

SHELLENBERGER, M. K. and DOMINO, E. F. (1967) Observations on intraventricular hemicholinium-3-induced EEG seizures. *Int. J. Neuropharmacol.* **6**: 283–91.

SLATER, P. (1968a) The effects of triethylcholine and hemicholinium-3 on the acetylcholine content of rat brain. *Int. J. Neuropharmacol.* **7**: 421–7.

SLATER, P. (1968b) The effects of triethylcholine, hemicholinium-3 and *N*-[4-diethyl-amino-2-butyryl]-succinimide on maze performance and brain acetylcholine in the rat. *Life Sci.* **7**: 833–7.

SLATER, P. and ROGERS, K. J. (1968) The effects of triethylcholine and hemicholinium-3 on tremor and brain acetylcholine. *Europ. J. Pharmacol.* **4**: 390–4.

SMITH, J. C., CAVALLITO, C. J. and FOLDES, F. F. (1966) The inhibition of choline acetylase (ChAc) by bisquaternary ammonium compounds. *Fed. Proc.* **25**: 320.

SMITH, J. C., CAVALLITO, C. J. and FOLDES, F. F. (1967) Choline acetyltransferase-inhibitors: a group of styryl-pyridine analogs. *Biochem. Pharmacol.* **16**: 2438–41.

STOVNER, J. (1957) The effect of low calcium and of tetraethylammonium (T.E.A.) on the rat diaphragm. *Acta. Physiol. Scand.* **40**: 285–96.

STOVNER, J. (1958) The anticurare activity of tetraethylammonium (TEA). *Acta Pharmacol.* **14**: 317–32.

SUNG, C. P. and JOHNSTONE, R. M. (1965) Evidence for active transport of choline in rat kidney cortex slices. *Canad. J. Biochem. Physiol.* **43**: 1111–18.

TAKAGI, H., KOJIMA, M., NAGATA, M. and KUROMI, H. (1970) On the site of action of hemicholinium-3 at the rat phrenic nerve-diaphragm preparation with special reference to its multiple presynaptic actions. *Neuropharmacol.* **9**: 359–67.

THAMPI, S. N., DOMER, F. R., HAARSTAD, V. B. and SCHUELER, F. W. (1966) Pharmacological studies of norphenyl hemicholinium-3. *J. Pharm. Sci.* **55**: 381–6.

THIES, R. E. and BROOKS, V. B. (1961) Postsynaptic neuromuscular block produced by hemicholinium No. 3. *Fed. Proc.* **20**: 569–78.

TUČEK, S. (1966) On the question of the localization of choline acetyltransferase in synaptic vesicles. *J. Neurochem.* **13**: 1329–34.

TUČEK, S. (1967a) Observations on the subcellular distribution of choline acetyltransferase in the brain tissue of mammals and comparisons of acetylcholine synthesis from acetate and citrate in homogenates and nerve-ending fractions. *J. Neurochem.* **14**: 519–29.

TuČEK, S. (1967b) Subcellular distribution of acetyl-CoA synthetase, ATP citrate lyase, citrate synthase, choline acetyltransferase, fumarate hydratase and lactate dehydrogenase in mammalian brain tissue. *J. Neurochem.* **14**: 531–45.

TuČEK, S. and CHENG, S.-C. (1970) Precursors of acetyl groups in acetylcholine in the brain *in vivo*. *Biochim. Biophys. Acta* **208**: 538–40.

VANDER, A. J. (1962) Renal excretion of choline in the dog. *Amer. J. Physiol.* **202**: 319–24.

VANOV, S. (1965) Responses of the rat urinary bladder *in situ* to drugs and to nerve stimulation. *Brit. J. Pharmacol.* **24,** 591–600.

VINCENZI, F. F. and WEST, T. C. (1965) Effect of hemicholinium on the release of autonomic mediators in the sino-atrial node. *Brit. J. Pharmacol.* **24**: 773–80.

WAELSCH, H. (1955) The turnover of components of the developing brain; the blood–brain barrier. In: *Biochemistry of the Developing Nervous System*, pp. 187–201. Waelsch, H. (ed.). Academic Press, New York.

WELLS, I. C. (1954) Oxidation of choline-like substances by rat liver preparation. Inhibitors of choline oxidase. *J. Biol. Chem.* **207**: 575–83.

WHITTAKER, V. P., MICHAELSON, I. A. and KIRKLAND, R. J. A. (1964) The separation of synaptic vesicles from nerve-ending particles ("synaptosomes"). *Biochem. J.* **90**: 293–303.

WILSON, H. and LONG, J. P. (1959) The effect of hemicholinium (HC-3) at various peripheral cholinergic transmitting sites. *Arch. Int. Pharmacodyn.* **120**: 343–52.

WOLFGRAM, F. J. (1954) Relative amounts of choline acetylase and cholinesterases in dorsal and ventral roots of cattle. *Amer. J. Physiol.* **176**: 505–7.

WONG, S. and LONG, J. P. (1967) Potentiation of actions of catecholamines by a derivative of hemicholinium. *J. Pharmacol. Exp. Ther.* **156**: 469–82.

WONG, S. and LONG, J. P. (1968) Antagonism of ganglionic stimulants by a,a'-bis-(dimethylammoniumacetaldehyde diethylacetal)-p,p'-diacetylbiphenyl bromide (DMAE). *J. Pharmacol. Exp. Ther.* **164**: 176–84.

WONG, S., LONG, J. P. and GROSS, E. G. (1968) Antagonism of the auricular stimulating action of nicotine by a,a'-bis-(dimethylammonium acetaldehyde diethylacetal)-p,p'-diacetylbiphenyl bromide (DMAE). *Arch. Int. Pharmacodyn.* **176**: 425–33.

ZAIMIS, E. (1960) *Ciba Foundation Symposium on Adrenergic Mechanisms*, p. 562. Churchill, London.

CHAPTER 14

INHIBITOR ION: MAGNESIUM

Lise Engbaek

Copenhagen

14.1. INTRODUCTION

Jolyet and Cahours (1869) were the first to demonstrate the blocking action of magnesium salts on the neuromuscular system; they localized the blocking effect to the neuromuscular junction. That Mg does not block nerve fibers was later confirmed by numerous workers, though nerve and muscle excitability was slightly depressed. The depressant action of Mg can be antagonized by calcium. Meltzer and Auer (1908) believed the action of Ca to be solely central; Bryant *et al.* (1939) demonstrated that Ca in addition counteracts the effect of Mg at the neuromuscular junction. The blocking action of Mg, like that of curare, was partly antagonized by acetylcholinesterase inhibitors (Brosnan and Boyd, 1937; Malorny and Ohnesorge, 1951). Experiments with repetitive stimulation of the motor nerve suggested that Mg and curare act on different sites at the neuromuscular junction; sustained stimulation of curarized muscle produced a rapid decrease in contraction, whereas Mg caused a rapid decrease followed by facilitation (Maaske *et al.*, 1938; Boyd *et al.*, 1938; Naess, 1952). When neuromuscular transmission was partially blocked by Mg the threshold to indirect stimulation decreased with frequency, whereas it was independent of frequency in partly curarized muscle (von Hof and Schneider, 1952). On the other hand, Mg decreased the sensitivity to acetylcholine (ACh) as does curare (Engbaek, 1948). Von Hof and Schneider (1952) showed that the concentration of Mg which antagonized ACh had to be 10 times that sufficient to block neuromuscular transmission. On the other hand, a blocking concentration of curarine also antagonized the effect of ACh, again suggesting different mechanisms of action. The site of action was clarified by recording end-plate potentials from Mg-blocked frog muscle (Del Castillo and Engbaek, 1954). The slight decrease in ACh

391

sensitivity of the postjunctional membrane could not account for the almost complete abolishment of the end-plate potential. The reduction in excitability of the muscle membrane was also of minor importance, since Ca antagonized the effect on the end-plate potential and relieved the block, and the effect of Mg and Ca on the muscle membrane was synergistic. Furthermore, Mg did not depolarize the postjunctional membrane. Thus the main action of Mg is prejunctional and is to reduce the amount of transmitter released by the nerve impulse.

The antagonistic action of Mg and Ca on ACh release was demonstrated directly in the mammalian sympathetic ganglion (Hutter and Kostial, 1954). It is less well known that the same effect has been shown in mammalian muscle by Straughan (1959). The Mg–Ca antagonism on the end-plate or junctional potentials in muscle has been found not only in the fast fibers of amphibian muscle but also in mammalian muscle (Boyd and Martin 1956b), human muscle (Elmqvist *et al.*, 1964), frog slow muscle (Burke, 1957), fish muscle (de Mello and Chang, 1966), insect "fast" muscle (Hoyle, 1955) and smooth muscle, probably adrenergic (Kuriyama, 1964).

The minimal concentration of Mg in the bathing solution necessary to block the neuromuscular transmission in frog muscle was 5 mM at room temperature (about 21°C, Del Castillo and Engbaek, 1954); in the rat diaphragm the minimal blocking concentration was 6 mM at 37°C, increasing to 10 mM at 22°C (Stovner, 1957).

The mechanism of the blocking action of Mg at the neuromuscular junction has been elucidated further in the last few years. The following sections deal mainly with the papers which have been published since 1963. For earlier references on the effect of Mg on neuromuscular transmission the reader is referred to reviews by Aubert (1963), Desmedt (1963) and Engbaek (1952).

14.2. THE EFFECT OF MAGNESIUM ON THE EVOKED AND SPONTANEOUS RELEASE OF TRANSMITTER

According to the quantum hypothesis of neuromuscular transmission (Del Castillo and Katz, 1954b) ACh is released by the nerve impulse in discrete units of the same size as the spontaneously liberated units which give rise to the randomly occurring miniature end-plate potentials (Fatt and Katz, 1952). The arrival of the nerve impulse normally results in a synchronous release of about 100 quanta in frog muscle (Martin, 1955; Takeuchi and Takeuchi, 1960) and 200–300 quanta in mammalian muscle

(Boyd and Martin, 1956b). Mg and Ca act oppositely on the evoked end-plate potential; an increase in the concentration of Mg ions or a reduction in concentration of Ca ions reduces the number of quanta released by a nerve impulse. At a suitable concentration ratio of Mg and Ca the end-plate potentials evoked by successive impulses fluctuate between total failure and one or a few unit potentials (Del Castillo and Katz, 1954b).

Recent evidence has placed the Mg and Ca effect in the process which couples the depolarization by the nerve impulse and the release of transmitter; recorded extracellularly, small diphasic all-or-none spike potentials precede the end-plate potentials in Mg-treated rat diaphragm. High concentrations of Mg cause intermittent failure of the end-plate potential without failure of the preceding spike potential (Hubbard and Schmidt, 1963). In frog muscle blocked by low Ca and high (about 6 mM) or low (about 0.8 mM) Mg, the release of transmitter is increased by local iontophoretic application of Ca while the extracellularly recorded spike in the terminal nerve fiber remains unaltered (Katz and Miledi, 1964, 1965).

Originally Del Castillo and Katz (1955, 1956) suggested that the ACh quantum might correspond to a synaptic vesicle inside the nerve endings. However, an acceleration of the quantum release by high concentrations of K and hypertonic solutions does not reduce the number of vesicles to an appreciable degree (Birks *et al.*, 1960). It has recently been shown that the number of synaptic vesicles which touch the axoplasmic membrane opposite the postjunctional folds decrease after depolarization for 2 hours in 20 mM K, known to increase the frequency of the miniature end-plate potentials. Addition of 12.5 mM Mg counteracts the acceleration of transmitter release and prevents the depletion of synaptic vesicles (Hubbard and Kwanbunbumpen, 1968).

Calcium is essential to the release of ACh from the nerve terminals subsequent to the arrival of the nerve impulse (Del Castillo and Stark, 1952), and the antagonism of Mg may be accounted for by the occupation of a site for attachment of Ca (Del Castillo and Katz, 1954a). The kinetics of the Ca–Mg antagonism are in agreement with a competitive action of Mg on the evoked end-plate potential (Jenkinson, 1957; Dodge and Rahamimoff, 1967; Hubbard *et al.*, 1968b).

An inward movement of Ca through the nerve terminal membrane has been suggested to be the first step in the evoked release of transmitter, the permeability to Ca being increased by the depolarization (Katz and Miledi, 1967a). The utilization of iontophoretically administered Ca stops immediately after the application of a depolarizing pulse to the nerve endings (Katz and Miledi, 1967b). The duration of the Mg effect is less certain, although there are indications that the competitive action of Mg takes place in the same brief period.

Depolarization of the nerve terminals by steady current or high external K concentration causes a striking increase in frequency of miniature end-plate potentials in amphibian and mammalian (including human) muscle. This increase in frequency is counteracted by Mg (Del Castillo and Katz, 1954d; Liley, 1956b; Elmqvist, 1965). Liley (1956b) suggested a similar mechanism for the release of ACh by the action potential and by a steady depolarizing current. The decrease in quantal content of the end-plate potential caused by a blocking concentration of Mg corresponds to the change in slope of the relation between the calculated depolarization by excess K and the extrapolated discharge frequency.

The supposition that the nerve impulse accelerates the spontaneous release of transmitter encounters a difficulty in the finding that the rate of spontaneous discharge does not decrease in blocking concentrations of Mg (Del Castillo and Katz, 1954a; Boyd and Martin, 1956a). Only in insect muscle does a small (15%) reduction in spontaneous frequency follow an increase in Mg concentration from 2 to 10 mM (Usherwood, 1963). On the other hand, the increase in discharge frequency with the concentration of Ca is consistent with the action of Ca on the evoked end-plate potential (Boyd and Martin, 1956a; Hubbard, 1961; Mambrini and Benoit, 1964).

Hubbard *et al.* (1968a) have clarified the action of Mg on the spontaneous release of transmitter. A fraction of the spontaneous release persists for up to 8 hours in Ca-depleted mammalian muscle; this basic release is accelerated by Ca and the acceleration is counteracted by 1 to 3 mM Mg (Hubbard, 1961). Higher concentrations of Mg, above 6 mM, increase the frequency, most markedly in low Ca (Hubbard *et al.*, 1968a). The difficulty still persists that the evoked release is depressed by Mg whereas the spontaneous release is both depressed and increased according to the concentration. Hubbard *et al.* (1968a, b) explain this discrepancy by a kinetic model assuming three different sites for the action of Ca and Mg.

In frog muscle at low concentrations of Ca the relation between the end-plate potential and the Ca concentration is nonlinear (Jenkinson, 1957). The course of this relationship suggests that the end-plate potential depends on a higher power of Ca. Dodge and Rahamimoff (1967) derived an exponential expression for the dependence of the end-plate potential on the external Ca and Mg concentration suggesting that four Ca ions are involved in the release of one quantum of transmitter. Magnesium (0.5–4 mM) does not change the slope of the relation between Ca and the end-plate potential, but shifts the line along the axis representing the concentration. In mammalian muscle the slope indicates a cooperation of 3 Ca ions (Hubbard *et al.*, 1968b).

In frog muscle a reduction in the Na concentration produces an increase in the quantal content of the evoked end-plate potential in the presence of low external Ca, suggesting a competition between Ca and Na for the binding sites in the presynaptic membrane (Birks and Cohen, 1965; Kelly, 1965). In mammalian muscle Na and Ca act competitively on the rate of spontaneous transmitter release in the presence of 15 mM K (Gage and Quastel, 1966). The increase in frequency produced by lowering of the concentration of Na is slightly enhanced in the presence of 15 mM Mg and 4 mM Ca, suggesting that Mg and Na do not compete with Ca at the same site or that Mg competes less effectively with Ca in lowered Na (Gage and Quastel, 1966). Since high concentrations of Mg increase the rate of spontaneous transmitter release the enhanced effect of reducing Na in the presence of Mg does not exclude that these ions act at the same site (Hubbard *et al.*, 1968a). In fact, the increase in quantal content of the evoked end-plate potential produced by a 40% reduction in Na concentration was significantly less pronounced when the concentration of Mg was raised from 1 to 8 mM, suggesting that Mg and Na compete with Ca for the same sites (Rahamimoff and Colomo, 1967).

14.2.1. REPETITIVE STIMULATION, DEPRESSION AND FACILITATION

Repetitive nerve stimulation gives rise to two opposite processes in neuromuscular transmission: depression of the end-plate potential, which prevails in mammalian muscle, and facilitation of the response, which predominates in amphibian muscle. The depression is due to a reduction and the facilitation to an increase in the number of normal-sized quanta released (Brooks and Thies, 1962; Del Castillo and Katz, 1954c; Liley, 1956a).

The depression was attributed to a depletion of transmitter in an immediately available store (Liley and North, 1953; Takeuchi, 1958a). Based on the early depression of transmitter release by nerve stimulation at high frequency Elmqvist and Quastel (1965) estimated the immediately available store to be 300–1000 quanta; the store is replenished by mobilization of ACh from a larger, less readily available store. The size of the immediately available store is the same whether Mg is present or not, whereas Mg reduces the fraction of transmitter released from the store; the quantum content of the first end-plate potential of a train was calculated to be reduced from 27% of the immediately available store to 13% in 4 mM Mg (Elmqvist and Quastel, 1965).

The facilitation produced by repetitive stimulation is present after a single impulse, even if this impulse fails to release transmitter in preparations blocked by high Mg and low Ca concentrations (Del Castillo and Katz, 1954c). Katz and Miledi (1965, 1968) suggested that this facilitation may be due to a residue of Ca at the critical sites on the inner surface of the membrane of the nerve terminals. In frog muscle facilitation is decreased by a rise in Ca or a reduction in Mg concentration (which is associated with an increase in the first response to double stimuli), even if the first response consists of very few quantal units due to reduced Ca and elevated Mg (Rahamimoff, 1968). This could be explained as due to a residue of Ca, since increase in Ca or decrease in Mg causes more sites to be occupied during the first impulse with a smaller fraction of unoccupied sites left for the second impulse. But if the transmitter release of the first impulse is kept constant by increasing Ca *and* Mg both the degree and duration of facilitation increase, suggesting that Ca and Mg have in addition some other effect on facilitation (Rahamimoff, 1968).

14.2.2. DEPOLARIZATION OF NERVE TERMINALS AND EVOKED RELEASE OF TRANSMITTER

The amplitude of the evoked end-plate potential in curarized mammalian muscle is depressed by depolarization of the nerve terminals (Hubbard and Willis, 1962a) due to a diminished quantum content, in this case presumably caused by a reduction in the available store and not, as in the case of high Mg, by a reduction in the fractional release (Hubbard and Willis, 1968). Strangely, the reduction of the end-plate potential by depolarizing current is completely counteracted by 12.5 mM Mg in the presence of 2 mM Ca (Hubbard and Willis, 1968). The amplitude of the terminal nerve action potential is reduced proportionately to the depolarizing current, and Hubbard and Willis (1968) suggested that this reduction (implying a reduction in the available store) is responsible for the decrease in transmitter release. However, in the presence of 12 mM Mg the end-plate potential is not reduced parallel to the reduction in nerve spike amplitude. A possible explanation is that depolarization of the nerve terminals reduces the rate of mobilization of transmitter into the immediately available store, the antagonism of Mg to the effect of depolarizing current being due to the reduction in the fractional release from this store produced by Mg.

14.2.3. MAGNESIUM AND MISCELLANEOUS FACTORS AFFECTING
SPONTANEOUS AND EVOKED RELEASE OF TRANSMITTER

Magnesium is without effect on the rise in frequency of spontaneous discharge caused by stretch (Hutter and Trautwein, 1956), repetitive stimulation (Liley, 1956a), ouabain (Elmqvist and Feldman, 1965), and an increase in temperature (Takeuchi, 1958b). The increase in frequency produced by hypertonicity is unaffected by the addition of Mg (6–14 mM) and simultaneous reduction of Ca (to 0.9–1.35 mM, Furshpan, 1956). The rise in frequency which occurs during hypoxia is suppressed by Mg, providing additional indirect evidence that the nerve terminals are depolarized (Hubbard and Løyning, 1966).

In mammalian muscle an increase in Mg concentration causes a rise in the discharge frequency to the original level when the frequency is reduced by applying hyperpolarizing current to the nerve terminals (Liley, 1956b; Hubbard and Willis, 1962b). In frog muscle weak hyperpolarizing current does not change the frequency; above a certain current strength bursts of miniature potentials occur and remain unchanged by a combined rise in Mg and a reduction in Ca (Del Castillo and Katz, 1954d).

The increase in discharge frequency in frog muscle produced by 3% ethyl alcohol in Ringer's solution is reduced by Mg and this effect is antagonized by Ca (Okada, 1967). The effect of ethyl alcohol on the miniature end-plate potential frequency might be due to its depolarizing action (Wright, 1947; Gallego, 1948; Posternak and Mangold, 1949) in agreement with the effect of Mg and Ca on the rise in frequency produced by depolarization (p. 396). But this is at variance with the facilitation of neuromuscular transmission produced by ethyl alcohol prejunctionally in the rat (Gage, 1965), since prolonged depolarization of the nerve terminals reduces the transmitter released by the action potential (Hubbard and Willis, 1962a).

In frog muscle the increase in evoked end-plate potential caused by stretch is more pronounced when the quantum release is reduced by Mg (Hutter and Trautwein, 1956). The effect of Mg on the temperature dependence of the end-plate potential amplitude differs in amphibian and in mammalian muscle. In curarized frog and mammalian muscle the end-plate potential increases with temperature. In frog muscle the increase is more pronounced in 16–20 mM Mg (Takeuchi, 1958b); in mammalian muscle the quantum content of the end-plate potential decreases when the temperature is raised in high Mg combined with low or high Ca (Boyd and Martin, 1956b; Hofmann *et al.*, 1966) in agreement with the finding

N.B.S.A.—O

of Stovner (1957) that the minimal blocking concentration of Mg is higher at 22°C than at 37°C.

14.3. THE EFFECT OF MAGNESIUM ON THE ACETYLCHOLINE SENSITIVITY OF THE POSTJUNCTIONAL MEMBRANE

In frog muscle 10–15 mM Mg reduces the depolarization of the postjunctional membrane caused by ACh by 20–40% (Del Castillo and Engbaek, 1954). Correspondingly the miniature end-plate potentials are diminished by about 40% in 16 mM Mg in frog and 9 mM Mg in cat muscle (Del Castillo and Katz, 1954a; Boyd and Martin, 1956a). The action of *d*-tubocurarine, which competitively blocks the postjunctional receptor, is antagonized by Mg (Del Castillo and Engbaek, 1954); the affinity of the receptor for *d*-tubocurarine is reduced by about 40% in the presence of 8.6 mM Mg (Jenkinson, 1960).

In normal Ringer's solution the postjunctional membrane at the neuromuscular junction is depolarized when transmitter is liberated and the negativity of the membrane potential exceeds -10 to -20 mV ("reversal potential"), whereas it is hyperpolarized when the negativity is less than the reversal potential (Del Castillo and Katz, 1954e). In frog muscle 30 mM Ca or 20 mM Mg increase the negativity of the reversal potential, consistent with a relative decrease in Na conductance (Takeuchi, 1963). Voltage clamp experiments indicated a reduction in Na conductance when the concentration of Ca is high (Takeuchi, 1963). It seems reasonable to assume that Mg has the same effect.

14.4. THE EFFECT OF MAGNESIUM ON THE MUSCLE MEMBRANE

The decrease in excitability of the muscle membrane caused by excess Mg and Ca has been investigated in voltage-clamped frog muscle fibers (Costantin, 1968). Both Mg and Ca increase the depolarization necessary to activate the specific increase in sodium permeability. The threshold membrane potential shifts from about -54 mV without Mg to about -32 mV in 18 mM Mg, indicating that Mg is about one-half as effective as Ca. The threshold depolarization to an increase in K conductance is also increased by Mg and Ca, but this threshold is less sensitive to excess Mg or Ca, and Mg and Ca seem to be equally effective.

14.5. THE EFFECT OF MAGNESIUM ON NERVE FIBERS

14.5.1. PERIPHERAL NERVE

Recent work has clarified the mechanism of the depressant action of Mg on the excitability of nerve. In concentrations which cause a complete block of neuromuscular transmission (18 mM) Mg reduces the excitability of the single myelinated nerve fiber of the frog by about 50% without changing the action current. Calcium and Mg act synergistically on nerve excitability, Mg being 2.4 times less active than Ca (Frankenhaeuser and Meves, 1958). In isolated fibers from the squid excess Ca or Mg increase the depolarizing current required to bring the Na conductance to the critical level, Mg being again less active than Ca (Frankenhaeuser and Hodgkin, 1957).

14.5.2. TERMINAL NERVE FIBERS

Several findings indicate that Mg also causes a reduction in excitability in the terminal nerve branches. In mammalian terminal fibers Mg increases the threshold in concentrations which block the neuromuscular transmission (Hubbard *et al.*, 1965), and in frog terminal fibers Mg facilitates post-tetanic conduction block (Braun and Schmidt, 1966). Magnesium antagonizes the decrease in the prejunctional spike during repetitive stimulation of frog nerve, explained as being due to subsiding depolarization (Braun and Schmidt 1966). However, this effect need not to be caused by a direct action of Mg on the depolarization of terminal branches; it can be due to diminished ACh release (Braun and Schmidt, 1966), since receptors for the depolarizing action of ACh have been demonstrated in the terminal nerve fibers (Hubbard *et al.*, 1965).

SUMMARY

The work of the past few years has clarified several aspects of the mechanism of action of Mg on neuromuscular transmission:

1. The Mg/Ca antagonism is related to the coupling between depolarization and transmitter release.

2. Magnesium acts competitively with Ca on the evoked release of transmitter.

3. Magnesium has a dual action in the spontaneous release of transmitter. Low concentrations of Mg diminish and high concentrations enhance the frequency of spontaneous activity.

4. Though Mg decreases the evoked transmitter release from an immediately available store, it does not affect the initial size of the store.

REFERENCES

AUBERT, X. (1963) Les ions alcalino-terreux et le muscle strié. In: *Handbuch der Experimentellen Pharmakologie*, suppl. 17, vol. 1, pp. 337–97. Bacq, Z. M. (ed.). Springer-Verlag, Berlin.

BIRKS, R. J. and COHEN, M. W. (1965) Effects of sodium on transmitter release from frog motor nerve terminals. In: *Muscle*, pp. 403–20. Paul, W. H., Daniel, E. E., Kay, C. M. and Monckton, G. (eds.). Pergamon Press, Oxford.

BIRKS, R., HUXLEY, H. E. and KATZ, B. (1960) The fine structure of the neuromuscular junction of the frog. *J. Physiol. (Lond.)* **150**: 134–44.

BOYD, I. A. and MARTIN, A. R. (1956a) Spontaneous subthreshold activity at mammalian neuromuscular junctions. *J. Physiol. (Lond.)* **132**: 61–73.

BOYD, I. A. and MARTIN, A. R. (1956b) The end-plate potential in mammalian muscle. *J. Physiol. (Lond.)* **132**: 74–91.

BOYD, T. E., BROSNAN, J. J. and MAASKE, C. A. (1938) The summation of facilitating and inhibitory effects at the mammalian neuromuscular junction. *J. Neurophysiol.* **1**: 497–507.

BRAUN, M. and SCHMIDT, R. F. (1966) Potential changes recorded from the frog motor nerve terminal during its activation. *Pflügers Arch. Ges. Physiol.* **287**: 56–80.

BROOKS, V. B. and THIES, R. E. (1962) Reduction of quantum content during neuromuscular transmission. *J. Physiol. (Lond.)* **162**: 298–310.

BROSNAN, J. J. and BOYD, T. E. (1937) Agents which antagonize the curare-like action of magnesium. *Amer. J. Physiol.* **119**: 281–2.

BRYANT, G. W., LEHMANN, G. and KNOEFEL, P. K. (1939) The action of magnesium on the central nervous system and its antagonism by calcium. *J. Pharmacol. Exp. Ther.* **65**: 318–21.

BURKE, W. (1957) Spontaneous potentials in slow muscle fibres of the frog. *J. Physiol. (Lond.)* **135**: 511–21.

DEL CASTILLO, J. and ENGBAEK, L. (1954) The nature of the neuromuscular block produced by magnesium. *J. Physiol. (Lond.)* **124**: 370–84.

DEL CASTILLO, J. and KATZ, B. (1954a) The effect of magnesium on the activity of motor nerve endings. *J. Physiol. (Lond.)* **124**: 553–9.

DEL CASTILLO, J. and KATZ, B. (1954b) Quantal components of the end-plate potential. *J. Physiol. (Lond.)* **124**: 560–73.

DEL CASTILLO, J. and KATZ, B. (1954c) Statistical factors involved in neuromuscular facilitation and depression. *J. Physiol. (Lond.)* **124**: 574–85.

DEL CASTILLO, J. and KATZ, B. (1954d) Changes in end-plate activity produced by pre-synaptic polarization. *J. Physiol. (Lond.)* **124**: 586–604.

DEL CASTILLO, J. and KATZ, B. (1954e) The membrane change produced by the neuromuscular transmitter. *J. Physiol. (Lond.)* **125**: 546–65.

DEL CASTILLO, J. and KATZ, B. (1955) Local activity at a depolarized nerve–muscle junction. *J. Physiol. (Lond.)* **128**: 396–411.

DEL CASTILLO, J. and KATZ, B. (1956) Biophysical aspects of neuro-muscular transmission. *Progr. Biophys. Chem.* **6**: 121–70.

DEL CASTILLO, J. and STARK, L. (1952) The effect of calcium ions on the motor end-plate potentials. *J. Physiol. (Lond.)* 116: 507–15.

COSTANTIN, L. L. (1968) The effect of calcium on contraction and conductance thresholds in the frog skeletal muscle. *J. Physiol. (Lond.)* 195: 119–32.

DESMEDT, J. E. (1963) L'action des cations alcalino-terreux sur les transmissions neuromusculaire et synaptiques. In: *Handbuch der Experimentellen Pharmakologie*, suppl. 17, vol. 1, pp. 295–336. Bacq, Z. M. (ed.). Springer-Verlag, Berlin.

DODGE, F. A. JR. and RAHAMIMOFF, R. (1967) Co-operative action of calcium ions in transmitter release at the neuromuscular junction. *J. Physiol. (Lond.)* 193: 419–32.

ELMQVIST, D. (1965) Potassium induced release of transmitter at the human neuro-muscular junction. *Acta Physiol. Scand.* 64: 340–4.

ELMQVIST, D. and FELDMAN, D. S. (1965) Effects of sodium pump inhibitors on spontane-ous acetylcholine release at the neuromuscular junction. *J. Physiol. (Lond.)* 181: 498–505.

ELMQVIST, D., HOFMANN, W. W., KUGELBERG, J. and QUASTEL, D. M. J. (1964) An electrophysiological investigation of neuromuscular transmission in myasthenia gravis. *J. Physiol. (Lond.)* 174: 417–34.

ELMQVIST, D. and QUASTEL, D. M. J. (1965) A quantitative study of end-plate potentials in isolated human muscles. *J. Physiol. (Lond.)* 178: 505–29.

ENGBAEK, L. (1948) Investigations on the course and localization of magnesium anesthesia. A comparison with ether anesthesia. *Acta Pharmacol. (Kobenhavn)* 4: suppl. 1, p. 189.

ENGBAEK, L. (1952) The pharmacological actions of magnesium ions with particular reference to the neuromuscular and the cardiovascular system. *Pharmacol. Rev.* 4: 396–414.

FATT, P. and KATZ, B. (1952) Spontaneous subthreshold activity at motor nerve endings. *J. Physiol. (Lond.)* 117: 109–28.

FRANKENHAEUSER, B. and HODGKIN, A. L. (1957) The action of calcium on the electrical properties of squid axons. *J. Physiol. (Lond.)* 137: 218–44.

FRANKENHAEUSER, B. and MEVES, H. (1958) The effect of magnesium and calcium on the frog myelinated nerve fibre. *J. Physiol. (Lond.)* 142: 360–5.

FURSHPAN, E. J. (1956) The effects of osmotic pressure changes on the spontaneous activity at motor nerve endings. *J. Physiol. (Lond.)* 134: 689–97.

GAGE, P. W. (1965) The effect of methyl, ethyl and n-propyl alcohol on neuromuscular transmission in the rat. *J. Pharmacol.* 150: 236–43.

GAGE, P. W. and QUASTEL, D. M. J. (1966) Competition between sodium and calcium ions in transmitter release at mammalian neuromuscular junctions. *J. Physiol. (Lond.)* 185: 95–123.

GALLEGO, A. (1948) On the effect of ethyl alcohol upon frog nerve. *J. Cell. Comp. Physiol.* 31: 97–106.

HOF, C. V. and SCHNEIDER, H. H. (1952) Über die Wirkungsweise von Magnesium im Gegensatz zu Curarin und Nicotin. *Naunyn-Schmiedeberg's Arch. Exp. Path. Pharmak.* 214: 176–84.

HOFMANN, W. W., PARSONS, R. L. and FEIGEN, G. A. (1966) Effects of temperature and drugs on mammalian motor nerve terminals. *Amer. J. Physiol.* 211: 135–40.

HOYLE, G. (1955) The effects of some common cations on neuromuscular transmission in insects. *J. Physiol. (Lond.)* 127: 90–103.

HUBBARD, J. I. (1961) The effect of calcium and magnesium on the spontaneous release of transmitter from mammalian motor nerve endings. *J. Physiol. (Lond.)* 159: 507–17.

HUBBARD, J. I., JONES, S. F. and LANDAU, E. M. (1968a) On the mechanism by which calcium and magnesium affect the spontaneous release of transmitter from mammalian motor nerve terminals. *J. Physiol. (Lond.)* 194: 355–80.

HUBBARD, J. I., JONES, S. F. and LANDAU, E. M. (1968b) On the mechanism by which calcium and magnesium affect the release of transmitter by nerve impulses. *J. Physiol. (Lond.)* **196**: 75–86.

HUBBARD, J. I. and KWANBUNBUMPEN, S. (1968) Evidence for the vesicle hypothesis. *J. Physiol. (Lond.)* **194**: 407–20.

HUBBARD, J. I. and LØYNING, Y. (1966) The effects of hypoxia on neuromuscular transmission in a mammalian preparation. *J. Physiol. (Lond.)* **185**: 205–23.

HUBBARD, J. I. and SCHMIDT, R. F. (1963) An electrophysiological investigation of mammalian motor nerve terminals. *J. Physiol. (Lond.)* **166**: 145–67.

HUBBARD, J. I., SCHMIDT, R. F. and YOKOTA, T. (1965) The effect of acetylcholine upon mammalian nerve terminals. *J. Physiol. (Lond.)* **181**: 810–29.

HUBBARD, J. I. and WILLIS, W. D. (1962a) Reduction of transmitter output by depolarization. *Nature (Lond.)* **193**: 1294–5.

HUBBARD, J. I. and WILLIS, W. D. (1962b) Hyperpolarization of mammalian nerve terminals. *J. Physiol. (Lond.)* **163**: 115–37.

HUBBARD, J. I. and WILLIS, W. D. (1968) The effects of depolarization of motor nerve terminals upon the release of transmitter by nerve impulses. *J. Physiol. (Lond.)* **194**: 381–405.

HUTTER, O. F. and KOSTIAL, K. (1954) Effect of magnesium and calcium ions on the release of acetylcholine. *J. Physiol. (Lond.)* **124**: 234–41.

HUTTER, O. F. and TRAUTWEIN, W. (1956) Neuromuscular facilitation by stretch of motor nerve-endings. *J. Physiol. (Lond.)* **133**: 610–25.

JENKINSON, D. H. (1957) The nature of the antagonism between calcium and magnesium ions at the neuromuscular junction. *J. Physiol. (Lond.)* **138**: 434–44.

JENKINSON, D. H. (1960) The antagonism between tubocurarine and substances which depolarize the motor end-plate. *J. Physiol. (Lond).* **152**: 309–24.

JOLYET, F. and CAHOURS, A. (1869) Sur l'action physiologique des sulfats de potasse, de soude et de magnesie en injection dans le sang. *Arch. Physiol. Norm. et Path.* **2**: 113–20.

KATZ, B. and MILEDI, R. (1964) Localization of calcium action at the nerve–muscle junction. *J. Physiol. (Lond.)* **171**: 10P–12P.

KATZ, B. and MILEDI, R. (1965) The effect of calcium on acetylcholine release from motor nerve terminals. *Proc. Roy. Soc. (Biol.)* **161**: 496–503.

KATZ, B. and MILEDI, R. (1967a) The release of acetylcholine from nerve endings by graded electric pulses. *Proc. Roy. Soc. (Biol.)* **167**: 23–38.

KATZ, B. and MILEDI, R. (1967b) The timing of calcium action during neuromuscular transmission. *J. Physiol. (Lond.)* **189**: 535–44.

KATZ, B. and MILEDI, R. (1968) The role of calcium in neuromuscular facilitation. *J. Physiol. (Lond.)* **195**: 481–92.

KELLY, J. S. (1965) Antagonism between Na^+ and Ca^{2+} at the neuromuscular junction. *Nature (Lond.)* **205**: 296–7.

KURIYAMA, H. (1964) Effect of calcium and magnesium on neuromuscular transmission in the hypogastric nerve–vas deferens preparation of the guinea pig. *J. Physiol. (Lond.)* **175**: 211–30.

LILEY, A. W. (1956a) The quantal components of the mammalian end-plate potential. *J. Physiol. (Lond.)* **133**: 571–87.

LILEY, A. W. (1956b) The effect of presynaptic polarization on the spontaneous activity at the mammalian neuromuscular junction. *J. Physiol. (Lond.)* **134**: 427–43.

LILEY, A. W. and NORTH, K. A. K. (1953) An electrical investigation of effects of repetitive stimulation on mammalian neuromuscular junction. *J. Neurophysiol.* **16**: 509–27.

MAASKE, C. A., BOYD, T. E. and BROSNAN, J. (1938) Inhibition and impulse summation at the mammalian neuromuscular junction. *J. Neurophysiol.* **1**: 332–41.

MALORNY, G. and OHNESORGE, F. K. (1951) Magnesium-Kalzium-Antagonismus bei Prüfung der neuromuskulären Erregbarkeit. *Naturwissenschaften* **38**: 481–2.

MAMBRINI, J. and BENOIT, P. R. (1964) Action du calcium sur la jonction neuro-musculaire chez la Grenouille. *C.R. Soc. Biol. (Paris)* **158**: 1454–8.

MARTIN, A. R. (1955) A further study of the statistical composition of the end-plate potential. *J. Physiol. (Lond.)* **130**: 114–22.

DE MELLO, W. C. and CHANG, Y. C. (1966). Neuromuscular transmission in *Electrophorus electricus* (L.). *Experientia* **22**: 680–1.

MELTZER, S. J. and AUER, J. (1908) The antagonistic action of calcium upon the inhibitory effect of magnesium. *Amer. J. Physiol.* **21**: 400–19.

NAESS, K. (1952) The peripheral effects of magnesium and curare. *Acta Pharmacol. (Kobenhavn)* **8**: 137–48.

OKADA, K. (1967) Effects of calcium and magnesium ions on the frequency of miniature end-plate potential discharges in amphibian muscle in the presence of ethyl alcohol. *Experientia* **23**: 363–4.

POSTERNAK, J. and MANGOLD, R. (1949) Action de narcotiques sur la conduction par les fibres nerveuses et sur leur potentiel de membrane. *Helv. Physiol. Pharmacol. Acta* **7**: C55–C56.

RAHAMIMOFF, R. (1968) A dual effect of calcium ions on neuromuscular facilitation. *J. Physiol. (Lond.)* **195**: 471–80.

RAHAMIMOFF, R. and COLOMO, F. (1967) Inhibitory action of sodium ions on transmitter release at the motor end-plate. *Nature (Lond.)* **215**: 1174–6.

STOVNER, J. (1957) The effect of tetraethylammonium (TEA) and temperature on the neuromuscular block produced by magnesium. *Acta Physiol. Scand.* **41**: 370–83.

STRAUGHAN, D. W. (1959) The effects of changes in temperature, ionic environment and of drugs on the release of acetylcholine from skeletal nerve-muscle preparations. Ph.D. Thesis, University of London.

TAKEUCHI, A. (1958a) The long lasting depression in neuromuscular transmission of frog. *Jap. J. Physiol.* **8**: 102–13.

TAKEUCHI, A. and TAKEUCHI, N. (1960) Further analysis of relationship between end-plate potential and end-plate current. *J. Neurophysiol.* **23**: 397–402.

TAKEUCHI, N. (1958b) The effect of temperature on the neuromuscular junction. *Jap. J. Physiol.* **8**: 391–404.

TAKEUCHI, N. (1963) Effects of calcium on the conductance change of the end-plate membrane during the action of transmitter. *J. Physiol. (Lond.)* **167**: 141–55.

USHERWOOD, P. N. R. (1963) Spontaneous miniature potentials from insect muscle fibres. *J. Physiol. (Lond.)* **169**: 149–60.

WRIGHT, E. B. (1947) The effect of asphyxiation and narcosis on peripheral nerve polarization and conduction. *Amer. J. Physiol.* **148**: 714–84.

SUPPLEMENTARY REFERENCES

Reference is not made to the following literature, most of which has appeared subsequently.

The effect of magnesium on the evoked and spontaneous release of transmitter

BLIOCH, Z. L., GLAGOLEVA, I. M., LIBERMAN, E. A. and NENASHEV, V. A. (1968) A study of the mechanism of quantal transmitter release at a chemical synapse. *J. Physiol. (Lond.)* **199**: 11–35.

COLOMO, F. and RAHAMIMOFF, R. (1968) Interaction between sodium and calcium ions in the process of transmitter release at the neuromuscular junction. *J. Physiol. (Lond.)* **198**: 203–18.

LANDAU, E. M. (1969) The interaction of presynaptic polarization with calcium and magnesium in modifying spontaneous transmitter release from mammalian motor nerve terminals. *J. Physiol. (Lond.)* **203**: 281–99.

ROSENTHAL, J. (1969) Post-tetanic potentiation at the neuromuscular junction of the frog. *J. Physiol. (Lond.)* **203**: 121–33.

USHERWOOD, P. N. R., MACHILI, P. and LEAF, G. (1968) L-glutamate at insect excitatory nerve-muscle synapses. *Nature (Lond.)* **219**: 1169–72.

Mg and miscellaneous factors affecting spontaneous and evoked release of transmitter

HUBBARD, J. J., JONES, S. F. and LANDAU, E. M. (1968) An examination of the effects of osmotic pressure changes upon transmitter release from mammalian motor nerve terminals. *J. Physiol. (Lond.)* **197**: 639–57.

SIMPSON, L. L. and TAPP, J. T. (1967) Actions of calcium and magnesium on the rate of onset of botulinum toxin paralysis of the rat diaphragm. *Int. J. Neuropharmacol.* **6**: 485–92.

The effect of magnesium on the acetylcholine sensitivity of the postjunctional membrane

FREEMAN, S. E. and TURNER, R. J. (1969) Ionic interactions in acetylcholine contraction of the denervated rat diaphragm. *Brit. J. Pharmacol.* **36**: 510–22.

FREEMAN, S. E. and TURNER, R. J. (1970) Facilitatory drug action on the isolated phrenic nerve-diaphragm preparation of the rat. *J. Pharmacol. Exp. Ther.* **174**: 550–9.

KATZ, B. and MILEDI, R. (1969) Spontaneous and evoked activity of motor nerve endings in calcium Ringer. *J. Physiol. (Lond.)* **203**: 689–706.

LAMBERT, D. H. and PARSONS, R. L. (1970) Influence of polyvalent cations on the activation of muscle end plate receptors. *J. Gen. Physiol.* **56**: 309–21.

MAGAZANIK, L. G. and VYSKOCIL, F. (1970) Dependence of acetylcholine desensitization on the membrane potential of frog muscle fibre and on the ionic changes in the medium. *J. Physiol. (Lond.)* **210**: 507–18.

NASTUK, W. L. (1967) Activation and inactivation of muscle postjunctional receptors. *Fed. Proc.* **26**: 1639–46.

NASTUK, W. L. and PARSONS, R. L. (1970) Factors in the inactivation of postjunctional membrane receptors of frog skeletal muscle. *J. Gen. Physiol.* **56**: 218–49.

The effect of magnesium on the muscle membrane

JENDEN, D. J. and REGER, J. F. (1963) The role of resting potential changes in the contractile failure of frog sartorius muscles during calcium deprivation. *J. Physiol. (Lond.)* **169**: 889–901.

The effect of magnesium on nerve fibers. Peripheral nerve

BLAUSTEIN, M. P. and HODGKIN, A. L. (1969) The effect of cyanide on the efflux of calcium from squid axons. *J. Physiol. (Lond.)* **200**: 497–527.

EVANS, M. H. (1969) The effects of saxitoxin and tetrodotoxin on nerve conduction in the presence of lithium ions and of magnesium ions. *Brit. J. Pharmacol.* **36**: 418–25.

ROJAS, E., TAYLOR, R. E., ATWATER, I. and BEZANILLA, F. (1969) Analysis of the effects of calcium and magnesium on voltage-clamp currents in perfused squid axons bathed in solutions of high potassium. *J. Gen. Physiol.* **54**: 532–52.

Terminal nerve fibers

RANDIĆ, M. and STRAUGHAN, D. W. (1964) Antidromic activity in the rat phrenic nerve-diaphragm preparation. *J. Physiol. (Lond.)* **173**: 130–48.

Miscellaneous

FREEMAN, S. E. (1968) Ionic influences on succinylcholine blockade of the mammalian neuromuscular junction. *Brit. J. Pharmacol.* **32**: 546–66.

FREEMAN, S. E. (1968) Antagonism of succinylcholine blockade of the mammalian neuromuscular junction. *J. Pharmacol. Exp. Ther.* **162**: 10–20.

GHONEIM, M. M. and LONG, J. P. (1970) The interaction between magnesium and other neuromuscular blocking agents. *Anesthesiology* **32**: 23–7.

D. METABOLISM

CHAPTER 15

SYNTHETIC NEUROMUSCULAR BLOCKING AGENTS: ABSORPTION— DISTRIBUTION—METABOLISM—EXCRETION

C. Chagas, L. Sollero and G. Suarez-Kurtz

Rio de Janeiro

15.1. ABSORPTION

Neuromuscular blocking agents are not absorbed through the intact skin; with the exception of the tertiary derivatives of β-erythroidine, they are relatively inactive when ingested orally, since the intestinal epithelium is an effective barrier to the penetration of organic ions, and in particular to the quaternary ammonium ion present in the great majority of neuromuscular blocking agents. Various salts of β-erythroidine and of dihydro-β-erythroidine are well absorbed orally since they form salts which are water soluble and also soluble in a variety of organic solvents. It has been shown that in the mouse, these substances are better absorbed following oral administration than subcutaneous injection (Unna *et al.*, 1944). Using dihydro-β-erythroidine in doses of 200 mg and of 6 mg/kg in man Murphree (1963) observed that the onset of the various systemic effects occurs 15 to 30 minutes after oral ingestion.

The studies of Erdei (1952) and Delay *et al.* (1952) and of Thuillier (1952) indicate that the buccal and anal mucosa readily absorb neuromuscular blocking agents. Erdei has verified that in man a sublingual dose of 2 to 12 mg of *d*-tubocurarine produces beneficial effects in spastic syndromes. This begins 2 to 3 minutes after application and lasts for 8 to 12 hours. Neuromuscular blocking agents are absorbed following parenteral administration and when the intramuscular route is utilized, the rate of absorption may be increased by the use of hyaluronidase.

The introduction of neuromuscular blocking agents into the lateral ventricles or into the cisterna magna does not produce muscular relaxation but a convulsive state resembling a grand mal epileptic convulsion. This is because these substances do not pass into the systemic circulation but produce an intense stimulation of the central nervous system.

The route of administration greatly alters the intensity of the muscular relaxation produced by curarizing agents. In the case of benzoquinonium, the acute toxicities (LD_{50}) in the mouse are: 140 mg/kg orally; 2.5 mg/kg subcutaneously; and 0.6 mg/kg intravenously. In the dog the neuromuscular effects of this drug following oral administration are even smaller. Thus the oral LD_{50} is 550 times larger than the intravenous LD_{50} (Hoppe, 1950). Decamethonium and gallamine are some 2 to 4 times less active by the subcutaneous or intramuscular route than by the intravenous route. Following oral administration of these drugs, doses of from 50 to 100 and 250 times the intravenous doses are required (Bovet, 1951; Paton and Zaimis, 1952).

15.2. DISTRIBUTION

The fate of *d*-tubocurarine in the body has been more extensively studied than that of other neuromuscular blocking agents. It appears that the distribution of other neuromuscular blocking agents is, in general terms, similar to that of *d*-tubocurarine.

The analysis of the plasma concentration curves for *d*-tubocurarine following intravenous administration in man has led Kalow (1959) to suggest that there are three phases in the process of distribution.

First phase. Distribution into the extracellular fluid and binding to plasma proteins.

During this phase, which lasts for 10 to 20 minutes, there is a rapid fall in the plasma concentration of *d*-tubocurarine (50% in 5 to 7 minutes). Similar results have been observed in the dog with gallamine and decamethonium labeled with radioactive carbon (Figs. 1 and 2) (Cole *et al.*, 1961; Suarez-Kurtz, 1967).

The onset of neuromuscular blockade probably corresponds to the first passage of the drug through the muscle. This makes it necessary to accept that diffusion of the drug from the capillaries to the site of action takes only a few seconds. According to Kalow, the motor end-plate is bombarded with the molecules of the curarizing agent which are present in the plasma even before an equilibrium is established with the interstitial fluid. Considering the great affinity of curarizing agents for the motor end-plate, this hypothesis is corroborated by the intimate anatomical relationships

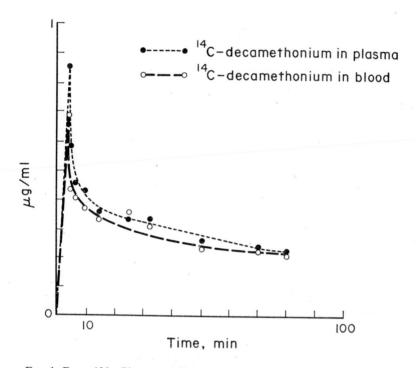

FIG. 1. Dog—12 kg. Plasma and blood concentrations of ^{14}C-labeled decame-thonium ($C_{10}C_{14}$) following intravenous injection of 100 mcg/kg.

between the motor end-plate and the capillaries of the systemic circulation. This has been well demonstrated by the work of Couteaux (1955) and of Benzley (cited by Kalow, 1959). Waser and Lüthi (1957) have demonstrated the specific binding of neuromuscular blocking agents (*c*-curarine and decamethonium) in the motor end-plate using autoradiographic techniques on the rat diaphragm.

That the onset of neuromuscular blockade is more rapid following dihydro-β-erythroidine than following any quaternary neuromuscular blocking agent suggests that there is a slowing of the passage of organic ions across the capillary endothelium and the axolema membrane. These membranes must be crossed by curarizing agents to reach their site of action in the neuromuscular junction.

During this first phase, an equilibrium is established between the curarizing molecules bound to plasma proteins and those in the extracellular liquid.

411

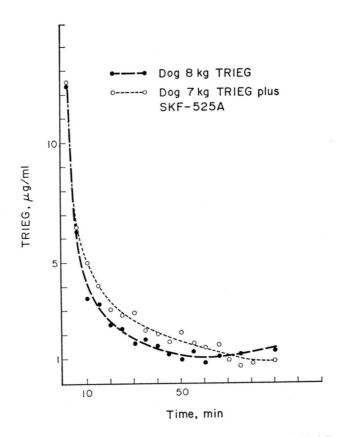

FIG. 2. Plasma concentration of ^{14}C-labeled gallamine (TRIEG) following intravenous injection of 1.5 mg/kg in a control dog and a dog pretreated with 10 mg/kg of SKF 525A.

Cohen *et al.* (1965) have verified that the binding of *d*-tubocurarine to plasma proteins is not specific for any fraction of the plasma proteins: i.e. albumin, gamma-globulin and fibrinogen bind curare. These authors have not been able to confirm that individual variation in protein affinity for *d*-tubocurarine was responsible for cases of resistance to its neuro-muscular blocking effects (Aladjemoff *et al.*, 1958).

Second phase. Redistribution and urinary excretion.

In the case of *d*-tubocurarine, the first phase has a duration of 2 to 3 hours during which there is a slow reduction in the plasma levels of the curarizing agent (5% reduction in plasma levels in 45 minutes, Kalow, 1959). Two factors contribute to the reduction in plasma concentration:

(a) *urinary excretion*—which in the case of *d*-tubocurarine amounts to 1/3 of the administered dose (Mahfouz, 1949; Marsh, 1952).

(b) *redistribution*—about 2/3 of a dose of *d*-tubocurarine is redistributed in the organism. Kalow states that the redistribution occurs in the body water.

The analogies which exist between the motor end-plate and the electric organ of *Electrophorus electricus* (L), both as regards the action of competitive and depolarizing neuromuscular blocking agents (Chagas *et al.*, 1952; Albe-Fessard and Chagas, 1951; Chagas, Bovet and Sollero, 1953; Chagas and Albe-Fessard, 1954), has aroused interest in the possibility that this organ could be used for the study of the binding of curarizing agents.

Chagas and his collaborators have used (1957-8) the curarizing agents gallamine triethiodide, dimethyl-*d*-isochondodendrine, dimethyl-*d*-tubocurarine labeled with carbon-14 and have been able to isolate from homogenates of the perfused and curarized electric organ a complex formed between the injected drug and a macromolecule.

These same authors have identified a component of this macromolecule

TABLE 1. VARIATION IN THE QUANTITY OF DIMETHYL-*d*-TUBOCURARINE BOUND TO VARIOUS TISSUES AS THE INJECTED DOSE IS INCREASED 10 TIMES

Tissue	DMDT bound (mcg/g tissue dry wt.)	Proportional increase in the amount of DMDT bound when the quantity of DMDT injected is increased 10 times	Uronic acid (mg/g tissue dry wt.)
Liver	0.45	10.5	0.33
Spleen	0.60	3.2	0.48
Muscle	0.13	4.4	0.13
Diaphragm	0.22	9.6	0.14
Cartilage	0.16	76.0	0.53
Vitreous humor	0.09	2.4	0.21
Adrenal	0.31	3.9	0.30
Ganglion chain	0.15	6.8	0.23
Heart	0.52	14.1	0.39
Lung	0.58	14.1	0.39

as an acid mucopolysaccharide rich in hexosamine. The analysis of the quantity and distribution of the mucopolysaccharide has led to the suggestion (Chagas, 1959) that this mucopolysaccharide represents the non-specific receptor or "acceptor". This interpretation is strengthened by the demonstration, by means of autoradiography, of the binding of curare to non-synaptic (anterior) structures as well as synaptic (posterior) structures of the electroplate. This may also provide an explanation for other experimental data such as the duration of curarization of the electric organ (Chagas *et al.*, 1953). The primary phenomenon is due to the binding of curare to the receptor; at the same time a certain quantity of the curare molecules become bound to the mucopolysaccharides present on the surface of the electroplate. As the curare molecules are removed from the synaptic site by competition with the chemical mediator, other curare molecules which were bound to the mucopolysaccharide diffuse into the specific receptors in the synaptic region. Thus the duration of neuromuscular blockade is prolonged.

The study of the binding of curarizing agents by tissue polysaccharides has been extended to mammals—A parallelism has been observed between the uronic acid of various tissues and their ability to bind dimethyl-*d*-tubocurarine (Table 1).

The most extensive binding seems to occur in areas where there is a large abundance of synapses. The specific activity (micrograms of curare per gram of tissue) for small doses of curare varies between 1.0 and 1.7 in synapse rich tissue, while the specific activity of areas poor in synapses is of the order of 0.5 (Chagas, 1962).

Contrasting results are obtained if a large dose is administered: Table 1 shows the amount of dimethyl-*d*-tubocurarine bound when the dose is 10 times larger.

Other molecules containing uronic acid as well as protein have been suggested as being capable of binding curarizing agents. Paton (1958) has shown that heparin is able to combine with *d*-tubocurarine. Muscular proteins also seem to have the ability of binding curarizing agents (Kalow, 1959). In view of their localization, it is difficult to determine their possible function in the phenomenon of redistribution.

The function of non-specific receptors in the intensity and duration of neuromuscular blockade has been pointed out by Bovet and his collaborators (1956) and by Bettschart *et al.* (1954) in order to explain the potentiation of the action of various neuromuscular blocking agents by β-diethylaminoethyl-diphenyl-propylacetate (SKF 525A). These authors have suggested that SKF 525A has the ability to displace the molecules of the curarizing agent bound to non-specific receptors, thus increasing the concentration of the inhibitor in the body fluids. The curarizing agent thus being in a pharmacologically active form can interact with the specific receptors and produce a response. This hypothesis has been supported by the observations of Waser (1958) that SKF 525A is able not only to increase the pharmacological activity but also the concentration of calabash curare on the motor end-plate.

Subsequent studies (Cole *et al.*, 1961; Sollero *et al.*, 1966; Suarez-Kurtz, 1967; Suarez-Kurtz and Paulo, 1968; Suarez-Kurtz and Bianchi, 1970) have led to an alternative hypothesis, not requiring a non-specific receptor, to explain the sensitizing action of SKF 525A on the effects of neuromuscular blocking agents.

Two further aspects of the distribution of curarizing agents remain to be discussed: placental transmission and the penetration into the central nervous system.

d-Tubocurarine does not seem to be able to pass across the placental barrier, either in women (Cohen *et al.*, 1953) or in experimental animals (Buller and Young, 1949).

Nevertheless the placental transmission of gallamine and of decamethonium has been shown in women by Crawford (1956) and by Spencer and Coakley (1955) respectively. However, in the rabbit and the guinea-pig decamethonium does not cross the placenta (Young, 1949). Thesleff has verified that succinylcholine does not cross the placental barrier in women and in experimental animals. Moya and Kuisselgaard (1961) have nevertheless been able to detect the presence of this curarizing agent in the blood of the fetus in spite of the fact that there was no sign of neuromuscular paralysis of the newborn in contrast to the profound curarization of the mother.

In contrast to the quaternary compounds, tertiary neuromuscular blocking agents are able to cross the blood–brain barrier and thus to penetrate into the central nervous system. This observation is partially confirmed by the sedative properties of dihydro-β-erythroidine and by its effects on Renshaw cells (Murphree, 1963). Paton (1959) has suggested that under certain conditions—asphyxia, anesthesia, dehydration, hemorrhage—which may alter the selectivity of the blood-brain barrier, quaternary neuromuscular blocking agents are able to exert a central effect. Cohen (1963) has been unable to prove experimentally this hypothesis.

Third phase. Destruction.

In this phase, the process of metabolism of the curarizing agent which began in the second phase is increased. The urinary excretion becomes less important in view of the concentrations of the substance in the extracellular fluid as a result of redistribution.

15.3. METABOLISM AND EXCRETION

15.3.1. *d*-TUBOCURARINE AND DIMETHYL-*d*-TUBOCURARINE

In man about 35% of the administered dose of *d*-tubocurarine is excreted unchanged in the urine in the first 10 hours (Kalow, 1953). There is species variation in the urinary excretion of this drug (Marsh, 1952). A greater proportion of dimethyl-*d*-tubocurarine than of *d*-tubocurarine is excreted by the kidneys: 60–70% of the injected dose can be recovered in the urine 3 to 6 hours after injection.

The excretion of these curarizing agents in the feces or by other routes is negligible.

Although the ligation of the renal vessels in the rat increases the duration of action of *d*-tubocurarine and its dimethyl derivatives (Collier *et al.*, 1948), in nephrectomized patients, Churchill-Davidson (1965) did not observe any increase in the duration of action of *d*-tubocurarine.

This latter fact emphasizes the importance of redistribution to the non-specific receptors in the duration of action of *d*-tubocurarine.

The role of the liver in the metabolism of *d*-tubocurarine is still a matter of uncertainty, the biotransformation of curarizing agents by the liver being claimed by some authors (Pick and Richards, 1948; Kelly and Shideman, 1949) and denied by others (Everett, 1947; Stead, 1957).

15.3.2. GALLAMINE

The elimination of gallamine triethiodide in the dog has been studied using the radio-labeled drug (Cole *et al.*, unpublished). Approximately one-quarter of the injected dose may be recovered in the urine in the first hour, and two-thirds in 5 hours. The substance is excreted unchanged, there being no metabolic transformation. The maximal excretion occurs between the 15th and 20th minute after injection of gallamine.

It has also been verified that, although SKF 525A clearly potentiates the neuromuscular blocking action of gallamine, it does not affect its over-all elimination. In some experiments, however, using animals pretreated with SKF 525A a delay in the onset and the point of maximal elimination was

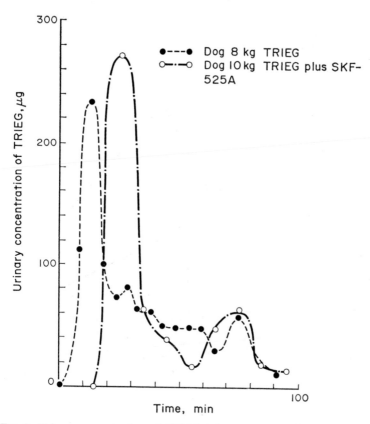

FIG. 3. Urinary concentration of ^{14}C-labeled gallamine (TRIEG) following intravenous injection of 1.5 mg/kg in a control animal and an animal pretreated with 10 mg/kg of SKF 525A.

observed. Maximal excretion occurred at the 30th minute (Fig. 3). These modifications have been attributed to the arterial hypotension and the oliguria produced by SKF 525A.

15.3.3.   DECAMETHONIUM

This substance undergoes little or no metabolic transformation and is eliminated unchanged in the urine. Paton and Zaimis (1952) were able to recover 80–90% of the administered dose in the first 24 hours. Lüthi and Waser (1962) obtained about 50% urinary excretion in the cat in the

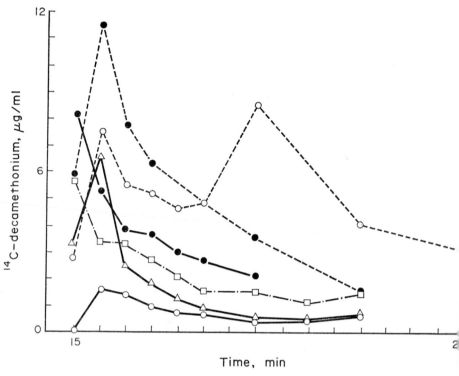

FIG. 4. Urinary concentration of ^{14}C-labeled decamethonium ($C_{10}C_{14}$) from six dogs to which 100 mcg/kg had been given intravenously.

first 60 minutes. In man, Churchill-Davidson and Richardson (1953) recovered some 40% of the injected dose in the urine in the first 3 hours following injection.

The urinary excretion of decamethonium labeled with ^{14}C has been studied in the dog, and the results obtained are shown in Table 2 (Suarez-Kurtz, 1967).

As can be seen from Fig. 4, the maximum urinary excretion of decamethonium occurs between 15 and 30 minutes after injection of the drug. Again, although SKF 525A markedly potentiates the neuromuscular blocking actions of decamethonium, it does not affect its overall rate of urinary excretion.

Renal ligation, which removes the only route for the excretion and detoxication of decamethonium may produce an increase in the duration of the curarizing action of the drug. This has been observed experimentally

TABLE 2. URINARY ELIMINATION OF
RADIOACTIVE DECAMETHONIUM
(100 mcg/kg i.v.) IN THE DOG

Time (min.)	% of total dose
15	5.51 (6)*
30	11.07 (6)
60	19.06 (6)
120	25.57 (6)
180	29.28 (6)

* Number of animals studied.

in the dog (Suarez-Kurtz, 1967). At the clinical level, however, there are no data to correlate the duration of action of the drug with renal function.

15.3.4. SUCCINYLCHOLINE

The short duration of action of succinylcholine *in vivo* is due to its rapid hydrolysis. The biotransformation of succinylcholine by plasma cholinesterase was demonstrated by Glick (1941) even before its neuromuscular blocking effects were described by Bovet *et al.* (1947). In 1952 Whittaker and Wijesundera demonstrated that the hydrolysis of succinylcholine takes place in two phases:

(a) The transformation of succinyl-dicholine into succinylmonocholine by the action of pseudo-cholinesterase. According to Fraser (1954) true cholinesterase does not take part in this reaction; 3% of the injected dose of succinylcholine may be recovered in the urine (Foldes *et al.*, 1955). This illustrates the importance of this first phase of metabolic reaction, the speed of which has been calculated by Tsuji *et al.* (1955) to be of the order of 4% of the rate of hydrolysis of acetylcholine. It has been confirmed that succinyl-monocholine also has a neuromuscular blocking action and may, therefore, maintain the neuromuscular blockade produced initially by the succinyl-dicholine. This is particularly true if large initial doses are used.

(b) Transformation of succinyl-monocholine into choline and succinyl acid. This reaction is slower (5–7 times slower than the first phase—Foldes and Tsuji, 1953). It is due to the action of a specific enzyme synthesized in the liver (Greenway and Quastel, 1955). Nevertheless, it is possible that pseudo-cholinesterase may also take part in this phase.

Succinyl-monocholine, choline and succinic acid have the property of inhibiting or slowing the rate of hydrolysis of succinyl-dicholine by plasma pseudo-cholinesterase.

A prolonged action of succinyl-dicholine may occur when it is not destroyed. This may result from a number of causes, such as a reduction in the synthesis of pseudo-cholinesterase by malnutrition or hepatic disorders, or by genetic causes. The latter is the case when the prolonged action may be attributed to the presence of an atypical cholinesterase as demonstrated by the method of Kalow and Genest (1957) to be of hereditary origin.

15.3.5. OTHER CURARIZING AGENTS

Waser and Lüthi (1966) have studied the distribution and elimination of diallyl-nortoxiferine in the cat using the tritium labeled drug. In the first 15–60 minutes following intravenous injection the greatest concentrations of radioactivity have been found in those tissues rich in acid mucopolysaccharides. Other authors have attributed the short duration of action of diallyl-nortoxiferine to this binding to nonspecific receptors. About 18% of the injected dose has been recovered unchanged in the urine in the first 30 minutes following injection, and approximately 50% in the first 4 hours.

Seventy per cent of the injected dose of hexamethylene carbomylcholine (Imbretil) may be recovered unchanged in the urine of experimental animals (Brüche *et al.*, 1954). In the case of benzoquinonium 80% may be recovered unchanged (Hoppe, 1951).

REFERENCES

ALADJEMOFF, L., DIKSTEIN, S. and SHAFIR, E. (1968) Binding of *d*-tubochloride to plasma proteins. *J. Pharmacol. Exp. Ther.* **123**: 43.

ALBE-FESSARD, D. and CHAGAS, C. (1951) Action d'une substance curàrisante sur la décharge electrique de l'*Electrophorus electricus* L. *Soc. Biol.* **145**: 248.

BETTSCHART, A., SCONAMIGLIO, W. and BOVET, D. (1954) Potenziamento degli effeti della Succinilcolina ad opera del β-dietilamminoetil-difenil propilacetato (SKF 525A). *Rendic. Ist. Sup. Sanità* **19**: 721.

BOVET, D. (1951) Some aspects of the relationship between chemical constitution and curare-like activity. *Ann. N.Y. Acad. Sci.* **54**: 407.

BOVET, D., BOVET-NITTI, F., BETTSCHART, A. and SONAMIGLIO, W. (1956) Mécanisme de la potentialisation par le chlorhydrate de diéthylamino-éthyl-diphénil propyl acetate des effets de quelques agents curarisants. *Helv. Physiol. Pharmacol. Acta* **14**: 430.

BOVET, D., DEPIERRE, F. and LESTRANGE, Y. (1947) Propriétés curarisantes des éthers phénoliques à fonctions ammonium quaternaires. *C.R. Acad. Sci.* (*Paris*) **225**:74.

BRÜCKE, H., KLUPP, H. and KRAUPP, O. (1954) A practice of anaesthesia. In: *A Practice of Anaesthesia*, p. 767. Wylie, W. D. and Churchill-Davidson, H. C. (eds.) Lloyd-Luke Ltd., London, 1966.

BULLER, A. J. and YOUNG, I. M. (1949) The action of *d*-tubocurarine chloride on foetal neuromuscular transmission and the placental transfer of this drug in the rabbit. *J. Physiol.* (*London*) **109**: 412.

CHAGAS, C. (1959) Studies on the mechanism of curarization. *Ann. N.Y. Acad. Sci.* **81**: 345.

CHAGAS, C. (1962) The fate of curare during curarization. In: *Curare and Curare-like Agents*. CIBA Foundation (ed.), Churchill, London, p. 2.

CHAGAS, C. and ALBE-FESSARD, D. (1954) Action de divers curarizants sur l'organe électrique de l'*Electrophorus electricus* L. *Acta Physiol. Lat. Amer.* **4**: 49.

CHAGAS, C., BOVET, D. and SOLLERO, L. (1953) Curarisation musculaire et curarisation électrique chez le poisson *Electrophorus electricus*. *Acad. Sci. Paris* **236**: 1997.

CHAGAS, C., PENNA-FRANCA, E., HASSON, A., CROCKER, C., NISHIE, K. and GARCIA, E. J. (1957) Studies of the mechanisms of curarization. *An. Acad. Bras. Ci.* **29**: 53.

CHAGAS, C., PENNA-FRANCA, E., NISHIE, K. and GARCIA, E. J. (1958) A study of the specificity of the complex formed by gallamine triethiodide with a macromolecular constituent of the electric organ. *Arch. Biochem. Biophys.* **75**: 251.

CHAGAS, C., SOLLERO, L. and MARTINS FERREIRA, H. (1952) On the utilization of acetylcholine during the discharge of the *Electrophorus electricus* L. *An. Acad. Brasil Ci.* **24**: 213.

CHURCHILL-DAVIDSON, H. C. and RICHARDSON, A. T. (1953) Neuromuscular transmission in myasthenia gravis. *J. Physiol.* (*London*) **122**: 252.

COHEN, E. (1963) Blood–brain barrier to *d*-tubocurarine. *J. Pharmacol. Exp. Ther.* **141**: 356.

COHEN, E., CORRASCIO, A. and FLEISCHLI, G. (1965) The distribution and fate of *d*-tubocurarine. *J. Pharmacol. Exp. Ther.* **147**: 120.

COHEN, E., PAULSON, W., WALL, J. and ELERT (1953) Thiopental, curare and nitrous oxide anesthesia for Cesarian section with studies on placental transmission. *Surg., Gynec. Obstet.* **97**: 456.

COLE, C., CHAGAS, C., SOLLERO, L. and MOURA, R. S. (1961) Estudos sôbre a eliminação do tri-iodo-etilato de Gallamina (TRIEG). *An. Acad. Bras. Ci.* **33**: xlvi.

COLLIER, H. O. J., PARIS, S. K. and WOOLF, L. I. (1945) Pharmacological activities in different rodent species of *d*-tubocurarine chloride and the dimethyl ether of *d*-tubocurarine chloride. *Nature* **161**: 817.

COUTEAUX, R. (1955) Localization of cholinesterase at neuromuscular junctions. *Int. Rev. Cytol.* **4**: 335.

CRAWFORD, J. S. (1956) Some aspects of obstetric anaesthesia. *Brit. J. Anesth.* **28**: 145.

DELAY, J., THUILLIER, J., MONTREMY, J. and TARDIEU, Y. (1952) Curarisation par voie rectale. *Presse Méd.* **60**: 1341.

ERDEI, A. (1952) Sub-lingual *d*-tubocurarine for muscular spasm. *Lancet* **253**: 1070.

EVERETT, G. M. (1947) Pharmacological studies of *d*-tubocurarine and other curare fractions. *J. Pharmacol. Exp. Ther.* **92**: 236.

FOLDES, F. F. and TSUJI, F. I. (1953) Enzymatic hydrolysis and neuromuscular activity of succinylmonocholine iodide. *Fed. Proc.* **12**: 321.

FOLDES, F. F., VANDERVORT, R. and SHANOR, S. (1955) The fats of succinylcholine in man. *Anesthesiology* **16**: 11.

FRASER, P. J. (1954) Hydrolysis of succinylcholine salts. *Brit. J. Pharmacol. Chem.* **9**: 429.

GLICK, D. (1941) Some additional observations on specificity of cholinesterase. *J. Biol. Chem.* **137**: 357.

GREENWAY, R. M. and QUASTEL, J. H. (1955) Hydrolysis of succinylmonocholine by liver esterase. *Proc. Soc. Exp. Biol.* (*N.Y.*) **90**: 72.

HOPPE, J. D. (1950) A pharmacological investigation of 2,5-bis-(3-diethylamine propylamine) benzoquinone-bis-benzylchloride (Win 2747). *J. Pharmacol. Exp. Ther.* **100**: 333.

HOPPE, J. O. (1951) New series of synthetic curare-like compounds. *An. N.Y. Acad. Sci.* **54**: 395.

KALOW, W. (1953) Urinary excretion of *d*-tubocurarine. *J. Pharmacol. Exp. Ther.* **109**: 79.

KALOW, W. (1959) The distribution, destruction and elimination of muscle relaxants. *Anesthesiology* **20**: 505.

KALOW, W. and GENEST, K. (1957) A method for the detection of atypical forms of human serum cholinesterase; determination of dibucaine numbers. *Canad. J. Biochem.* **35**: 339.

KELLY, A. R. and SHIDEMAN, F. E. (1949) The relative role of the liver and kidneys in the detoxification of a standardized curare preparation (Intocostrin). *J. Pharmacol. Exp. Ther.* **97**: 292.

LÜTHI, U. and WASER, P. (1965) Verteilung und Metabolismus von ^{14}C-Decamethonium in Katzen. *Arch. Int. Pharmacodyn.* **156**: 319.

MAHFOOL, D. (1949) Fate of *d*-tubocurarine in body. *Brit. J. Pharmacol. Chem.* **4**: 295.

MARSH, D. F. (1952) Distribution, metabolism and excretion of *d*-tubocurarine chloride and related compounds in man and other animals. *J. Pharmacol. Exp. Ther.* **105**: 299.

MOYA, D. D. B. and KVISELGAARD, N. (1961) The placental transmission of succinylcholine. *Anesthesiology* **22**: 1.

MURPHREE, H. B. (1963) Effects in human volunteers of sub-paralytic doses of dihydro-β-erythroidine. *Clin. Pharmacol.* **4**: 304.

PATON, W. D. M. (1958) Central and synaptic transmission in nervous system. *Ann. Rev. Physiol.* **20**: 431.

PATON, W. D. M. (1959) The effects of muscle relaxants other than muscular relaxation. *Anesthesiology* **20**: 453.

PATON, W. D. M. and ZAIMIS, E. (1952) The methonium compounds. *Pharmacol. Rev.* **4**: 219.

PICK, E. P. and RICHARDS, G. V. (1948) Action of curare alkaloids and erythrine alkaloids on morphinized mice. *Arch. Int. Pharmacodyn.* **76**: 183.

SOLLERO, L., CHAGAS, C., SUAREZ-KURTZ, G., NESRALLA, H. and BUENO, J. R. (1966) Absorption and excretion of labelled neuromuscular blocking agents. *Abstracts III Int. Pharmacol. Congress, São Paulo, Brasil*, p. 110.

SPENCER, C. H. and COAKLEY, L. S. (1955) Clinical evaluation of syncurine. *Anesthesiology* **16**: 125.

STEAD, A. L. (1957) The role of the canine liver in the detoxication of *d*-tubocurarine chloride, gallamine triethiodide and laudexium. *Brit. J. Anaesth.* **29**: 151.

SUAREZ-KURTZ, G. (1967) Thesis: Ações e efeitos do cloridrato de difenil-propilacetato de β-dietil-aminoetila (SKF 525A) na transmissão neuromuscular. Oficina Gràfica da UFRJ, Rio de Janeiro, Brasil.

SUAREZ-KURTZ, G. and BIANCHI, C. P. (1970) Sites of action of SKF 525A in nerve and muscle. *J. Pharmacol. Exp. Ther.* **172**: 33.

SUAREZ-KURTZ, G. and PAULO, L. G. (1968) Studies on the neuromuscular effect of β-diethyl amino-ethyl-diphenyl propylacetate (SKF 525A). *Arch. Int. Pharmacodyn.* **173**: 133.

THUILLIER, J. (1952) Curarisation par voie rectale. *Anesth. Analg.* **9**: 405.

TSUJI, F. A., FOLDES, F. F. and RHODES, D. H. (1955) The hydrolysis of succinyl-choline chloride in human plasma. *Arch. Int. Pharmacodyn.* **104**: 146.

UNNA, K., KNIAZUK, M. and GRESLIN, J. G. (1944) Pharmacological action of erythrine alkaloids. β-Erythroidine and substances derived from it. *J. Pharmacol. Exp. Ther.* **80**: 39.

WASER, P. (1958) Autoradiographie von Endplatten mit Radiocurarin nach Denervierung Prostigmin oder SKF 525A. *Helv. Physiol. Acta* **16**: 171.

WASER, P. and LUTHI, U. (1957) Autoradiographische Lokalisation von C¹⁴-calabassen-curarine I und decamethonium in der motorischen end platte. *Arch. Int. Pharmacodyn.* **112**: 272.

WASER, P. and LÜTHI, U. (1966) Verteilung, metabolismus und elimination von H-diallyl-nor-toxiferin (Alloferin) bei katzen. *Helv. Physiol. Acta* **24**: 259.

WHITTAKER, V. P. and WIJESUNDERA, S. (1952) Hydrolysis of succinylcholine by cholinesterase. *Biochem. J.* **52**: 475.

YOUNG, I. M. (1949) The action of decamethonium iodide (C-10) on foetal neuromuscular transmission and its transfer across the placenta. *J. Physiol.* (*London*) **109**: 31 P.

AUTHOR INDEX

xiii

SUBJECT INDEX